The Cancer Fighting Diet

The
Cancer
Fighting
Diet

Diet and Nutrition Strategies to Help Weaken Cancer Cells and Improve Treatment Results

Dr. Johannes F. Coy
Maren Franz

Robert
ROSE

For complete cataloguing information, see page 352.

Disclaimer

This book is a general guide only and should never be a substitute for the skill, knowledge and experience of a qualified medical professional dealing with the facts, circumstances and symptoms of a particular case. The nutritional, medical and health information presented in this book is based on the research, training and professional experience of the authors, and is true and complete to the best of their knowledge. However, this book is intended only as an informative guide for those wishing to know more about health, nutrition, and medicine; it is not intended to replace or countermand the advice given by the reader's personal physician. Because each person and situation is unique, the author and the publisher urge the reader to check with a qualified health care professional before using any procedure where there is a question as to its appropriateness. A physician should be consulted before beginning any exercise program. The authors and the publisher are not responsible for any adverse effects or consequences resulting from the use of the information in this book. It is the responsibility of the reader to consult a physician or other qualified health care professional regarding his or her personal care.

This book contains references to products that may not be available everywhere. The intent of the information provided is to be helpful; however, there is no guarantee of results associated with the information provided. Use of brand names is for educational purposes only and does not imply endorsement. The recipes in this book have been carefully tested. To the best of our knowledge, they are safe and nutritious for ordinary use and users. For those people with food or other allergies, or who have special food requirements or special health issues, please read the suggested contents of each recipe or formula carefully and determine whether or not they may create a problem for you. All recipes or formulas are used at the risk of the consumer.

We cannot be responsible for any hazards, loss or damage that may occur as a result of any recipe use. For those with special needs, allergies, requirements or health problems, in the event of any doubt, please contact your medical adviser prior to the use of any recipe.

Design and production: Martina Hwang/PageWave Graphics Inc.
Editor: Tina Anson Mine
Copy editor/proofreader: Marnie Lamb
Indexer: Beth Zabloski
Translator: Sylvia Goulding
Illustrations: Niloofar Bijanzadeh, except for page 71 (Therry Whelan)

Cover and part opener images: Red cabbage, cucumber, tomato, artichoke and orange © iStockphoto.com/Dimitris66

The publisher gratefully acknowledges the financial support of our publishing program by the Government of Canada through the Canada Book Fund.

Published by Robert Rose Inc.
120 Eglinton Avenue East, Suite 800, Toronto, Ontario, Canada M4P 1E2
Tel: (416) 322-6552 Fax: (416) 322-6936
www.robertrose.ca

Printed and bound in USA

1 2 3 4 5 6 7 8 9 CKV 23 22 21 20 19 18 17 16 15

Contents

Introduction

As it is for many people, eating used to be merely a means to an end for me. I ate because I was hungry, and I ate what I enjoyed. Although I had gained extensive, specialized knowledge about genetics and human biochemistry through my biological studies, this had no effect on my own diet whatsoever. It changed only once I discovered the TKTL1 gene during the course of my 11 years of research at the German Cancer Research Center in Heidelberg, Germany.

This unusual gene, initially regarded as defective, so ignited my appetite for research that I founded several companies. I have now been researching this gene for more than two decades in order to better understand and successfully treat cancer. Meanwhile, international studies have demonstrated that the TKTL1 gene performs a key function in cancer cells. More than that, the TKTL1 sugar metabolism has been shown to play a major protective role in our cells by helping them overcome difficult and dangerous situations. In addition, TKTL1 represents one of the five most important genes in humans, enabling the evolution of cognitive performance in the modern human being.

When the first edition of this book was published in September 2009, many laypeople and scientists alike vehemently doubted that nutrition could help achieve anything in the fight against cancer. Now, six years later, it has become clear that diet plays an important role in the development and recurrence of cancer. We also know that the correct diet is decisive in how effective a cancer therapy is.

It is not possible to simply starve cancer cells to death. However, we can change their metabolism before treatment in such a way that their sensitivity to radiation and chemotherapy is increased, thus clearly improving the chances of a full recovery. The way to do this is to avoid the intake of carbohydrates for a few days before the start of radiation or chemotherapy in order to shift the body into a ketogenic metabolic state.

Similarly, it makes sense to continue to reduce the amount of carbohydrate intake after successful treatment and to favor those carbohydrates that do not significantly increase blood sugar levels, because raised blood sugar and insulin levels increase the risk of redeveloping cancer and the likelihood of death from cancer. For healthy people, too, stable blood sugar levels and moderate carbohydrate intake are recommended; in addition to reducing the chances of developing cancer, these will also reduce the risk of obesity, metabolic syndrome, diabetes, cardiovascular disease and Alzheimer's disease.

A strict cancer-fighting diet is, therefore, not only sensible but also essential to good health. You can read all about how this diet works in this book, then take the opportunity to get active and protect your own good health.

I wish you all the best and good luck.

— Dr. Johannes F. Coy

How Can I Help?

Imagine there was a way you could actively support your treatment. Imagine there was a book that could not only give you basic information about cancer, but also provide detailed advice and a fully worked-out diet plan that would help you fight your personal battle against cancer and significantly improve your chances of conquering the disease. The search for such a book is over — you are holding it in your hands.

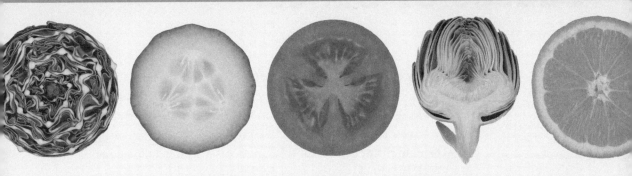

PART 1

Cancer Basics and Strategies for Healing

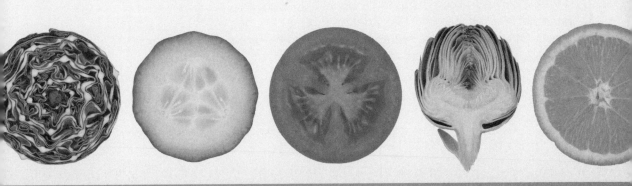

Understanding the Causes of Cancer

A cancer diagnosis often hits people like a bolt of lightning out of a blue sky. Those affected find themselves suddenly faced with a gravely serious condition that they do not understand yet are asked to surrender to. Although a physician will usually explain the next medical steps, patients are often left to cope with the shocking diagnosis on their own.

The most potent weapon in the fight against cancer is knowledge, and it is important to learn how to effectively employ it. Therefore, you'll find out all about the complex processes inside your body in the following pages. You'll come to understand the mechanisms that lead to the development and spread of cancer cells. Understanding the causes for what is happening inside your body helps you better implement the recommendations in this guide. Once you realize the immense importance of diet for your health, you'll be more active in your fight against cancer, and feel more energetic and healthier after only a few days. And you won't have to starve or forgo the pleasures of eating.

How Cells Are Replaced: A Real-World Example

Imagine you fall off your bike and scrape your knee. To ensure rapid healing of the wound, the abraded, damaged skin must be re-formed. In this case, a skin cell on the knee "reports" that its neighboring cell has suddenly gone missing. It then receives the command to divide and close the gap as quickly as possible. In response, the cell divides and forms new, healthy tissue, a process that continues until the damaged tissue is completely replaced, and the skin cells are again in immediate contact with one another.

The Body Rebuilds Itself

Our bodies continuously renew and regenerate themselves (see box, opposite). Used or damaged cells are replaced with fresh and fully functional cells, which counteracts the natural aging process. Cells are pure anti-aging structures.

Like multidimensional construction sites, cells in our bodies are checked around the clock, demolished and rebuilt. While you are relaxing on the sofa, perhaps with a glass of red wine and a good book, your cells regenerate nonstop, keeping you young and healthy. Depending on their load and task, some cells renew themselves quickly and often, while others do so very slowly.

Perfect Organization

Every second, the human body destroys somewhere between 10 and 50 million cells and replaces them with newly formed ones. While some areas hardly renew themselves at all, others overhaul themselves around the clock. By the end of our lives, we have, in essence, completely rebuilt ourselves several times over. Only very few cells accompany us throughout our lives — for example, germ cells, which are crucial for the formation of sperm and egg cells.

How Young Are Your Cells?

- Healthy liver cells reproduce so frequently that, in theory, our largest detoxifying organ rebuilds itself 17 times a year. This is why the liver is able to regenerate so quickly after partial surgical removal.

- Skin takes about 14 days for complete, all-around renewal. The worse the damage caused by ultraviolet (UV) radiation to the outer skin cells, the faster regeneration occurs. When you get sunburned, you can easily see this process in action — as the skin peels, the old, dead skin cells are shed.

- Fingernails grow throughout your life; generally, they take about six months to grow from the root to the tip.

- White blood cells (called leukocytes) are vital for your immune system. They live for only a few days, because they die in action while defending your health.

- In contrast with all of the previous cell types, heart cells regenerate very slowly, at a rate of about 1% per year in 25-year-olds and 0.45% per year in 75-year-olds.

- Brain and nerve cells regenerate so slowly that they hardly regrow at all.

DNA: The Book of Life

DNA, or the genetic strand, is created using four components; each is identified by its first letter: adenine, cytosine, guanine and thymine. This four-letter alphabet is used to link and code about three billion of these letters in a clearly defined sequence in a person's DNA. The sequence of the letters contains all the information necessary for life.

The most important subunit of information is the gene. It usually provides the blueprint for creating proteins, the body's building blocks. The body takes good care during cell division to ensure that no error creeps in when cells reproduce these long letter sequences; however, incorrect duplicates may be created while copying these codes (see box, at left).

How Cells Reproduce

Cell division always follows the same routine. Regardless of their specific tasks in the body, all cells divide in the same manner; a hair follicle cell, for example, does it the same way a skeletal muscle cell or a liver cell does.

For cell division to occur, all cell structures and cell contents, including the nuclear DNA (the carrier of genetic information) first have to duplicate themselves. Then, the identical copy moves away from the original to the opposite side of the parent cell, which then divides itself in half to create two daughter cells.

It's All in the Details

As unbelievable as it may sound, your entire genetic blueprint is stored inside this tiny strand of DNA, which is organized in the form of a double helix (also called the genetic strand). Since all these data are required to ensure your very survival,

A Written Analogy for Mutations

An incorrectly copied DNA sequence can wreak havoc, just as a single wrongly copied letter can change or destroy the meaning of a whole sentence. For example, if the letter "i" is changed to "x" in one word, the following sentence loses its meaning: "The mother breastfeeds her child" becomes "The mother breastfeeds her chxld." Thus, you can see how a seemingly tiny error can have major consequences.

they are backed up on a second DNA strand. If an error occurs on one of the two strands, the error-free strand can, as a rule, compensate for this deficit. In a way, the double helix is the book of your life. In it is stored all the necessary information to create your body down to the smallest details, such as the color of your eyes, the shape of your nose or the size of your feet.

Mutation Allows Tumor Cells to Develop

During cell division, if a mutation occurs in gene segments that are responsible for a cell's growth control, this copying error will cause the uncontrolled growth of a tumor cell. This type of mutation is relatively common in a healthy body. In addition, there are a number of external factors, such as radiation exposure, viruses or cigarette smoke, that trigger the formation of cells that grow uncontrollably.

As dramatic as a mutation like this may sound, our bodies are usually well prepared for it. Using special mechanisms, the cell ensures that it stops growing as soon as it touches a neighboring cell. This process is known as contact inhibition.

Important Carcinogenic Factors

The development of a cancer cell is encouraged by a person's exposure to the following environmental and physical factors:

- Cancer-causing chemicals (such as certain coloring agents, plasticizers and pesticides)
- Radioactive materials
- Electromagnetic waves (such as radar waves)
- UV radiation
- Certain viruses and bacteria (such as human papillomavirus or *Helicobacter pylori*)
- Moldy food (aflatoxins)
- Carcinogenic substances in food (nitrosamines)
- Cigarette smoke
- DNA mutations

The Faulty Copy Self-Destructs

In tumor cells, the healthy, harmonious cycle of growth, division and dissolution within the cell structure is suspended. When the growth-control switch is damaged during cell duplication, the cell's regulatory signals can be neither recognized nor executed. For this reason, our bodies are provided with a further safety device: a kind of self-destruction program for cells that grow without restraint. This auto-destruction program is referred to as programmed cell death, or apoptosis.

Normally, the problem of unchecked growth is solved when the cell touches its neighbor and dies. However, if mutation affects the very genes that control apoptosis (such as the p53 gene), this mechanism is deactivated. The mutated cell becomes immortal in the truest sense of the word, because the self-destruct program can no longer be set in motion.

The Six Universal Signs of Cancer

In order to harmonize the concept of the term *cancer*, scientists have established the following six criteria. Only once all criteria are met do we speak of a cell as cancerous. The cell must exhibit

- Independence from external growth signals
- Insensitivity to growth-inhibitory signals
- Blockade of programmed cell death
- Ongoing formation of new blood vessels
- Unlimited proliferative potential
- Tissue invasion and metastasis

A Tumor Does Not Always Mean Cancer

When a cell's growth control and self-destruction functions are deactivated by a mutation, it begins to grow in an unchecked manner, leading to cell proliferation. The cluster of cells created is called a benign tumor. While dividing in an uncontrolled manner, it displaces its healthy neighboring cells by pushing them to the side, so to speak. Only when the tumor cells gain the ability to actively dissolve the surrounding, healthy tissue and grow into it has this relatively harmless accumulation of tumor cells turned into a malignant cancer.

Is My Tumor Cancerous?

Only malignant tumors that have the six universal signs of cancer (see box, opposite) are called cancerous growths, or cancers. Tumors that simply displace surrounding tissue are benign and are not called cancer. However, it is not easy to look at the outside of a mass and determine whether tissue proliferation is due to a benign or a malignant tumor. Only an accurate analysis of the tissue within can determine that. For this reason, when there is a suspicion of cancer, the suspect tissue is surgically removed and systematically investigated. This allows for the tumor to be accurately classified.

How the Immune System Fights Internal Enemies

Unnoticed by us, every day, our bodies form several hundred cells that have mutations leading to uncontrolled growth. But we don't all have cancer. While tumor or cancer cells constantly form within the body, they face a mighty opponent: the body's immune system, which rapidly detects abnormal cells and immediately disables them.

For the immune system to effectively destroy degenerate cells in the body, these cells have to first be identified as the enemy. Tumor and cancer cells reveal themselves through certain structures on the surface of their cell membranes. But because they originate from the body's healthy cells and closely resemble them, they can be extremely difficult for the immune system to recognize and attack. Plus, some cancer cells may fool the immune system and use a "shield" to defend themselves from attack.

DID YOU KNOW?

Metastasis
The transformation of a benign tumor into an invasive one often causes the tumor cells to expand well beyond their point of origin in the body, a process known as spread, or metastasis. It is only when this dangerous state of invasiveness and spread is achieved that we speak of a malignant tumor, or cancer.

DID YOU KNOW?

Protect Your Immune System
A healthy, powerful immune system is the best tool for protecting you every day against the growth of mutated cells.

Testing to Determine Whether a Tumor Is Cancerous

If your health care provider suspects that you have cancer, it is often possible to take a small tissue sample during a minimally invasive procedure (such as surgery that causes the smallest possible damage to the skin and soft tissues). This method is used, for example, in the biopsy of suspicious breast lumps or suspected prostate cancer. If, during the analysis of the retrieved tissue sample, the pathologist determines that there is a tumor or cancerous tissue, the mass is usually surgically removed. In addition, the patient with cancer is treated using chemotherapy and/or radiation to help kill tumor or cancer cells that were not (or could not be) removed during surgery.

The Earlier, the Better

Generally speaking, the earlier a degenerate cell cluster is detected, the better your chances of recovery. Make sure, therefore, that you take advantage of regular cancer screenings offered by health insurance programs.

Unfortunately, however, even with regular testing, it is not always possible to discover all precursors or small cell clusters. It, therefore, becomes ever more important for scientists to develop better cancer-screening tests that will, on one hand, detect degenerate cell groups as early as possible and, on the other hand, check on the progress of specific therapies. A series of new tests, such as the EDIM-TKTL1 blood test (see diagram, page 21), are likely to considerably improve cancer screening in the near future. They will help detect cancerous growths and tumor recurrences, and monitor the success of cancer-fighting therapies.

Why Do We Get Cancer?

Whether we will suffer from cancer at some point in our lives depends on many factors. Usually, a combination of circumstances encourages a cancer to develop and, eventually, leads to the outbreak of the disease. These factors include inherited genetic defects, viral infections, chemical poisoning, exposure to DNA-damaging radiation and — last but not least — an unhealthy lifestyle. Increasingly, however, this insidious disease affects people who follow a seemingly healthy diet, exercise regularly, maintain a healthy weight,

---

DID YOU KNOW?

Early Detection of Adenomas

Early discovery is especially helpful in the case of adenomas, the precursors of colon tumors; they are usually benign. Through the use of cancer-screening tests and/or a colonoscopy, these precancerous lesions can usually be easily detected and removed via a minimally invasive procedure. In most cases, this means that the patient has beaten the cancer.

---

and do not smoke or drink heavily. How, then, can this massive increase in cancers in supposedly healthy people be explained?

Recent Research into the Causes

Only in rare cases can the occurrence of a carcinoma be explained by a single cause, such as an inherited genetic defect (see box, below). But even if there are various reasons for the formation of cancer cells — and not all causes have been explored — it has become increasingly apparent that there is one crucial factor that plays a greater role in the emergence and spread of cancer cells than previously thought: the metabolism of the cancer cell and the direct impact of diet on cancer growth.

BRCA1 or BRCA2: Should You Have a Mastectomy if You're at Risk?

In the United States, there has been much publicity surrounding the high risk of breast cancer in women who have inherited a defect in their BRCA1 or BRCA2 genes. This has led to an extremely dubious situation, in which women with these mutations choose to preventively have their breasts removed. Even prepubescent girls have been advised to opt for this surgery.

Although women who have these mutations do have a predisposition to the disease, the fact is that the development of breast cancer is not a foregone conclusion for them. In other words, not every person who carries the mutation actually develops cancer (in scientific language, this is called an incomplete penetrance of the mutation). The probability of developing cancer for those with the inherited gene defect is, however, significantly higher than in those without the mutation. Affected women should, therefore, ensure they have earlier and more frequent checkups and cancer-screening tests.

Is Each Cancer Unique?

Current teaching assumes that there is no common denominator for all malignant cancer cells. Rather, each cancer cell — depending on its point of origin, type and localization — is said to have its own form, therefore requiring its own specific therapy.

Now, however, we have proof that it is neither the type nor the localization of cancer cells that decides their malignancy. Instead, it is the way in which cancer cells metabolize glucose. A normal cell burns glucose to release energy. A cancer cell ferments glucose, producing lactic acid, to sustain its energy supply and to help it proliferate inside the body.

Rogue cells occur in the body every now and then; they continue to divide, yet they do not actively destroy their surroundings. However, if a cluster of malignant cells changes its metabolism, it quickly turns into a predator, mercilessly invading the adjacent tissue and destroying it in order to make room for itself. This mechanism, when the cell's metabolism switches from combustion to fermentation, is identical in all aggressive cancer cells.

The Discovery of the TKTL1 Metabolism

Until recently, this change in the metabolism of cancer cells was largely ignored. Now, it may bring about a decisive breakthrough in cancer therapy.

TKTL1 is the abbreviation for transketolase-like-1. It is a gene, or rather a protein, that resembles transketolase (TKT). TKT is an enzyme that occurs in all living beings and permits the conversion of sugars into other forms — for example, when the body turns glucose into a sugar called deoxyribose, which forms part of the DNA strand.

Scientific Recognition

Renowned scientific institutions have confirmed the importance of TKTL1 in the formation of aggressive cancer cells, and have included this information in their research. In recent studies by Johns Hopkins University, the German Cancer Research Center and other international research groups, one aspect in particular has been demonstrated: the vital importance of the activation of sugar fermentation in cancer cells via the TKTL1 metabolism. Scientists examined

TKTL1 in Different Types of Tumors

The activation of TKTL1 fermentation has been demonstrated in every type of cancer that has been tested for it. It is a general phenomenon of cancer — and, therefore, the common denominator in all types of cancer, which scientists had previously searched for in vain. Researchers from Johns Hopkins University in Baltimore, MD, have identified the TKTL1 gene as an especially important gene (called a proto-oncogene) for head and neck tumors, which lead to malignant cancer by activating glucose metabolism.

the presence of the TKTL1 protein in tumors and cancerous growths (see box, opposite). In their analysis of the results, they took into account both the number of TKTL1-positive tumor cells and the concentration (known as the expression) of TKTL1 in the tumorous cells.

New Diagnostic Methods

Evidence of TKTL1 fermentation offers diagnostic and therapeutic options that were not previously available. There is now a test that can prove whether the TKTL1 gene in tumor or cancer cells has been activated, independent of the type of tumor or cancer in question. The EDIM-TKTL1 blood test (see diagram, page 21) is a procedure that uses a laser-based technology called flow cytometry (see box, at right). The test uses the body's immune system to demonstrate the presence of tumor-specific structures that are consumed by macrophages (the body's own scavenger cells). Laser light passes through the blood sample, revealing these structures and enabling the identification of macrophages that have invaded tumorous tissue and consumed tumorous cells. As they devour these structures, macrophages show up as the laser light passes through the blood.

If the test results are positive — that is, fermenting TKTL1-positive cancer cells have been found to be present — the patient should insist that the results be taken into account when a treatment plan is devised. Below are details on how TKTL1 affects specific types of cancer.

- **Bladder Cancer.** In this type of tumor, a correlation was found between the presence and concentration of the TKTL1 protein and the invasiveness of tumors, as well as the imminence of death in patients. The more tumor cells showed the presence of the TKTL1 protein and the higher the concentration of TKTL1 in the tumor cells, the faster the victims died.
- **Colorectal Cancer.** In patients with colorectal cancer, the presence and concentration of the TKTL1 protein also correlated with tumor invasiveness. Here, too, patients with large amounts of TKTL1 in their tumors died significantly sooner than those who had little or no TKTL1. Furthermore, patients with activated TKTL1 in rectal tumors have been shown to be resistant to radiation and chemotherapy, which causes those patients to die very quickly.

DID YOU KNOW?

Flow Cytometry
This laser-based technique allows doctors to count and identify specific types of cells. They are suspended in liquid, sometimes marked with fluorescent dye, and passed through a strong beam of laser light. There, the amount of light they scatter is measured, which identifies the types of cells or specific characteristics of those cells.

- **Ovarian and Cervical Cancers.** Studies of patients with ovarian cancer and cervical cancer showed that there is a clear connection between TKTL1 expression and the formation of metastases.

- **Laryngeal Cancer.** In patients with laryngeal cancer, TKTL1 expression was also associated with the occurrence of metastases.

- **Nasopharyngeal and Thyroid Cancers.** In nasopharyngeal and thyroid carcinomas, TKTL1 expression was associated with the occurrence of metastases in lymph nodes.

- **Kidney Cancer.** In kidney cancer, TKTL1 expression correlated with disease progression and the formation of metastases. In addition, it was possible to identify a group of TKTL1-positive renal tumors that had been classified by standard diagnostic procedures as tumors having a good prognosis, but that actually were highly aggressive and caused death quickly. These aggressive, malignant tumors had simply been missed by previously available diagnostic methods; today, they can be identified by detecting the presence of TKTL1 and treated aggressively.

- **Brain Cancer.** Relatively benign brain tumors called astrocytomas were found to exhibit no or low expression of the TKTL1 protein, while aggressive brain tumors called glioblastomas showed very high TKTL1 expression.

- **Lung Cancer.** Patients who have lung tumors with high levels of TKTL1 experienced shorter survival times compared with patients whose lung tumors had low amounts of TKTL1.

- **Children's Cancers.** An analysis of tumors revealed that the switch to TKTL1 fermentation is of great importance in both adults and children with cancer. In the case of nephroblastoma (also known as Wilms' tumor, the most common malignant kidney cancer in children), TKTL1 expression was specifically detected in aggressive and chemotherapy-resistant tumors.

The EDIM-TKTL1 Blood Test

In this diagnostic examination, macrophages are tested for increased levels of TKTL1 antigen. A positive result indicates energy production by fermentation, and, thus, the presence of aggressive cancer cells, increased resistance to radiation and chemotherapy, and increased risk of metastases.

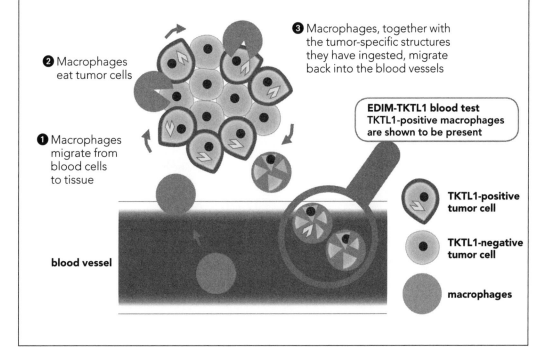

❷ Macrophages eat tumor cells

❸ Macrophages, together with the tumor-specific structures they have ingested, migrate back into the blood vessels

❶ Macrophages migrate from blood cells to tissue

EDIM-TKTL1 blood test TKTL1-positive macrophages are shown to be present

blood vessel

TKTL1-positive tumor cell

TKTL1-negative tumor cell

macrophages

Dr. Johannes F. Coy on Discovering the TKTL1 Metabolism

Q: Once you got your doctorate in biology with a focus on molecular genetics and biochemistry, what made you decide to engage so intensively in the study of cancer?

A: For more than 80 years, there has been an intense search for the causes of and therapies for cancer. Despite some successes, researchers have not yet found all the answers. Cancer is still a leading cause of death, and it creates much suffering and pain. In the late 20th century, people had high hopes for the human genome project. By determining the complete sequence of the human genome and all the genes encrypted therein, we hoped it would finally be possible to reveal the causes of diseases. It was hoped that new, successful therapies could be developed as a result. The human genome sequence was decrypted, thanks to great financial and technological efforts. But in the eyes of many researchers, the hopes that had been placed on this project were not fulfilled.

Q: What was the German Cancer Research Center's goal in its genome research?

A: When I started my job at the German Cancer Research Center (DKFZ) in Heidelberg in 1990, genome research was still in its infancy. Our research group, for example, focused on a special section of the X chromosome (Xq28). You have to imagine a chromosome as a very long thread, which is built using only four letters: A, G, T and C. In the case of the X chromosome, this is a thread of 240 million letters. With a pair of chemical "scissors" called a restriction enzyme, the thread was cut into many small pieces.

At the time, I was developing a new method that exploited the similarity of gene sequences between different mammals. I went to a butcher shop and took tissue samples from a slaughtered pig, then compared these with human DNA pieces. I was able to identify a piece of DNA that I suspected contained a gene; then, a group of researchers from England who worked with us determined the complete sequence of this piece of DNA. Using computer analysis, we were able to demonstrate that the selected DNA sequence had similarities with the transketolase (TKT) gene.

The TKT gene in humans had been discovered only a few years prior. It forms a protein, the TKT enzyme, which is able to transform sugar. These TKT enzyme reactions are so important that all forms of life on Earth depend on them, from simple bacteria and yeasts to complex plant and animal cells. Among other things, the TKT enzyme creates an enzymatic reaction, during which glucose is converted into a sugar that is required to build DNA letters. Because of its similarities to the known TKT gene, I called the gene that I had discovered transketolase-like-1 (TKTL1).

Q: Is TKTL1 an absolutely new discovery?

A: Yes. Discovering and decrypting a previously unknown gene made me feel a bit like an explorer finding a new continent, or at least a new island. I can still remember how excited I felt when it became clear that I had made this discovery. Unfortunately, it was not long before my euphoria was reduced to zero by bad news: a short time later, an English research group declared that because the TKTL1 gene contained a serious fault, it did not constitute a functional gene.

Q: Was this a serious setback?

A: Not really. My experiments were able to prove that although this fault was, indeed, present, it had been cleverly corrected. I want to explain this using an image. The previously known transketolase gene was like the blueprint for a four-wheeled car. In the TKTL1 gene, one of those wheels was altered and could no longer turn. At first glance, researchers assumed that the entire car would not be able to run. However, I was able to show that while the wheel was broken, it was no longer needed. To clarify the image: Normally, cars have four wheels. If you remove the right front wheel, it can no longer run because it's unbalanced. If, however, you reposition the functioning left front wheel to the middle of the car, it will run like a tricycle. In my opinion, the fault in the TKTL1 gene, therefore, did not deactivate the gene but rather changed it.

Q: Was the TKTL1 gene recognized at this point?

A: Unfortunately not. I published my research results in 1996, pointing out that the TKTL1 gene is, indeed, an altered transketolase gene, but one that could still be fully functional. But nobody was interested.

Q: What led you to continue your research into the TKTL1 gene despite these setbacks?

A: After another five years of research at the DKFZ, I moved to a small biotech company in 2001. This company was developing a test for the early diagnosis of cervical cancer and bringing this test to the market. My task was to identify additional genes that would be suitable for the early detection of other cancers. Besides my actual research, I also studied "my" already discovered gene, to see whether it also played a role in cancer. I found that the TKTL1 gene was activated in some of the cancer tissue I examined. When it became clear that the activation occurred in all cancers under investigation, the company filed a patent on the TKTL1 gene.

Q: Was this the first step to success?

A: Initially, yes. But after a year and a half, the company had to decide whether to pursue the patent, and they stopped research into the TKTL1 gene. At the same time, I was told that the patents to protect the TKTL1 gene would be abandoned. Legally, I had the right to continue with the patent application myself. So I was faced with an important decision: forfeit the patent or pay for the patent application out of my own pocket.

Q: How did you face this difficult decision?

A: I knew that I could take over the TKTL1 patent application, but that I could not continue for long. The financial requirements for the maintenance of an international patent application are immense. Despite the high costs, I took over the TKTL1 and two other patent applications the company no longer wanted to pursue. This process was vastly expensive, and I was often overcome by doubt. Was it a huge mistake to invest my life savings in such a risky undertaking? At the time, I did not know whether the TKTL1 gene represented a functional gene at all.

Q: How did you overcome this situation?

A: In 2004, I convinced a diagnostics company that worked in the field of food, animal feed and serology to get involved in the field of tumor diagnosis, and to conduct research on my projects. They hired me as an employee for this newly created department. Due to the company's focus, as well as its existing research and development projects, I could not conduct cancer research in the way that I was accustomed to. All I could do was instigate further experiments and studies in collaboration with other laboratories, and to advance testing within the company. Meanwhile, I established an antibody for demonstrating the presence of the TKTL1 protein. With the help of a hospital, I succeeded in testing the antibody, and I finally had the proof I needed. It was a moment I will never forget: I had goosebumps, and tears of joy welled up in my eyes. For a moment, time stood still.

Q: You had proven the existence of the TKTL1 gene, but were you also able to ascertain its function?

A: That was the next difficult step. Night after night, I read papers on the subject of transketolase and cancer. At that time, literature on the topic was sparse. It was known, however, that the inhibition of TKT (using oxythiamine) also inhibited tumor growth in mice. This effect was credited to the previously known TKT enzyme, and researchers concluded that it played an important role in tumor growth. As a result, several pharmaceutical companies began to develop a drug to inhibit the TKT enzyme — without success. Apparently, no one had checked whether the TKT gene was, indeed, the bad guy. My tests demonstrated, however, that it was exclusively the TKTL1 gene that was activated in tumors; neither the normal TKT gene nor the TKTL2 gene (a kind of lesser-known identical twin brother of the TKTL1 gene) were more active in tumors than in corresponding healthy tissue. So I was absolutely certain that TKTL1 was the only transketolase or transketolase-like gene that was important for tumor growth.

Q: Had no one else realized this before?

A: Amazingly, neither researchers nor pharmaceutical companies believed in the existence of a functioning TKTL1 gene. And due to increasing specialization in research, hardly anyone has an overview anymore or is able to position his or her own results within an overall picture. Scientists have ever-more detailed knowledge, but hardly anyone understands the connections between the puzzle pieces. Except for the TKTL1 gene, all the pieces were already at hand, but the missing link still eluded us. It was only with TKTL1 that I managed to put the entire picture together. During my studies, I came across a review article from 1998, which pointed out that uncertainties still existed concerning transketolases and their related metabolic pathways. Intrigued, I studied more literature on this topic. And I soon realized that for more than 50 years, certain reaction equations had been presented as fact in standard textbooks around the world, although research had shown as early as 1954 that further reactions occur which might still be beyond our knowledge. I wondered how we could understand the interaction of nutrition and human metabolism correctly when the foundations of teaching were incorrect.

Q: Were you surprised that no one had pursued this any further?

A: Yes, I was more than surprised at this state of affairs. I think my literature research on the topic of transketolases is as exciting and captivating as a Hitchcock thriller. The next important piece of the puzzle, which I came across in my search for the truth about transketolases, was a publication by a Hungarian research group, which dealt with vitamin C metabolism. At first glance, it seemed like an insignificant paper, but the researchers demonstrated, almost in passing, that oxythiamine inhibited the production of lactic acid in cancer cells. Since oxythiamine is also an inhibitor of transketolases, this meant, in my opinion, that transketolases were instrumental in the formation of lactic acid in cancer cells. So, aside from the lactic acid fermentation we already knew about, production of lactic acid done with the help of transketolases also had to exist.

Q: So, instead of investigating this yourself, you essentially reinterpreted "old" results?

A: I had no other way of doing it. My tools consisted of a desk, a laptop with Internet access and time to think. Lacking in both means and equipment, I could not do any active research. But maybe that was a good thing. Perhaps it was exactly this identification of interconnections and imagining new, unknown pathways led me to the target.

The Cancer Cell's Metabolism

When life developed on Earth millions of years ago, conditions were entirely different than they are today. The atmosphere did not yet contain oxygen, and it, therefore, did not support any form of life as we know it. Chemical compounds were the only available energy source for microorganisms, which were able to use them to live. This type of oxygen-independent energy creation is called **fermentation.** In ecological niches, such as sulfur hot springs, microorganisms still use this type of energy production today.

Oxygen Fills the Atmosphere

Eventually, thanks to photosynthesis, the first bacteria made use of the energy contained in sunlight and succeeded in splitting water into its atomic parts. The hydrogen that they formed was stored in the form of sugar molecules and used as an energy source. As they split water molecules, in addition to hydrogen, oxygen was created as a "waste product." Primeval bacteria produced so much oxygen that, over time, this gas enriched the oceans, then the atmosphere.

Once that occurred, microorganisms developed. These evolved into larger creatures, who used oxygen to release the energy stored in food. In humans, hydrogen is separated from carbon and oxidized as water by the body's own fuel cells, the mitochondria (see box, below). The energy stored

---

Mitochondria, Our Power Generators

The main energy suppliers for most types of cells in our bodies are the mitochondria. These structures basically work like small fuel cells, releasing energy by burning hydrogen with the help of oxygen to make water. This combustion is a highly effective form of energy release, because it completely metabolizes the fuel and maximizes energy gain. Much of the energy needed to maintain vital body functions is efficiently released in this way.

---

in hydrocarbon compounds is again released, and the waste products water and carbon dioxide are formed. This process of energy production is called **combustion.**

A Hybrid Form Appears

For a time, fermenting and direct-combustion microorganisms existed side by side. Over time, the two forms of life fused. They formed a hybrid from a fermented primordial cell (archaea) and a combusted bacterium (mitochondrion). This created the first cell of higher organisms.

Today, every cell of the human body still carries these "swallowed" primitive bacteria within itself, and, thus, employs both methods of energy release:

- Oxygen-dependent (aerobic) energy release by combustion in the mitochondria (see box, opposite)
- Oxygen-independent (anaerobic) energy release by fermentation and the formation of lactic acid (see page 28)

Oxygen Is Life

Around the clock, countless metabolic activities take place in the body. For the cells to be able to release sufficient energy in the mitochondria, they need oxygen continuously. This is why we need to breathe in and out all the time.

Without air to breathe, our bodies would collapse within a few minutes and our lives would be snuffed out like a flame under a glass dome. Even when we breathe quickly, pumping lots of oxygen into the lungs (hyperventilation), a short-term lack of oxygen may occur within the body. This is the case when we run very fast, and insufficient oxygen reaches the muscles. They simply require more energy than is released via direct combustion, and oxygen is the limiting factor.

Turbo Drive to Escape

Over the course of millennia, our ancestors had to cope with exactly this type of situation. For example, when they had to run away from or fight an animal, they found themselves in a life-threatening situation; due to hyperventilation, they had only limited amounts of oxygen available.

But thanks to a trick played by the body, they could manage to at least partially overcome this limitation. As soon as muscle

> **DID YOU KNOW?**
>
> **Energy Generation**
> The way we create and use energy has hardly changed since the first humans appeared. We ingest as food the solar energy stored in plants, then split this into its smallest components. These components are either used immediately to supply power to the body or stored for later use.

cells had insufficient or no oxygen at their disposal and their performance became impaired, a fermentation "emergency program" would kick in. This method of delivering energy to the cells without using oxygen was a type of "turbo drive" that provided additional reserves. The cells were instantly able to call up more energy, allowing the muscles to achieve greater performance. These dual options for energy generation still exist in our cells today.

Fermentation's Waste Product: Lactic Acid

During fermentation in normal cells (when they need a lot of energy quickly), lactic acid is created and transported from muscle cells via blood vessels to the liver. There, using energy, it is converted back into glucose (sugar), then rereleased into the bloodstream and transported back to the muscles.

For as long as a fight-or-flight situation persists, the muscles conduct this hybrid form of combustion and fermentation of glucose. As soon as the muscles are at rest and have sufficient oxygen at their disposal, the fermentation reaction stops and the cells burn energy as usual.

Glucose Is Ideal Energy for Cells

Whenever large amounts of strength are required, glucose is the ideal form of energy. It has one major advantage over fat (the body's other main source of energy): cells can release the energy glucose contains through both combustion and fermentation. Fatty acids, however, can be burned only if there is sufficient oxygen present. This is why sports scientists always recommend aerobic exercise for weight loss during endurance training. The muscles stay supplied with enough oxygen, which melts fat. For our ancestors, it was vital to constantly fill up with both forms of stored energy: glucose for speedy energy release (especially in emergencies) and fat for a long-term supply.

DID YOU KNOW?

Muscle Acidosis
At some point, you have probably suffered from muscle acidosis, the consequences of this hybrid process of fermentation and combustion in stressed muscles. If you exercise anaerobically (such as when you exert great strength, as in weight lifting), the lactic acid created during fermentation, together with microtears in the muscle fibers, causes sore muscles.

Energy Generation: Tumor Cells vs. Cancer Cells

In benign tumor cells (TKTL1-negative tumor cells), sugar consumed in food is burned through combustion. In TKTL1-positive tumor cells (cancer cells), combustion in the mitochondria is switched off, and fermentation via the TKTL1 enzyme is switched on. During fermentation, the cancer cell produces lactic acid from sugar. The lactic acid keeps the immune system from attacking and simultaneously dissolves the surrounding tissue. The cancer cells begin to spread.

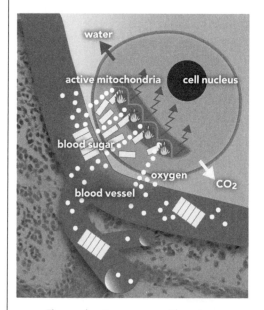

The combustion process with oxygen

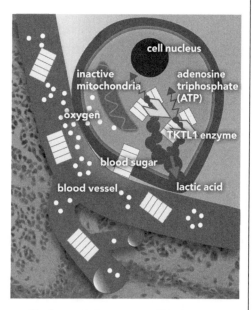

The fermentation process without oxygen

Cancer Cells Ferment, Too

Renowned scientists from around the world have repeatedly reported increased concentrations of lactic acid surrounding cancer cells. They have also concluded that cancer cells have a different metabolism than healthy cells. Otto Heinrich Warburg (1883–1970), a Nobel Prize–winning scientist, observed fermentation in cancer cells as early as 1924 and called it the real cause of the disease. But little significance was attached to this discovery until recently.

The Warburg Hypothesis

In 1931, Warburg, the founder and director of the Kaiser Wilhelm Institute for Cell Physiology in Berlin (renamed the Max Planck Institute for Cell Physiology in 1953), was awarded the Nobel Prize in Medicine for his "discovery of the nature and mode of action of the respiratory enzyme."[1] Warburg discovered that cancer cells do not combust glucose, creating water and carbon dioxide, but instead ferment it into lactic acid — even when sufficient oxygen is present to allow direct combustion. As early as 1924, he deduced from this fact his hypothesis: a disruption in the function of the mitochondria and the release of energy via fermentation were the actual causes for the development of cancer cells within the body. The Warburg Hypothesis has been repeatedly confirmed in recent studies.

Not All Fermentation Is Alike

Fermentation in cancer cells differs fundamentally from that in muscle and some other tissues. In muscles, it is used as a backup form of energy generation for times when oxygen is scarce. It is similar to the fermentation that occurs in healthy cells in the retinas, testes and nerves, which generates energy even when sufficient oxygen is present and protects these cells from damaging oxygen radicals (also called reactive oxygen species). The product is the same in both fermentation processes: the formation of lactic acid. The twist: cancer cells abuse this energy-generating process to protect themselves from harm.

Before the discovery of the TKTL1 gene, no one knew about an alternative pathway that allowed fermentation even in the presence of oxygen. Researchers concluded that the lactic acid produced by cancer cells was formed via the Embden-Meyerhof-Parnas (EMP) pathway, which muscle cells use when oxygen deficiency occurs. This pathway causes sugar to split into two parts; after a series of chemical reactions, the hydrogen splits off and is burned in the mitochondria, releasing energy and creating lactic acid as a waste product. Then, the muscle cells switch back to direct combustion as usual once oxygen is available again. Cancer cells, however, don't switch back but continue to ferment.

[1] "The Nobel Prize in Physiology or Medicine 1931." *Nobelprize.org.* Nobel Media AB 2015. Web. 12 Jan. 2015.

The hypothesis that the EMP pathway was the only fermentation route was finally seen as flawed when the TKTL1 enzyme was discovered. This enzyme causes a reaction that connects the pentose phosphate pathway directly to lactic acid (and fatty acid) production. Via this pathway, sugar is converted to lactic acid, releasing energy without damaging the cell. Since it is not suppressed by oxygen, it does not constitute an emergency response. Instead, it is a specifically chosen way of generating energy — in both healthy cells (such as those in the retinas, testes and nerves) and cancer cells, it is used to avoid oxygen radicals and the DNA damage they cause. However, when cancer cells generate energy this way, they make themselves almost invincible.

Fermenting Cancer Cells Can Grow Without Oxygen

Oxygen is often the factor that limits growth. A dangerous oxygen deficiency exists as soon as a cell is even one-tenth of a millimeter away from an oxygen-carrying capillary (a small blood vessel). So even in small tumors, the oxygen supply of cells located inside the tumor and away from blood vessels is a major problem.

Unfortunately, however, the tumor's inner cells do not die off completely due to this oxygen deficiency, as scientists had previously thought. The tumor's innermost cells do die due to absence of oxygen and glucose. But the cells in the medial layer still have access to glucose, and they switch to anaerobic fermentation, which produces less energy but can occur without the presence of oxygen. This is the fermentation process that happens via the TKTL1 gene. The affected tumor cells create an advantage for themselves over their oxygen-dependent relatives.

When Lactic Acid Becomes Dangerous

The metabolic switch to TKTL1 fermentation means cancer cells begin to create lactic acid, which destroys the surrounding healthy tissue (a process called matrix degradation). These fermenting cancer cells are then more malignant because they grow into these surrounding free spaces and can spread throughout the body, causing distant metastases.

The Missing Piece of the Puzzle

Discovering the TKTL1 gene and its significance in fermentation allowed scientists to appreciate the importance of the Warburg Hypothesis (see page 30) for the first time. The missing piece of the puzzle, this discovery solves the apparent contradiction between Warburg's concept of mitochondrial disorder and the activation of fermentation, and current teachings about DNA mutations being at the root of cancer development. The two theories are not mutually exclusive, but rather component parts of the overall way that cancer cells form. The importance of Warburg's theory of cancer development becomes particularly apparent if you think about how fermentation benefits the cancer cell.

How Cancer Cells Protect Themselves

A quick review: cancer cells start as a result of mutations in genes that control, among other things, the growth and death of cells. These abnormal cells grow in an uncontrolled manner. Initially, they obtain energy — just like most healthy cells — from active mitochondria; that is, they convert hydrogen to water. Further mutations switch off healthy combustion and enable fermentation via the TKTL1 enzyme. These cancer cells do not burn glucose normally, but rather ferment it into lactic acid, even when there is sufficient oxygen present to allow normal direct combustion.

Lactic Acid Forms a Protective Shield

At first glance, this appears to make no sense. Glucose fermentation is not a very efficient source of energy, and a lot of energy in the lactic acid remains untapped. The cancer cell, however, turns this apparent shortcoming to its advantage and uses the lactic acid as a shield. Here's how: the output of lactic acid blocks attacks by the so-called natural killer cells, creating a kind of barrier and inhibiting the immune system. This is because lactic acid transforms the area immediately surrounding the cancer cell into an extremely acidic environment. This abnormal acidity (of up to 2 on the pH scale) prevents immune system cells from actively attacking the cancer cells. The lactic acid surrounds the cancer cell like a shield, disabling the otherwise very powerful immune system.

Tumor Size Doesn't Guarantee Aggressiveness

There are some very large benign tumors that do not spread, despite reaching a weight of 6½ to 8¾ lbs (3 to 4 kg). On the other hand, there are very small malignant tumors that start spreading immediately. Size alone, therefore, is not an indication of a tumor's aggressiveness. Tumors that push aside other tissues and grow only locally are not a deadly problem. They become life threatening only once they change their metabolisms to fermentation and turn into invasively growing cancers, which take over healthy tissue and metastasize.

Lactic Acid Also Destroys Neighboring Healthy Cells

Human tissue is not simply a loose accumulation of cells. It is firmly connected by sophisticated cell-to-cell contact. The individual cells within these associations are in constant, close contact and share information in the fastest possible way.

However, the lactic acid generated by a cancer cell destroys this cell-to-cell contact like a sword. The tissue structure gets increasingly broken up and eventually dissolves completely; this process is called matrix degradation. In addition, the acidic environment around cancer cells causes major damage to adjacent healthy cells, eventually triggering their programmed death.

Put simply, a fermenting cancer cell, with the help of lactic acid, drives its healthy neighboring cells to "voluntary" suicide. Because of the cancer cell's mutation, this cell death trigger does not function in the cancer cell, so it is absolutely immune to the program of destruction that it has triggered in its neighbors. Using this dirty trick, the cancer cell simply dissolves its surroundings by producing lactic acid and slashes its way without hindrance through healthy tissue in order to conquer new territory.

This process is called the invasive growth behavior of a malignant tumor cell. The cancer cell is now free to spread throughout the body without local restrictions and to form metastases. Studies have shown that the higher the lactic acid production of a tumor, the greater the likelihood it will metastasize.

How the Fermentation Metabolism Obstructs Cancer Treatment

Cancer cells often divide at an extremely high rate. The principle of chemotherapy and radiation is to take advantage of exactly this fact and to kill cells during their growth phase. However, the free radicals (aggressive oxygen molecules) formed by irradiation are neutralized by the metabolic products of fermentation in cancer cells; therefore, programmed cell death is not triggered in the cancer cells.

Chemotherapy is similarly hampered by fermentation. Because fermentation leads to a shutdown of the mitochondria and blocks the cell-destruction program, the cancer-killing substances delivered during chemotherapy are not allowed to trigger cancer cell death. Chemotherapy works only in tumor cells that do not ferment and are not invasive.

Research Study:
Fermentation Helps Cancer Cells Repair Themselves

It is well known that glucose-fermenting tumors are resistant to radiation and chemotherapy (see above). Now, a 2014 study conducted by Dr. Anant Narayan Bhatt and his colleagues at the Institute of Nuclear Medicine and Allied Sciences in Delhi, India, has demonstrated *how* glucose fermentation plays a role in radiation resistance.

This new study confirms that when a cell switches from combustion to fermentation, it becomes resistant to radiation because the switch activates two independent mechanisms that repair DNA damage. These mechanisms fix both single- and double-strand DNA damage induced by radiation. This means that a fermenting cancer cell can actually repair the damage caused by radiation, allowing the cell to survive and rebuild itself.

Many standard chemotherapy drugs — including platins (such as cisplatin, carboplatin and oxaliplatin), alkylating agents (such as cyclophosphamide), intercalating agents (such as doxorubicin) and topoisomerase inhibitors (such as irinotecan and topotecan) — also induce DNA damage. So this discovery shows how the cancer-killing effects of most chemotherapy drugs can also be hampered by glucose fermentation in cancer cells. This revelation means that it is crucial for people with cancer to avoid a diet rich in starch and glucose, as you will learn on the following pages.

Research Study:
Blocking the TKTL1 Gene

In studies published by Johns Hopkins University (2009; 2010) and the German Cancer Research Center (2009), the role of the TKTL1 gene in cancer cells was investigated. When the TKTL1 gene was inhibited by blocking the formation of TKTL1 protein, it led to an inhibition of glucose uptake and lactic acid production. At the same time, cancer cell growth slowed down and cell division was inhibited; the cancer cells were also considerably more responsive to free radicals and therapies that induced cell death.

Furthermore, inhibiting the TKTL1 gene was shown to reduce cancer cell invasiveness and limit tumor growth. TKTL1 was also demonstrated to activate a signal called hypoxia-induced-factor-1-alpha, which leads to invasive growth and resistance to radiation and chemotherapy. The results impressively demonstrated how important the role of the TKTL1 gene is in cancer. They also show that its inhibition is a promising strategy to break through fermenting cancer cells' resistance to chemotherapy and radiation.

Resistant to Radiation

Both healthy cells and benign tumor cells die when exposed to radiation, but a fermenting cancer cell cheats death. Why? The activation of the pentose phosphate pathway (see page 31) and TKTL1 in the cancer cell prevents treatment from triggering programmed cell death. As soon as the cell's metabolism switches, a byproduct called nicotinamide adenine dinucleotide phosphate (NADPH) forms. This hydrogen compound reduces glutathione, one of the most important antioxidants produced by the body, which protects cells from damage by free radicals and oxidation. A compound called cytochrome c released by the mitochondria is also reduced by NADPH, which in turn suppresses programmed cell death. So a fermenting cancer cell loses the ability to destroy itself. The result is that fermenting cancer cells become significantly more resistant to radiation than healthy cells.

Besides lactic acid, fermentation also produces a metabolite called pyruvate, which efficiently neutralizes the free radicals formed during irradiation. Together with the prevention of the self-destruction program, this increases the resistance of cancer cells even more. Put simply, this means that radiation has exactly the opposite effect of what it is meant to achieve: healthy tissue and less harmful tumor tissue dies, while aggressive cancer cells survive.

DID YOU KNOW?

Radiation
During irradiation with gamma rays (X-rays), free radicals are produced in the target tissue; these cause changes in the DNA and kill irradiated cells. The aim of localized irradiation is to destroy as few healthy cells and as many cancer cells as possible. However, as X-rays traverse healthy tissue on their way to cancer cells, normal cells are always damaged, too.

Tumor cells that continue to release energy through combustion in the mitochondria die more easily after radiation. They can neither reduce glutathione nor make pyruvate to protect themselves. Unlike a cancer that consists of fermenting cells, tumor cells that generate energy through combustion can be treated successfully with radiation.

Resistant to Chemotherapy, Too

It is especially galling for patients with cancer that a fermenting cancer cell makes use of the same mechanism to fight destruction by chemotherapy as it does to fight destruction by radiation. A research group in the United States proved this in 2005. However, on the positive side, the same scientists also demonstrated that the removal of glucose kills aggressive cancer cells — an important tool that increases the effectiveness of cancer treatments.

In 2011, oncologists at the University of Mannheim in Germany demonstrated that TKTL1 gene activation led to radiation and chemotherapy resistance. However, on the positive side, several studies also demonstrated that aggressive cancer cells could be resensitized to radiation and chemotherapy through a strict reduction in the amount of glucose and carbohydrates in the diet, or by using drugs to inhibit TKTL1 fermentation. This knowledge is an incredibly important tool that increases the effectiveness of treatments for radiation- and chemo-resistant cancers.

What Fermenting Tumors Do

By switching to the TKTL1 metabolism, cancer cells enjoy several important advantages at once. When their metabolism changes and they ferment sugar, cancer cells are able to do the following:

- Build a shield, using the lactic acid that they have formed, against the immune system when it attacks them

- Grow whether or not sufficient oxygen is present, making them resistant to drugs that inhibit blood vessel formation (angiogenesis)

- Dissolve adjacent tissue with the help of lactic acid, grow invasively and metastasize

- Become resistant to therapies that form cancer-killing free radicals, such as radiation

- Develop resistance to chemotherapy, which normally triggers cell death

How Does Metastasis Occur?

Imagine cancer cells separating from the original tumor (called the primary tumor). First, they create space for themselves by using lactic acid to destroy the surrounding healthy cells. Next, they try to work their way through to a lymph node or blood vessel. When they reach it, the cancer cells migrate through the vessel wall into the bloodstream or through the lymph node into the lymphatic system so that they can spread to another location in the body.

The result is a metastasis, or a cancerous tumor in a lymph node or a distant piece of solid tissue, such as the liver or brain. Once they arrive at their new destination, the cancer cells again permeate the lymph node or blood vessel wall, and begin dissolving the cell-to-cell contact between healthy cells in this new location. The cells divide and grow while invading fresh territory. Not even hard bone structures are protected against this invasive growth; the lactic acid in cancer cells dissolves bone just like other tissue.

Sugar: The Engine of Aggression

Like most healthy cells, developing tumor or cancer cells are initially able to switch energy generation back and forth between combustion and fermentation. However, once they have a continuous, sufficient sugar supply, they lose the ability to reactivate the combustion process. They become totally dependent on sugar as their only source of energy. Plus, a cancer cell uses fermentation to its advantage in order to defend itself against standard anti-cancer treatments.

Fermentation is much less efficient than combustion in terms of energy yield, so a cancer cell has to absorb about 20 to 30 times more glucose than it would for normal combustion. That means a fermenting cancer cell requires an extremely large amount of glucose; it can carry out fermentation and generate energy only when enough is available. This makes the cancer cell directly and totally dependent on its main energy supplier, sugar. That means that the cancer cell has a major weakness that you can exploit to your advantage.

A New Therapeutic Approach

When you use radiation or chemotherapy, you provide fermenting cancer cells with a clear advantage. While healthy and direct-combusting cells die from these treatments, the unharmed fermenting cells can freely expand into the former's space. Plus, they no longer have to share their glucose supply.

With each subsequent radiation or chemotherapy treatment, the balance shifts further in favor of the fermenting cancer cells; finally, they are the only ones that remain — with fatal consequences. The cancer is now protected against attacks by both the immune system and cancer-fighting treatments.

A Strict Reduction in Glucose and Carbohydrates

Aggressive cancer cells can survive only if sufficient glucose is available for fermentation. So if standard treatment is combined with an appropriate diet that greatly reduces your intake of glucose (and carbohydrates, which can be converted to glucose), the cells can, in essence, be "starved" to death. When fermentation is inhibited, cancer cells are forced to switch back to direct combustion and to reactivate the mitochondria. A "young" cancer cell can, when there is no sugar available, switch back to oxidative energy production in the mitochondria in order to survive. And the bonus is that this cell is then susceptible to the usual anti-cancer therapies, such as chemotherapy and radiation.

There's another way reducing glucose helps. If a cancer cell is certain of a long-term ongoing supply of sufficient sugar, it will gradually loses its ability to reactivate the mitochondria in the event of an emergency. If the energy-producing sugar supply is absent, the cell will die. This is also great news because you can use this knowledge to fight your cancer even more aggressively with simple changes in your diet.

Glucose: The Nutritional Staple of Cancer Cells

It's probably not news to you that common sugars — such as glucose, fructose and table sugar (sucrose) — aren't particularly good for you and your teeth. Dentists have been ringing alarm bells for years, warning us that foods (and especially drinks) made with these sugars destroy teeth, unlike those that contain healthy sugars — such as galactose, trehalose and tagatose (see page 159) — which protect your teeth.

Glucose, fructose and sucrose (as well as starch, which is converted to glucose in the mouth) are the staple foods of acid-forming bacteria in the mouth, which lead to tooth decay. It's easy to understand, then, that you should avoid them in beverages and foods (think chocolate and ice cream), and choose foods and drinks that contain tooth-friendly sugars.

However, you might not realize that you ingest sugar in forms other than table sugar. The body converts all foods that contain carbohydrates (such as potatoes, pasta and bread) to glucose. Pasta, for example, is converted into about 80% sugar. The amount of carbohydrates (and with it, of sugars) that we ingest daily not only affects the condition of our teeth, but also can have catastrophic consequences for our entire metabolism.

> **DID YOU KNOW?**
>
> **How to Spot Sugar**
> Scientific terms for sugar often end in -ose. Check ingredient labels for these words to see what kind of sugar has been added to packaged foods. The type and amount of sugar you consume are both important.

The Source of Energy

Glucose plays a central role in the human metabolism, because cells can use it to create energy through both combustion and fermentation (see page 28). A cell's function within the body and its diet determine whether it uses glucose for its energy supply, or fats and ketone bodies (a byproduct of fat burning in the liver cells, caused by low blood sugar levels). Nerve and brain cells, for example, prefer glucose as their energy supplier. Indeed, they need a certain amount of glucose in order to remain functional. If you ingest too little glucose, this need is initially met by the body's glycogen stores (see box, page 41).

The metabolism switches to an austerity program only once this stock has been exhausted. When this occurs, all cells that do not absolutely need glucose are reset to reduce glucose consumption and, ultimately, stop using it altogether. The valuable glucose is now available exclusively to those cells that really need it. A sort of ranking determines which cells have priority; at the top of the list are nerve and brain cells.

Glucose Transport in Humans

In the human body, blood and the glucose it carries are like an irrigation system (see box, below). The cells may extract glucose from the blood with the help of sugar pumps called glucose transporters. Thanks to this sophisticated mechanism, high-priority cells are still supplied with glucose even when little is available, whereas low-priority cells are forced to switch to fats and ketone bodies as a source of energy.

How Glucose Distribution Works

To understand glucose distribution in the body, imagine an irrigation system. Picture it as a reservoir, with several openings along the side, through which water flows into irrigation channels. Imagine that each of these openings is at a different height.

Let's assume the reservoir is a total of 40 inches (1 m) high and outlet openings exist at heights of 35 inches (90 cm), 20 inches (50 cm) and 4 inches (10 cm). If the tank is completely filled with water, water drains through each opening into the irrigation channels. When the water level in the basin is reduced to 30 inches (80 cm), the water flows only into the two channels whose openings are below the water level, and so on.

Therefore, the height of the openings can correspond to the priority of water needs in specific plants. Plants that need little water can be irrigated via a water channel whose outlet opening is located at the height of 35 inches (90 cm). They will be watered only when the basin is nearly full. When the water level sinks, no more water feeds into this channel. Plants that need a lot of water would, therefore, be supplied via irrigation channels whose openings are positioned at the lowest level. These plants will still be watered even when only a small amount of water is available in the tank. So the higher the water needs of the plants, the lower the opening has to be for the water. The body prioritizes cells' glucose needs in a similar manner.

Glucose Is Poison As Well As Medicine

Glucose is distributed throughout the body via the bloodstream so that any cell that needs this vital energy source can access it. So when a deficiency occurs, such as during a period of fasting, the body is perfectly equipped to keep functioning.

However, the body is not prepared for the opposite situation: overeating. After a large meal, the blood sugar level rises quickly and very high, requiring a large release of the hormone insulin. Insulin helps pump sugar from the blood into the cells as quickly as possible, which is dangerous. If a cell's sugar stores are already filled, this high sugar concentration damages sensitive structures and causes the cell to try to rapidly convert the sugar into another form. The extra sugar is turned into a nonreactive, safe form for energy storage: fat.

High blood sugar levels and the accompanying insulin release literally feed up fat cells. More and more nutritionists and researchers, therefore, refer to insulin as the "fattening hormone."

The Dose Makes the Poison

At the start of the early modern period, the famous Renaissance physician Paracelsus (1493–1541) said, "All substances are poisons: there is none which is not a poison. The right dose differentiates a poison and a remedy." This is no different for sugar. Unlike water and salt — two other vital substances that can cause death in high doses — sugar molecules also have chemical properties that cause adverse reactions with other molecules within cells, thereby seriously damaging the cell structure. Sugar has two faces: on one hand, it is an energy source and a basic material for the synthesis of important substances; on the other hand, an excess of it can cause significant cell damage and serious diseases.

High-Risk Cells

Some tissues and cells in the human body are particularly affected by the risks associated with excessively high glucose concentration. They are the tissues that are first supplied with glucose in an emergency. Accordingly, they are allocated the largest dose of sugar even when there is a surplus.

How Sugar Creates Fat: An Animal Example

The principle of sugar-induced fat formation is exploited in the production of foie gras from geese. Over a period of time, the birds are force-fed large amounts of high-starch cereals. During digestion, glucose is released, then insulin is released to accelerate the absorption of glucose from the blood into the fat cells, particularly in the liver. There, the glucose is converted to fat. This creates the enlarged, super-fatty liver that is sold as foie gras.

Unknowingly, many people crank up this cycle in themselves by eating a large amount of starchy and sugary foods. And their unhealthy diet isn't just reflected on a scale in the form of extra pounds. The liver also accumulates excess fat — a malady called nonalcoholic fatty liver — which significantly affects health and well-being.

The retinas, the nerve cells (neurons) and the blood vessel cells (endothelial cells) are the first victims of a consistently excessive blood sugar level. Blood sugar that is too high frequently and over a longer period of time leads to chronic damage from a number of diseases (see box, opposite). In the worst-case scenario, constant sugar consumption can lead to blindness, nerve damage, foot amputations and heart attacks. Several recent studies have shown that high blood glucose levels can also lead to memory loss and Alzheimer's disease.

Stored Energy

As you've discovered, glucose supplies energy to cells in two ways: they can burn it and ferment it. But there are some cells and tissues in the human body that voluntarily do without glucose and prefer to cover their energy needs using fatty acids and ketone bodies, even there is sufficient glucose available.

This happens because these cells and tissues have a limited capacity for storing glucose. The body's sugar stores (in the form of glycogen) last for only a day or two — and then only if we hardly move or work. If the body needs to achieve peak physical performance, those stores will be depleted after only about 30 minutes. So this one energy source has never been sufficient on its own. For our ancestors to achieve top performance despite empty glycogen stores — to hunt, fight or escape — they had to be able to tap into additional energy sources.

Fat Burning: An Emergency Solution

Once glycogen stores are gone, burning fat is the only way the body can generate energy. People without fat reserves can't perform. As fat stores are depleted, mostly fatty acids are released. Only a small part (one-sixteenth) of the fat molecule is released in the form of glycerin, which can be converted into glucose and used to maintain the blood sugar level. Fatty acids, however, are available to the body to burn or to form ketone bodies (see box, at right). When there is a glucose deficiency, the brain can switch into a type of conservation mode, in which only basic glucose needs are met and the remaining energy comes from ketone bodies.

The Heart Does Not Depend on Glucose

The heart muscle always requires large quantities of energy. In case of an emergency, the body's own production of sugar molecules is insufficient to meet its enormous energy needs. This is why, during the course of evolution, our most important muscle developed the sensible survival strategy of concentrating on fat as an easy-to-store, glucose-independent energy source. The heart, therefore, takes its energy supply from fatty acids, ketone bodies and lactic acid even when there is enough glucose to cover its needs.

For this very reason, when the body reacts to an emergency case of oxygen deficiency, fermentation does not play a role as an energy generator for the heart, as it does for other organs and tissues. Thanks to the heart muscle's autonomous energy supply, it is also protected from fermenting cancer cells.

DID YOU KNOW?

Ketone Bodies
The body forms ketone bodies, such as acetone, acetoacetate and alpha-hydroxybutyrate, from fatty acids to serve as a source of energy. The latter two ketone bodies serve as fuel sources for the brain and heart muscle.

Too Much Sugar Causes Disease

When you have too much sugar in your bloodstream on a consistent, long-term basis, you are at higher risk for certain diseases, such as

- Diabetes
- Retinopathy, or damage to the retinas caused by diabetes
- Nephropathies, or types of kidney damage
- Neuropathies, or nerve diseases caused by diabetes
- Damage to blood vessels
- Memory loss
- Alzheimer's disease

The Heart Actively Protects Itself from Cancer Cells

By forming lactic acid, metastasizing cancer cells are able to proliferate in the surrounding tissue and to form new colonies at various locations in the human body (see page 37). Cancer cells circulating in the blood can settle in large organs, such as the brain, liver or lungs, and even in solid structures, such as bones. In the process, cancer cells come into contact with the heart muscle several times via the bloodstream. While there are benign tumors that grow invasively (primarily around the margins of the heart), as a rule, malignant cancer cells generally cannot colonize the heart muscle. Nor have scientists identified any invasive cancers that emanate from the heart.

From this, we can conclude that aggressive cancer cells can colonize new tissues only when they are able to ferment sufficient glucose into lactic acid. Because of the heart's combustion action and the lack of sugar supply, this fermentation strategy does not work; the cancer cells that end up there soon lack a food source, die and are dissolved by the immune system.

Go Back to Your Roots?

For the first time in history, a large part of the population in the developed world is confronted not with hunger and insufficiency, but with surplus food. It's something every single one of us needs to take into account when we choose what and how much we eat. It's time to return to a diet and lifestyle that promise health and well-being into a ripe old age.

Our bodies adapt to fundamental changes in diet slowly, over many generations. Today, people's bodies are completely overwhelmed by ongoing changes, and are reacting with unpleasant symptoms and chronic diseases. These are, quite rightly, referred to as lifestyle diseases: cardiovascular disease, diabetes, dementia and, of course, cancer.

But don't worry. In order to eat a healthy diet, you won't have to return to long-forgotten times; you'll just have to rigorously rethink your diet. You won't have to give up too many things, and you'll be able to eat a large variety of foods, just like you do now. The key is to not wait. Take control of your health, starting today.

The Diet of TKTL1-Negative and TKTL1-Positive Tumor Cells

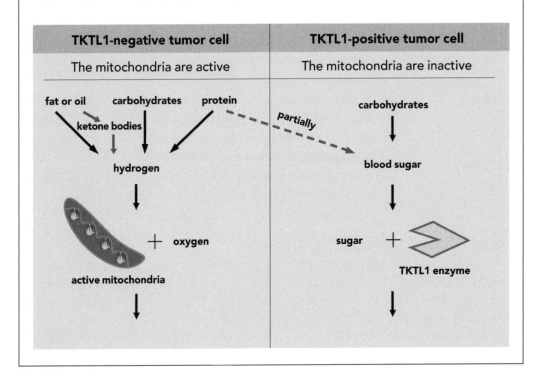

An Effective Strategy

Looking at the heart example on page 46, you can see that age alone cannot play a decisive role in the development of a malignant tumor. The only logical explanation is that the heart's fixation on combustion and renunciation of glucose as an energy supply protects the heart muscle from fermentation, thereby protecting it from cancer, as well.

The good news is that you can adopt the same strategy throughout your body by following the cancer-fighting diet. By depriving fermenting cancer cells of glucose in a targeted way, you force them to reactivate their combustion metabolism. In the best case, the cancer cells will "starve" to death (see page 38) and help make your cancer treatments more effective.

Humans as a Special Case

Unlike wild animals, humans mostly consume a mixture of plants and meat. Our diet consists of proteins, fats and carbohydrates. In our digestive tracts, unlike those of animals, the majority of the carbohydrates are converted into sugars. The indigestible parts (fiber) now only play a subordinate role, at least in the Western diet.

Most of the carbohydrates we humans ingest are monosaccharides, such as glucose (dextrose) or fructose; disaccharides, such as granulated sugar, lactose and maltose; and polysaccharides, such as starch. All of these glucose-based compounds are known generally as sugars. They are typically water soluble and, except for starch, taste sweet. (Read more on the different types of sugar starting on page 72.)

Can You Get Heart Cancer?

Have you ever heard of anyone who suffers, or has died, from heart cancer? No. Yet you read and hear everywhere that cancer is on the rise because people are living longer. True, the probability of cancer-causing mutations does increase with the age of the cell. The older the cell, the greater the likelihood that mutations may lead to degeneration. However, is this really the explanation for the increasing number of cancer cases?

The example of the heart clearly shows that the old-age hypothesis cannot be correct. The heart is the organ that is most reliant on the release of energy via combustion and that is least inclined to ferment glucose. During acute oxygen deficiency, such as in a myocardial infarction caused by vascular occlusion (in layperson's terms, a heart attack caused by a blocked blood vessel), a heart cell cannot switch exclusively to the oxygen-independent form of energy generation. Instead, it dies immediately.

And while this situation can, in an acute case, prove lethal, the heart's dependence on this source of energy is still beneficial in the long term because the commitment to oxygen-dependent energy release protects heart muscle cells from mutating into fermenting cancer cells. Additionally, cancer cells that circulate in the bloodstream are generally unable to migrate into the heart muscle and form dangerous metastases there.

The Danger of Hidden Sugars

Unfortunately, not all sugars are recognizable at first glance (or bite). Many staple foods contain a high proportion of starch; these include bread, pasta, rice and potatoes. The glucose in these foods is released into the intestine during digestion, absorbed through the intestinal mucosa and very quickly delivered into the bloodstream. There, it causes a rapid rise in the blood sugar level. In reaction to this danger, the pancreas releases insulin. This hormone docks in cell membranes and ensures that glucose is actively transported from the blood to the cells so that the blood sugar level can return to normal (see diagram, page 71).

Only humans, and domesticated animals to whom we feed an inappropriate diet, have to cope with severe fluctuations in blood sugar levels. We and our pets experience a rapid, powerful increase in glucose in the bloodstream after a meal. And it is this high blood sugar level that is ultimately responsible for the outbreak of so-called lifestyle diseases, including obesity, Alzheimer's disease, cardiovascular disease, diabetes and cancer. After all, a frequent, sharp rise in blood sugar is the best energy source for proliferating cancer cells and promotes their growth accordingly.

Did Prehistoric Humans Get Cancer?

When human beings set out to conquer the Earth about 2.5 million years ago, their diet did not differ fundamentally from that of other mammals in their environment. Humans ate what they could gather, pick or capture. Their bill of fare included wild fruits, tubers, berries and nuts, as well as insects, reptiles and small mammals.

Humans have nourished themselves this way for most of their existence. The prehistoric humans' menu was dictated by the seasons and the weather, and consisted of animal proteins and fats as well as fiber-rich plant parts, such as leaves. Carbohydrates, on the other hand, so coveted and revered by us today, played only a minor role in the primeval diet.

Whether people of that era got cancer is hard to know for certain. However, excavated bones give no indication of cancers that might have manifested in the form of bone metastases.

Cancer in the Animal World

The currently accepted doctrine on cancer says that the number of cell mutations increases with advancing age, and that this leads to an increase in the number of cancers (see page 46). The logical conclusion, then, would be that creatures that consist of more cells would also have a higher incidence of cancers. The more cells in an animal, the greater the likelihood that mutation will occur in one of those cells.

If this theory were true, a blue whale that weighs 264,000 lbs (120,000 kg, or 120 million grams) would have a two million–fold increase in the incidence of cancer compared with a house mouse that weighs a mere 2 oz (60 g) — all because the whale has more cells. In addition, if we factor in the life expectancy of the mouse (two years) and the whale (50 years), the statistical probability of cancer in the whale as opposed to the mouse increases 50 million fold. So this is the theory; but what about the facts?

Do Animals Get Cancer?

If whales really did have a two million–fold higher probability of contracting cancer than mice did, they would have had little or no chance of long-term survival over the course of evolution. Typically, this phenomenon — just like the lack of patients with heart cancer — has been recognized and questioned, not by cancer researchers, but by researchers in other areas of biology.

The ingenious Nobel Prize–winning bacterial geneticist Joshua Lederberg (1925–2008) answered a key question in the field of cancer research with a remarkable counter-question: "How do whales and giant octopuses avoid a single neoplastic event in their vast biomass?" (Neoplasia is a synonym for tumor.) He was amazed that creatures of such enormous size had no problems with cancer. Is cancer also a problem for animals? Data show that domesticated animals — pets such as dogs and cats — that are fed carbohydrates die of cancer, exactly like laboratory mice and rats. But what about cows, horses, goats and sheep? Do these animals get cancer?

No Animal Cancer Statistics

There is no register of cancers and no study of the number of cancer cases in livestock. Nevertheless, thanks to general observation, it is possible to find parallels. For livestock animals, such as cows and sheep that are raised for meat, slaughter is basically a postmortem examination. Were workers to discover a larger number of cancerous growths during slaughter, the meat most likely would not be used as food.

Herbivores and Indigestible Carbohydrates

Cows, horses, goats and sheep, however, live on a completely different diet than humans, dogs and cats do. The former mostly eat plants, which consist primarily of indigestible carbohydrates.

As the animal chews, the plant particles are mechanically chopped into smaller parts. Then the carbohydrates, which are indigestible as is, are broken down by bacteria in the digestive tract. A cow, for example, hardly digests anything itself but instead leaves all the work to bacteria and *Protozoa* in its gut. In the digestive tract, these organisms ferment the carbohydrates in the food into fatty acids and the waste product methane gas. These bacteria are digested by the cow, as well, and form an important source of protein. The cow also absorbs the fatty acids created by the bacteria and exploits them further.

As you can see, although the cow ingests only carbohydrates, it nourishes itself exclusively with fatty acids and proteins. This is why, immediately after eating, cows experience neither a rapid increase in blood sugar levels nor an increased release of insulin. The ruminants' method of feeding leads to a stable blood sugar level. The same is true for other plant eaters.

What About Carnivores?

Just like plant eaters that nourish themselves exclusively on fatty acids and protein, as explained above, pure carnivores, such as wild cats, supply their bodies with these same food components via the prey they've killed. Because they eat no glucose-releasing carbohydrates, they also do not experience an automatic increase in blood sugar and insulin levels after feeding.

Agriculture Changed the Human Diet

When prehistoric humans settled down and became less nomadic, a dramatic change took place in their eating habits that has significant medical consequences today. With the transition to a farming lifestyle, the ratio of hunted animals in the human diet fell drastically, and meat consumption plummeted. Agriculture provided a simple means of obtaining energy, in the form of carbohydrate-rich foods that rapidly released plenty of glucose and insulin. Archaeological finds show that this new diet brought not only benefits, but also clear disadvantages, such as reduced height and the development of diseases that left marks (caries) on bones.

What We Eat Makes Us Sick

An increasing number of studies demonstrate the direct link between the consumption of foods rich in glucose and starch, and the development of diseases. But since our eating behavior is learned, it is strongly influenced — and passed on — by role models, societal rules of conduct and family environment. Parents transfer their unhealthy eating habits to their children. They can't help that they pass on the potential presence of an organic disease or a genetic predisposition to cancer, but they can keep from teaching their children risk-promoting behaviors and food preferences.

The Role of Nutrition

Foods that rapidly release plenty of glucose during digestion — such as bread, pasta, potatoes, rice and, of course, pure table sugar — have long been suspected of contributing to the emergence of so-called lifestyle diseases, such as diabetes, Alzheimer's disease and heart disease. The latest scientific findings show that our "normal" diet is also significantly implicated in the emergence and growth of cancer cells.

The Curse of Abundance

The daily oversupply of foods rich in sugars and starches, as well as the fear of supposedly fattening fats, has long driven many people to consume a diet that is no longer attuned to humans' natural physical needs. The modern diet is designed to fill us up quickly without a great expenditure of time or money, and, at the same time, provide an intense flavor experience. The problem lies in the "outdated" genetic and biochemical programming of our cells, which has not adjusted to this modern diet.

So How Do You "Fix" Cancer?

Modern cancer treatments regard cancer cells as dangerous entities that must be killed in order to successfully cure a patient — no matter what happens to the healthy surrounding cells. However, since this strategy is not always successful, cancer researchers have begun to rethink the problem.

Researchers now regard both healthy cells and cancer cells as parts of an ecosystem (the body) where they compete for food and resources. If you think of healthy cells as beneficial entities and cancer cells as pests, you should opt for treatments that stop the pests from getting out of hand. This requires you to weaken the pests as well as strengthen the beneficial cells. It is, in fact, not necessary to completely eradicate these cancerous pests; it is sufficient simply to control them.

Achieving this balance is best accomplished by significantly limiting the enormous sugar requirements of the cancer cells, thus inhibiting their growth. If the glucose supply is lacking, the tumor cell cannot switch permanently to fermentation. As a result, it will be very hard for the cell to protect itself from attacks by the immune system, and it will not be able to build distant metastases. There are several more strategies you can employ that will help you prevent cancer or, if you already have cancer, make cancer treatments be more effective and have fewer side effects.

Set Up a Protective Shield

Avoid anything that leads to DNA mutations in normal cells (see box, page 13). These mutations cause the formation of tumors and cancer cells in the first place. One important contribution in the fight against cancer is giving up smoking (both first- and secondhand). You should also avoid consuming fruits, vegetables and leafy greens contaminated with pesticides. And keep an eye on the quality of the meat you eat, choosing sustainably and ethically raised options.

Strengthen Your Immune System

The transition from healthy cell to tumor cell to cancer cell is gradual, so cancer cells are not invincible. Increased DNA mutations within the cell lead to changes on the surface of the cell membrane. Once that happens, the immune system can recognize from the outside that something is wrong, and trigger the dissolution of the unwanted cell. Anything that strengthens the body's defenses, therefore, helps prevents cancer. Get adequate sleep, exercise in the fresh air, eat a balanced diet and make regular visits to a sauna to sweat out toxins. Minimizing stress is also important (see box, opposite).

Avoid Inflammation

Inflammatory diseases can be precursors of cancer. Chronic inflammation of the pancreas (pancreatitis), for example, can lead to pancreatic cancer. Gastritis triggered by the bacteria *Helicobacter pylori* in the gastric mucosa contributes to the development of gastric cancer. And people with inflammatory bowel disease (ulcerative colitis) have a significantly increased risk of colon cancer.

Why is this the case? Because tumor cells co-opt the body's healing processes; they give off inflammatory signals to attract immune cells, which they abuse for their own purposes. A particularly important type of immune cell, called a macrophage, produces growth factors that can be used by tumor cells to help them grow faster. The proliferating tumor cells then form more and more inflammatory signals, attracting ever more macrophages and creating a vicious circle.

That's why it is so important to prevent or track down and reverse inflammatory reactions in your body. For example, go to the dentist if you have inflamed, painful tooth roots. Avoid chronic intestinal inflammation by preventing the growth of unwanted or toxic bacteria and yeasts. (The good news is that restricting glucose and starch in your diet counteracts the growth of harmful yeasts, such as *Candida*.) Consume the correct ratio of omega-3 to omega-6 fatty acids (see page 87). Avoid foods that cause inflammatory reactions specific to you; these foods can be identified by a blood test. Ask your doctor which test is most appropriate for you.

Exercise

Regular physical exercise empties the body's glycogen stores and deprives fermenting cancer cells of their energy supply. In addition, aerobic exercise activates the immune system, and body tissues are better supplied with blood and oxygen. It also suppresses the switch from combustion to fermentation in cancer cells. If you eat a low-carb diet and exercise regularly, your body also forms ketone bodies (such as acetoacetate), which inhibit tumor cells without harming normal cells. Turn to page 124 for all the information you need on exercising properly while fighting cancer.

Eat According to the Dr. Coy Principles

An important part of cancer prevention is consuming a diet low in glucose and carbohydrates. By pursuing a consistently healthy diet and lifestyle, like the one described in this book, you can help prevent the metabolism of tumor cells from switching to cancer-promoting fermentation.

By reducing your sugar intake to a reasonable level, you have a very simple and effective way to positively influence your health and your aging process. And you won't have to forgo the pleasures of eating. Turn to page 168 and you'll see how varied — and delicious! — the cancer-fighting diet can be.

Stay the Course

Each day that you eat the right amount of carbohydrates, that you are moderately active and that you enjoy life is a success for you and for your health. But don't worry if you go a little wild at a party or get-together with family and friends once in a while. Even if cancerous cells form at exactly those moments, you'll still be able to keep them in check (or even kill them) by adhering to the cancer-fighting diet the rest of the time.

DID YOU KNOW?

Best Stress Reducers
The best way to banish stress is to practice a mind-body technique, such as yoga, qigong or progressive muscle relaxation. For more on these and other stress-reducing practices, turn to page 120.

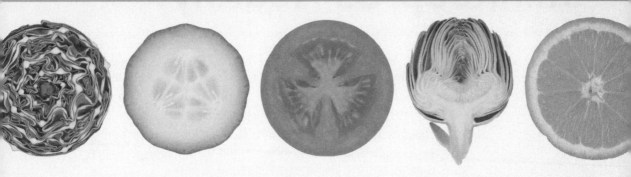

PART 2

The Principles of the Cancer-Fighting Diet and Lifestyle

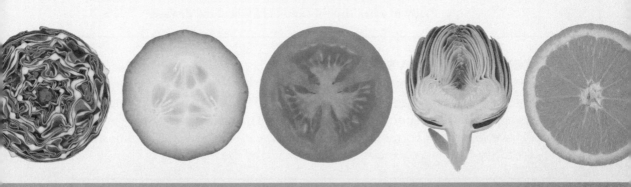

Does the Modern Diet Still Keep Us Healthy?

The first traces of human life date back about seven million years. Ever since, humans have continuously evolved, genetically adapting to diverse climatic and ecological changes. It is only in the last roughly 40,000 years that our genes have not altered noticeably, and the human species has only marginally adapted to its environment through genetic changes; instead, our ancestors survived simply by adapting their behavior to diverse habitats and varied conditions.

In addition to droughts, famines, natural catastrophes and wars, there have also been technological innovations that have caused our species to adapt. This external adaptation happens faster and faster as a result of these innovations, right up to the present day. Humans have never been richer or less dependent on nature.

Viewed in a certain light, society in the developed world is getting ever closer to the medieval ideal of paradise: the fairy-tale land of Cockaigne, a land with an unbelievable abundance of food, where grilled geese fly directly into people's mouths, and there are rivers of milk and honey. Yet, while our dreams seem to be coming true, we are also realizing with dismay that this paradisiacal fulfillment is precisely what is making us sick. Excessive intake of carbohydrates, in particular, increasingly affects our health and well-being — and not beneficially. Fortunately, however, you are free to choose from this dizzying array of modern dishes exactly those foods that nourish your body in a healthy way and help you avoid disease.

Faster Isn't Always Better

In the modern world, many people are beginning to believe that they can no longer keep up with the speed of development. It's no wonder. At no time in history have so many important inventions been created in such a short time as they are today. People are exhausted and stressed by the rapid rate of change.

The Curse of Convenience

Our diet isn't the only thing that has changed. Our activity level has also been transformed dramatically in modern society. Just a few generations ago, most people earned their daily bread through hard physical labor. The human body, and all its genes, is ideally suited to that type of activity-rich lifestyle.

Today, technological developments have made us increasingly sedentary. Most of us spend the day seated, and we're usually stressed out, concentrating very hard and, all too often, under considerable time pressure. In addition, activity has become less important in the remainder of our everyday lives. Our parents and grandparents often went to work or went shopping by bicycle or on foot, but today, we sit on buses or in our cars. It's no surprise, since people's homes and workplaces are often a great distance from each other in modern society, and there are fewer local, mom-and-pop shops left in most towns. And thanks to washing machines and other gadgets, the need to do physical labor at home has been greatly reduced.

There's no question: no one wants to turn back the clock on modern conveniences. Thanks to them, we have plenty of leisure time. But perhaps we shouldn't laze away these hours on the couch in front of the TV or at the computer. Instead, we should occasionally try to achieve the physical balance that is lacking in the rest of our everyday lives. Use your leisure time to reintroduce your body to the natural joy of movement and activity.

Restoring Balance

Genetically, human beings are programmed to move. Activity, diet and metabolism form a harmonious balance. If this balance is neglected, as it often is today, the needle on the scale will move up steadily.

Few of us change our eating habits despite being less active, and this triggers imbalance. To change that, you need to take your lifestyle into account and develop strategies to reduce the danger that this poses to your health. The solution is a combination of regular, gentle endurance exercise and a consistently low-carb diet.

DID YOU KNOW?

Burn Calories Doing Chores
Standing at the sink washing dishes burns more calories than sitting on the couch listening to the dishwasher run. Try including more manual labor in your day to keep your metabolism humming so your body can efficiently burn up glucose. Use a reel mower instead of a gas-powered one, or shovel snow (carefully!) instead of depending on a snowblower. Your body will thank you for the extra activity. Just go slowly and build up your endurance gradually.

Set a Good Example for Your Kids

Many adults are becoming aware of the importance of physical activity in maintaining good health. Unfortunately, it's a very different story for children and adolescents: in this age group, the tendency is to drastically reduce physical activity. Therefore, it's up to parents to use their position as role models and encourage their children to be more active. Frolicking, running and climbing are all keys to the healthy development of children's motor skills. Plus, if kids don't do these things, their risk of developing lifestyle diseases and eating disorders increases significantly.

We Burn Less Energy

Performing hard physical labor, as our ancestors had to do for thousands of years, meant that active muscles had to consume plenty of energy. This energy was supplied to the body in the form of fats, proteins and carbohydrates.

Prehistoric hunter-gatherers covered most of their needs with fats and proteins. Later, farmers, who also worked hard physically, increasingly fell back on starchy staple foods, such as cereals, bread and, later, potatoes. Their diet was, however, always rich in water and fiber, and, therefore, had low energy density. This means that in humans' early days, their diet contained fewer calories per volume unit than it does today. People had to eat larger portions to fill themselves up, and they burned more total energy.

It's a very different situation today. The energy content of modern ready-made foods and snacks is often staggering. And we're eating these foods even though we need considerably fewer calories, because we do less physical labor and have the decreased muscle mass that goes with it.

The consequence? People who continue to eat their fill will, necessarily, put on weight. And this can be fatal, because this consumption — particularly of carbohydrates that quickly release lots of glucose — creates the feeling of satiety for only a short time. After blood sugar peaks, it falls again just as quickly. You fall into a hunger hole and get cravings, often for something sweet. If, however, you fill yourself up on a low-carb diet, you can avoid this trap and feel satisfied for longer.

Nutrition Is More than Just Food Intake

In the long run, the modern diet combined with declining physical activity will lead to a constantly overloaded metabolism. The metabolism is inherently flexible, so it will adapt to a certain degree; but today's diet sometimes far exceeds this tolerance. More and more scientists are warning that too little physical exercise combined with the wrong diet is making us sick.

It is good to reflect on what we eat, but often diet is discussed only in one context: obesity. (We focus on it so much that some children know the calorie content of various foods better than the multiplication tables.) But one thing is much more important than simply counting calories: to focus on the content, quality and composition of our daily meals. By concentrating on these characteristics, you can enjoy your meals and relax without any regrets — while, at the same time, protecting your body from lifestyle diseases, such as cancer, diabetes, Alzheimer's disease and other dementias.

Can Food Really Make You Sick?

In the last 100 years or so, certain health problems have dramatically increased in the Western world; these are known as lifestyle diseases. Cardiovascular diseases, neurodegenerative diseases (such as Alzheimer's disease), diabetes and cancer occur only in modern industrial societies, and scientists now agree that this increase must be connected to changes in lifestyle and diet in the affected countries. But what exactly makes people ill? Is it the fault of artificial additives, such as aroma and flavor enhancers, in our modern meals? Or is it the composition of the foods themselves that harms us?

The answer to this question can be found by looking at the changes that occurred when the original human gatherers turned into hunter-gatherers and, finally, into farmers. It was not until after the Ice Age that resources became scarce enough in barren areas to force prehistoric humans to look for new food sources. Primitive humans supplemented their vegetarian diet with maggots, insects and, later, small animals.

For much of their evolutionary existence, humans fed themselves in this primitive manner. Their diet consisted of high-quality meals that were rich in protein, fat and fiber. Game meat and fish were as rich in natural omega-3 fatty acids as many nuts and green plants. It is only in the last 10,000 years, a mere blip on the historical time line, that some humans began to grow cereal grains. As farming spread, the human diet became rich in carbohydrates, and moved far away from its primitive origins.

DID YOU KNOW?

Packed with Calories
Modern snacks can be real sugar and calorie traps. A single energy bar can contain as many calories as a complete meal.

Our ancestors' metabolisms were perfectly adapted to the natural rhythm of activity, hunger and satiety. Their bodies were optimally adjusted to the available foods, and their specific protein-, fat- and fiber-rich compositions. In good times, the body made use of abundantly available energy by storing it in the form of fat, with the help of the hormone insulin (see diagram, page 71). In lean times, such as winter or periods of famine, these fat reserves were used up.

In terms of metabolism, modern humans are still much more like hunter-gatherers than you might think. And this results in an organo-biochemical problem: our bodies' cells are simply not programmed to cope with the excessive sugar and starch content of our daily diet. They have not been able to adapt to the excesses we consume via our modern food choices, and so they are damaged.

From Hunter to Farmer

Overcoming periods of food shortage was an important aspect of survival for our ancestors. One way to live through dangerous famines was to create stocks of food. But some foods were difficult to preserve, especially meat, the main food of hunters. Salt for preserving was scarce, and in many regions, humidity or cool temperatures made it barely possible or downright impossible to dry food.

In contrast, agriculture and the cultivation of fruit and vegetables meant that foods would be available over a relatively predictable time frame. Plus, farmers could function independently of the migration patterns of the animals they had previously hunted; they were able to settle in one location. The conscious search for larger grass seeds and tastier kinds of fruits also led to early selection, and more productive varieties were bred. So increasing numbers of communities changed from hunter-gatherers to farmers, growing cereal grains and storing the plants' starchy kernels as both food and seeds for future crops.

Settlers quickly realized that it was much easier to supervise a herd of animals than to hunt them in the wild, especially because supervising guaranteed that meat would always be available, even in winter. Over time, settlers discovered an additional source of food: the milk yielded by their livestock could be drunk and processed to make storable foods, such as cheese, butter and yogurt. This further encouraged them to stay put and switch to a farming lifestyle.

DID YOU KNOW?

Smart Enough to Hunt

It took human beings almost 2.5 million years to develop sufficient cognitive abilities to catch enough animals to cover the majority of their nutritional needs.

What Is Gluten?

Gluten is a protein found in many cereal grains. It is a vital component of flour used in baking, because it combines with water to form a sticky dough and helps breads rise. For many people, however, gluten causes an intolerance reaction, with symptoms such as diarrhea, nausea and flatulence. If a genetic predisposition is present, this can lead to the onset of an inflammatory disease of the intestinal mucosa known as celiac disease. Gluten is also suspected of encouraging the onset of type 1 diabetes; approximately 30% of all people who suffer from this type of diabetes also suffer from celiac disease.

One interesting fact: the gluten in ancient grains, such as einkorn, emmer and spelt, causes far fewer reactions than the gluten in modern wheat. Other grains, such as amaranth, millet and quinoa, are completely gluten free. However, even these types of grains contain starch, which affects blood glucose levels as much as wheat. They should, therefore, be included in the diet only in small quantities. Corn, which is also gluten free but very rich in sugars, is not recommended for the cancer-fighting diet.

Seeds and Starch

Most plants cultivated as food crops have one thing in common: the parts that are used for food, such as the tuber of the potato plant or the seeds of cereal grains, contain energy in the form of glucose, which is stored as starch. The real purpose of starchy seeds, especially those of grasses, is not to serve as human food, but to ensure the reproduction of the plant itself.

How Healthy Are Cereals?

For thousands of years, humans ate only seeds that were surrounded by tasty, sweet flesh. Some, such as beans, contain toxins that protect them from foraging animals, but humans can render them less bothersome through cooking. Cereal grains, however, contain a combination of protective, toxic components in the husk (such as lectins) and a high concentration of sugars (in the form of starch) inside each kernel, which was new to humans. The seed-protecting toxins may inflame the intestines and other organs, and the lectins are only partially neutralized by cooking or baking.

Separating grain from chaff is time consuming and costly, so naked cereal grains, such as wheat, are more profitable (see box, page 62). In addition to the toxins in the husk, wheat causes another problem: the gluten it contains makes it great for baking, but can also cause severe intolerances

Cereal seeds with easily removed husks (chaff), such as wheat, are referred to as free-threshing, or naked, cereals. They lack a physical barrier and are more palatable to animals, and, therefore, contain more toxins to protect them from being eaten. This is why easier-to-remove wheat hulls contain more toxins than the better-protected seeds of spelt, emmer and einkorn. These primitive cereals are considerably easier to digest, and cause few or no inflammatory reactions in the human intestines.

DID YOU KNOW?

Top Foods
After corn and rice, wheat is the third most common source of food for the world's population today.

and lead to serious health problems in some people. Wheat gluten intolerance is also much more common than gluten intolerance caused by eating ancient grains (einkorn, emmer and spelt), oats and barley.

To make matters more complicated, gluten proteins in various wheat varieties carry different degrees of intolerance risk. This is at least partially because, in recent decades, much effort has been expended in breeding higher-yield wheat varieties with better baking properties — without concern for the health-threatening components of these hybrid grains.

The Cost of Billowing Wheat Fields

White flour made from modern wheat varieties consists mostly of sugar, and has hardly any health-promoting phytochemicals (such as carotenoids). This is why it is said to contain empty calories. Besides its caloric content and taste, white flour offers neither nutritious nor health-promoting components.

Higher-yield varieties of wheat have been bred to contain a higher proportion of starch at the expense of important secondary compounds and valuable proteins. This is why einkorn, a primitive type of wheat, contains approximately twice the amount of protein as modern wheat varieties, as well as healthy secondary nutrients. The protein content of spelt, another ancient grain, is also about 50% higher than that of modern wheat.

Another disadvantage of modern wheat hybrids is that they are much more susceptible to attack by pests and diseases. To cultivate them successfully, pesticides are needed. To further increase yields, fields are heavily fertilized — and with that come all sorts of negative environmental consequences.

Carbohydrates Are Bad for the Intestines

The intestines play not only a vital role in digestion but also an extremely important part in the immune system. The intestinal mucosa (the mucous membranes) contain more than 70% of the body's total defense cells; that means the colon is the largest organ in the human immune system. Certain antibodies are produced there, such as immunoglobulin A (IgA), that help the body ward off intruders.

Nutrition and Colonic Function

Diet and lifestyle greatly affect how well the colon's defense system works. Foods that are recognized as enemies can lead to intolerance reactions, which can sometimes have serious side effects, such as severe diarrhea. Whether a food triggers an intolerance reaction essentially depends on whether its components reach the bloodstream. In a damaged colon, disturbances in the mucosa and bad intestinal flora (microorganisms) markedly increase permeability, and insufficiently digested food components can enter the bloodstream and trigger inflammatory reactions.

How Can I Clean Up My Colon?

The intestines can function properly only if the right bacteria grow inside them, and if the intestinal mucosa is intact. This makes it worthwhile to try an intestinal rehabilitation program, which includes the following:

- **Fasting.** This complete renunciation of solid food is a classic method of bowel cleansing. Patients with cancer should fast only in the initial stages of the disease, before the use of chemotherapy. By following the cancer-fighting diet, which is low in carbohydrates and rich in proteins and oils, you'll achieve almost the same biochemical results in the body as fasting (see page 82).

- **Enema.** This is a fast, effective method of bowel care. Only a few minutes after filling the colon with a watery solution, the liquid and the colon's contents are evacuated. Beneficial intestinal flora find a healthy, clean place to grow.

- **Colon Hydrotherapy.** This modern variant of colonic irrigation takes longer than a conventional enema, but evacuation involves fewer spasms and less discomfort. In colon hydrotherapy, up to 6½ gallons (25 L) of water are flushed through the colon. The water is about 106°F (41°C), which decreases spasms. An accompanying abdominal massage aids relaxation.

- **Digestion Stimulants.** Flax seeds and psyllium husks are good examples of these compounds, which contribute to regularity. Psyllium husks also soften waste, allowing it to pass more easily and cleansing the colon in a very gentle way. When you switch to the cancer-fighting diet, you will automatically ingest more fiber, which also helps. One caution: do not forget to drink plenty of fluids (8½ to 12½ cups/2 to 3 L a day) to keep these compounds moving.

- **Probiotics.** Treatment with probiotic bacteria, which colonize the gut and promote its healthy activities, is recommended. Take probiotics with a large amount of dietary fiber to protect them from other microorganisms.

- **Lactic Acid–Fermented Foods.** Among the intestine's health-promoting bacteria are lactic acid bacteria. These organisms form lactic acid, which helps maintain a healthy acidic pH in the colon. Eat and drink lacto-fermented foods as often as possible (see page 93).

Sugar Promotes Fungi Growth

A diet rich in sugars and starch suppresses the growth of healthy, acid-forming intestinal bacteria, and encourages the growth of fungi. Yeasts, such as *Candida*, especially love sugar, which they ferment into poisonous fusel alcohols that circulate through the body. Fungi may also damage the intestinal mucosa so severely that they trigger inflammation, which can significantly and negatively affect the immune system.

The decline of good, lactic acid–forming intestinal bacteria and the growth of fungi also lead to a more alkaline pH value in the body. When this happens, ammonia can no longer be excreted by the intestine in the form of non-hazardous ammonium ions (NH_4+), but must be detoxified in the kidneys. This toxic, cell-damaging ammonia inhibits mitochondrial energy generation and encourages the conversion of benign tumor cells into cancer cells. All the while, this ammonia also stresses the metabolism and promotes inflammation.

But you can fight fungi. By reducing your carbohydrate intake, you fight cancer, encourage healthy intestinal flora, and prevent fungi growth and ammonia buildup. This promotes healthy intestinal function, reduces inflammatory processes and strengthens your immune system.

Why Heirloom Crops Are Best

The move toward breeding crops without regard to their biological value and purely in terms of higher yields has intensified in recent decades. In addition to new high-performance grains, there are also significant changes being made to fruit varieties to enhance their appeal and profitability.

Breeders started with plants such as wild apples and wild cherries, modifying and hybridizing the original species to increase yield, without worrying that the biological value of the fruit decreased dramatically. In the hybridization process, sweet and good-looking fruits are preferred, and more and more of the original nutrients are lost while the sugar content steadily increases. Compared with newer hybrids, heritage cherry varieties and heirloom apples (such as Alkmene/Early Windsor, Gravenstein, James Grieve and Belle de Boskoop) boast both valuable nutrients and only a moderate sugar content.

It's good to buy these old fruit varieties as often as possible. When buying heirloom apples, don't be put off by apple scab and other imperfections. Apple scab is a sign that the fruit was not treated with pesticides. The fruits are healthier than their shiny, hybrid relatives. Wildcrafted berries, such as wild blueberries, wild blackberries and wild strawberries, are also particularly good for you. But cultivated heirloom varieties of strawberries, raspberries, gooseberries and currants also contain lots of valuable nutrients.

Katrin B. on Life and Breast Cancer — and What Comes Next

Q: How did you realize that you had breast cancer?

A: It all started with a queasy feeling. I'd had a bad dream and woken up with vague fears that had to do with my breast. During my stressful day at work, these fears receded, and I almost forgot about them. But in the evening, I felt a strong need to thoroughly examine my breast. I sat down on my bed and touched my breast. Suddenly, I literally stopped breathing. I felt hot and cold at the same time. With my examining fingers, I could quite clearly make out a small lump. Again and again, in all kinds of postures, I felt for the spot, and nothing changed — the lump remained. It was inconspicuous, like a small pea, but stubbornly frightening. At first, I tried to talk myself out of the fears and calm down. OK, I thought, this is probably a cyst or some hardened tissue just before my period. For a few days, I felt every morning to see whether the lump had disappeared. Finally, reason got the better of fear, and I made an appointment with my gynecologist.

Q: Did your gynecologist give you a firm diagnosis right away?

A: No, quite the contrary. I anxiously told the doctor about my accidental discovery and asked for a thorough examination. Instead, he tried to convince me that I was probably approaching menopause and might be slightly oversensitive. My discovery was unremarkable, and there was no need for a mammogram. But a subsequent ultrasound examination clearly showed a dark shadow on the right side. When I pointed this out to the doctor, he suggested that it might be better to let him decide, then dismissed me with a few soothing words.

Q: Did this calm your fears?

A: No, of course not. I waited for a few days, confused by the gynecologist's assessment, before taking the initiative myself, and asking for an appointment at the breast center of a major hospital. My gut feeling simply couldn't let his diagnosis stand.

Q: Did the lump turn out to be harmless, after all?

A: No, it was anything but. Instead of an arrogant rejection, I was offered the entire range of diagnostics at the breast center: ultrasound, palpation and mammography. The doctor was very friendly, but she was a bit worried when she saw the first results, so she advised me to have a biopsy.

Q: What was the result?

A: A text came the following day: " … punch biopsy right breast at 10 o'clock, histologically a fibrotic parenchyma can be made out in the right mammary gland with formations of a malignant epithelial … " This cryptic text left no doubts: breast cancer. The doctor was very helpful on the phone at this awful moment and was able to calm me down somewhat. I had called from the office, so I kept working, feeling like I was wrapped in cotton. My body seemed to say, "You have to function now." I went home and Googled all night. What diagnoses were available, what treatments? And above all: what were the chances of survival? I had only one aim: to survive. My world view completely shifted at that point. My life was more precious than ever.

Q: What did you do after the diagnosis?

A: I functioned like a machine, consulted my family doctor of many years, checked out some clinics, finally selected one and researched all forms of treatment on the Internet. I also confided in a therapist whom I knew well. She was a great help in those days — and still is today. I got even more support from a self-help group called Mamazone. Extensive phone conversations with a counselor who was also a patient gave me a lot of courage. Four weeks after the diagnosis, I had an appointment for the operation I needed. The more I looked into the topic, the more my fears gave way to understanding.

Q: What was treatment like?

A: The surgery went very well. The surgeon told me right away that I could have breast-conserving surgery that would not completely remove my breast. That was very reassuring. After the surgery, I felt relatively well; I walked down the corridor the same evening. I came home after five days, which I had not expected. But I still had to wait a week for test results and a treatment plan. During that time, I continued to find out all the information I could about nutrition, lifestyle, psychology, etc. I had decided not to go for chemotherapy under any circumstances. I was terrified of this treatment, and I had been treated exclusively with naturopathic medicine for the last 10 years. At the end of November, I finally received the good news from the hospital: there were no lymph nodes involved, there was no infection at the tumor margins and I had positive hormone receptor status [the tumor had been encouraged by hormones]. I was delirious with happiness. But the hospital, nevertheless, recommended radiation, chemotherapy and anti-hormonal therapy, which was a shock.

Q: So they recommended the full program, after all?

A: Yes. My first thought was, "My God, after these treatments, you'll be an old woman. Nothing will ever be the same again. Life is finished." I was angry, sad and frustrated. A few days later, I had an appointment to discuss the details of the treatment. I asked why I should undergo such an ordeal when the lymph nodes were not affected. The doctor looked at me, confused, and said, "Mrs. B., we only want the best for you. You are still a young woman, and you should really take every opportunity to become healthy again."

Q: What did you do?

A: That was when the fear and panic really hit home. I had sleepless nights and didn't know anymore what I wanted. No one could make that decision for me. Those were upsetting weeks. I used the time to get a second opinion and to research on the Internet, so I could make up my mind for or against chemotherapy. Making this decision really took a lot out of me. After all, it was vital, in the truest sense of the word. One morning, shortly after waking up, I was sure that I wanted to go for the entire treatment plan.

Q: How was your treatment experience?

A: On the whole, I coped well with the treatments, and did not, in fact, become a gray old woman, as I had feared. This I owe mainly to the fact that I took a critical look at my diet, which I had previously thought was healthy by commonly accepted standards.

Q: What made you decide to do that?

A: I started chemotherapy after the New Year. At Christmastime, I wanted to eat everything I loved without restraint and in large quantities. Maybe my body wanted to create a stockpile of nutrients or to be compensated. But when chemotherapy began, I very consciously ate only those foods that were rich in vital nutrients and low in carbohydrates. Amazingly, during the course of the treatments, I had no desire for sweets, alcohol, potatoes, pasta or pizza. Apart from the first three or four days after each treatment, when I felt bloated and uncomfortable, I felt really well at times. My doctor had prepared a very good plan for me: high doses of selenium; coenzyme Q10, an agent that protects the mucous membranes in the body; and some homeopathic essences. I spent a lot of time in the fresh air, and I even took saunas. I painted and, all in all, was in a good frame of mind. I met many people and went out a bit. I just avoided large crowds. Otherwise, there were not many restrictions. I firmly believe that a person's attitude to treatment, diet and lifestyle can significantly contribute to the success of the therapies.

Q: What happened next?

A: A newsletter from Mamazone alerted me to an interesting research and therapeutic approach regarding cancers: the discovery of an enzyme named TKTL1, which can be detected in a tumor. During chemotherapy, with the help of my physician, I found out I could have a special test for the TKTL1 enzyme. We had the tumor that had been removed sent to a laboratory. The result: 77% of my cancer cells showed the presence of the TKTL1 enzyme, so they were TKTL1 positive. Luckily, my doctor reacted right away. He told me to immediately and severely restrict the consumption of all "sugar generators." So I had to stop, as much as possible, eating foods that the body converts to glucose. It's a strategy that may seem unusual at first glance but, ultimately, it makes sense.

Q: Was the transition hard for you?

A: No, not at all. I knew what was at stake. I introduced foods that were specifically tailored to this type of diet, and I drastically reduced my intake of carbohydrates overnight. Overall, I ate no more than 60 grams a day. I even completely gave up candy. During this time, I also contacted Dr. Coy, who gave me very good advice on the cancer-fighting diet.

Q: Did you ever feel you had to give up too much?

A: No, quite the contrary. I had a good feeling from the start. The chemotherapy was almost complete at that point. After the sixth and final treatment, contrary to all expectations, I was feeling relatively well. At the same time, I was so happy to have finally gotten through everything. I now know that this success was due in large part to the change in my diet. All the time, however, I had to listen to the doubts of my family, friends and acquaintances: "Do you really think your diet makes a difference?" or "But that's ridiculous; cancer doesn't come from the diet. What nonsense!" or "Yes, go ahead, live healthily — you'll see what good it does for you." Acceptance was, unfortunately, rather low. How I felt and looked did not seem to count.

Q: What do you eat today, years after the therapy?

A: To this day, I don't find it difficult to restrict my carbohydrate intake. My well-being is very good, despite having had a serious illness. I'm fit and can even play sports. And I also tolerate well the anti-hormone treatment I have been taking for years. After four weeks of rehabilitation post-treatment, I went back to work. Although it may seem unbelievable to many, I'm healthy. I am really convinced of the importance of nutrition during and after cancer treatment. And I have noticed that my knowledge about the disease and my attitude toward its management play a major role. I must mention therapeutic support, as well. Unfortunately, many women are ashamed to consult a psychologist at this difficult time. But it is essential. I want to encourage every woman who develops breast cancer, and say, "There is life after this awful diagnosis. One that, if seen from another point of view, is even better, liberated and not so cramped." Today, I can very clearly feel the changes: I've become much more open and tolerant, I am more aware of myself, and I no longer put as much stock in the judgment of others.

Q: How are you now?

A: It's now seven years after my breast cancer diagnosis, and I feel good. I am once more fully immersed in my life and work. Before and during my chemotherapy treatments, I followed Dr. Coy's ketogenic diet plan, and in my chemotherapy-free periods I ate low-carbohydrate meals. I still eat a healthy, low-sugar diet, and am very cautious about my carbohydrate intake. If I had to do it all over again, I would do it the same way. I am very glad that I used all the conventional medical therapies while maintaining a strong focus on natural healing. At this point in my life, I owe a very big thank-you to Dr. Coy.

Glucose Is Poison for Cell Structures

You've already read the first part of this book, so you know that your blood sugar level plays a major role in the development and spread of cancer cells. The more sugar there is in the blood, the easier it is for the cancer cell to capture it, to ferment the dissolved glucose and to start deadly lactic acid production. Luckily, however, this mechanism is fairly easy to stop. You simply need to deprive the malignant cells of their vital food.

Why Slower Is Better

When it comes to your blood sugar level, the most important aspect is the speed at which sugar appears in the bloodstream. If glucose is released into it quickly, the level shoots up rapidly and cells gobble it up. The speed at which the blood sugar level increases after a meal depends on the type and quantity of sugar you have ingested, and what other foods it was combined with. In addition, two other major factors determine spikes in the blood sugar level:

- The insulin sensitivity of the glucose-receiving cells
- The level of glycogen in the individual cells

How to Control Blood Sugar Spikes

You can positively influence insulin sensitivity and glycogen levels (see above). How? By exercising regularly and restricting your carbohydrate intake.

Limit your daily intake of carbohydrates to about 1 g per 2.2 lbs (1 kg) of body weight. That means if you weigh 132 lbs (60 kg), you can eat 60 g of carbohydrates per day. This is equivalent to having Strawberry Quark with Flaxseed Crunchies (20 g carbohydrates; page 180) for breakfast; a slice of Bacon and Leek Quiche (18 g carbohydrates; page 267) for lunch; Jerusalem Artichoke Gratin (11 g carbohydrates; page 238) for dinner; and Ginger Panna Cotta on Papaya Purée (11 g carbohydrates; page 331) for dessert. If you consume more carbohydrates (which covert into more glucose), make up for the excess by getting additional physical activity and burning them off.

Sugar Damages Even Healthy Cells

Your main meals of the day, especially if they are rich in sugar and starch, are not the only things that make your blood sugar level rise dramatically (these are called postprandial blood glucose peaks). Snacks (such as cake, candy and ice cream) and sugary drinks (such as soft drinks) also drive up blood sugar. To counteract these dangerous spikes, the pancreas secretes the hormone insulin. It opens the cells so they can use the increased blood sugar, and plays a decisive role in carbohydrate metabolism (see diagram, opposite).

If your blood sugar level is regularly high, the pancreas constantly produces new insulin to lower it. Initially, this helps the body keep the amount of sugar in the blood relatively constant. However, this does not really solve the problem; it just shifts it to another location. Insulin does not dissolve sugar molecules, but rather repeatedly pushes them into cells, which are already full to bursting.

Under this constant stress, the cells, at some point, withdraw their insulin receptors to protect themselves. Now that they are closed to sugar, this leads to what doctors call insulin resistance: the sugar is disposed of by converting it to fat and storing it in fatty tissue. And because the excess sugar is no longer transported into cells, the pancreas tries to produce ever more insulin. It's a losing battle that results in the onset of type 2 diabetes.

Adult-Onset Diabetes Isn't Just for Adults Anymore

For our grandparents and great-grandparents, the pancreas lasted at least until their pensions began. This is why type 2 diabetes used to be known as old-age diabetes.

In the last 50 years, however, people's consumption of sugar and starch has increased dramatically. The pancreas is under far more pressure than ever before. This is why, today, young people increasingly suffer from type 2, or adult-onset, diabetes; in children, the rate has increased a thousandfold.

Why? Many children and young adults nourish themselves predominantly with carbohydrates and consume sugary drinks. They are also less active; many partake passively in sports, such as watching a soccer game on TV or playing a video game version of it, rather than kicking a ball around a field with their friends.

The Insulin System

In order to use the energy in food, the pancreas produces insulin, which "jams" cells open and allows them to take in glucose. If the insulin system is not functioning properly, cells become resistant to the hormone. In the worst-case scenario, this can cause diabetes.

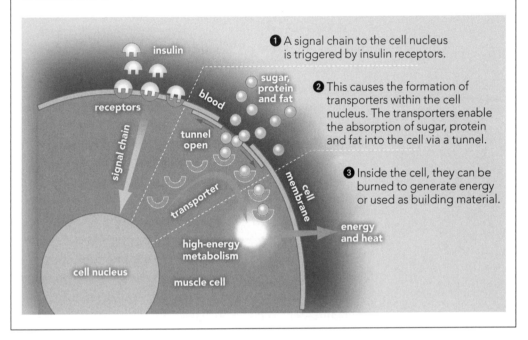

❶ A signal chain to the cell nucleus is triggered by insulin receptors.

❷ This causes the formation of transporters within the cell nucleus. The transporters enable the absorption of sugar, protein and fat into the cell via a tunnel.

❸ Inside the cell, they can be burned to generate energy or used as building material.

What Happens in Type 2 Diabetes

In patients with type 2 diabetes, either a lack of insulin or insulin insensitivity (insulin resistance) can be observed — sometimes both. The most common medical treatment for diabetes today is to constantly replace the missing insulin. Many people with diabetes, therefore, inject insulin before a meal; this allows the glucose consumed in the food to move from the bloodstream into the cells in order to counteract the rise in blood sugar.

This conventional treatment relieves the symptoms of diabetes without recognizing their causes and curing the underlying problem. In addition, insulin offers a virtual "free pass" to continue unhealthy diet and lifestyle habits. It might sound overly simple, but the root cause of the diabetes problem in modern society is the excessive consumption of sugar and starch.

The Consequences for Cells

For the body's cells, the recurring, forced intake of excess glucose has serious consequences. Sugar molecules start an irreversible chemical reaction with the protein molecules in the cell, destroying it in the process. High blood sugar levels cause the worst damage in the very tissues that normally like to take up glucose, such as brain and nerve cells; cells in the retinas; and endothelial cells, which line the blood vessels.

These glucose-loving cells are the ones that suffer first and that are eventually destroyed. Damage to the retinas can cause sight impairment and blindness, and the destruction of nerve cells can lead to extremely painful neuropathies (diseases of the nerves, which cause pain, numbness or weakness). Finally, damage to the endothelial cells leads to arteriosclerosis and narrowing of the blood vessels, which in the worst case can trigger a heart attack.

Sugar: The Happy Drug

When your blood sugar level spikes, your brain absorbs a large amount of glucose. This leads to increased activity in your nerve cells, which makes you perceive pleasant feelings more intensely. When blood sugar drops due to the release

Research Study: Looking at Sugar's Role in Cancer

Carbohydrates that lead to a rapid and strong rise in blood sugar levels — and, consequently, induce the release of hormones (such as insulin) and growth factors (such as insulin-like growth factor 1, or IGF-1) — have been found to promote the growth of cancer cells. A study of more than 1.2 million patients showed that elevated blood sugar levels on an empty stomach significantly increased the incidence of cancer. A further study demonstrated that those with elevated blood sugar levels (such as people with prediabetes or diabetes) had a higher risk of developing cancer, and that the death rate from cancer increased in direct proportion to the rise in blood sugar levels. A third study showed that raised concentrations of IGF-1 in the blood also correlated with the incidence of cancer. These three studies, taken together, demonstrate that a person's blood sugar level, plus the hormones (insulin) and growth factors (IGF-1) it induces, promotes cancer and influences the course of the disease.

of insulin, the nerve cells begin to feel the symptoms of withdrawal. They do not want to go without their cherished sugar. The brain, therefore, orders the body to resupply it with sugar as quickly as possible. The body reacts to this command by making you crave sweet and/or carbohydrate-rich foods, such as cake or potato chips.

Giving in to these desires has consequences, and not just when you step on a scale. When your blood sugar level experiences continual upward and downward swings, you'll find yourself on an emotional roller coaster. The sudden burst of energy and happiness at the peak is quickly reversed: tiredness, lack of energy and bad moods occur in the valley.

Starch Is Just Another Form of Sugar

Wheat flour, in the form of white flour, is one of the main staples in the Western diet. For many people, bread, rolls, pasta, pizza and baked goods made from it are part of their daily diet. What they don't realize is that the starch in wheat is just another form of pure sugar. Immediately after you eat refined wheat products, your blood sugar level increases rapidly and powerfully. Today, the main source of glucose in the Western diet is not granulated sugar but starch. This is the main factor to consider if you want to change your diet.

A Possible Contradiction?

At first glance, it seems surprising that starch gets into the bloodstream faster than granulated sugar. After all, starch is a complex carbohydrate that needs to be broken down before it can be used. Right?

Starch consists of many long, branched dextrose chains called amylopectin. These chains are broken down very

Add It Up

When compared with granulated sugar, the same amount of wheat flour causes blood sugar levels to rise even more rapidly. Say you eat a slice of white bread with normal sugary jam. Both the sugar in the jam — which includes added sugar as well as natural sugar in the fruit — and the sugar released by the starch in the bread will cause a fast, significant rise in blood sugar. And while you may think the jam is the culprit, it is worth noting that the branched starch in the white bread is even more dangerous to your blood sugar than the sugar in the jam.

quickly after a meal and enter the bloodstream just as fast. The first sugar molecules are broken down by enzymes in the mouth; this is why bread tastes sweet if you chew it long enough. Granulated sugar (sucrose), on the other hand, is a disaccharide, which is broken down into two halves inside the digestive tract: glucose and fructose. Only the glucose half enters the bloodstream directly and immediately raises the blood sugar level. The fructose half needs to be converted into glucose by the liver before it can enter the bloodstream; it, therefore, does not have an immediate effect on blood sugar. This means that starchy foods, such as white bread or pasta, are actually *more* dangerous than refined sugar because they cause an undesirably high spike in blood sugar.

Carbs Are Not All the Same

All sugars are not created equal; their composition has a decisive influence on how they affect blood sugar. Nutrition labels list carbohydrates, but due to the types of sugars they contain, they, too, are not all the same. Inulin-containing tubers, such as Jerusalem artichokes (see box, below) and parsnips, are excellent for low-carbohydrate diets, whereas wheat or potatoes are not. The term *carbohydrate* is appropriate only to a limited degree, because different types are metabolized differently.

Nearly Forgotten Superfood: Jerusalem Artichokes

Jerusalem artichokes originated in North and Central America. These tubers were an important foodstuff and fodder in the 18th century — in their native lands and in Europe. Over time, due to the emphasis on creating heavy-yield, starch-rich foods, the consumption of this valuable crop has declined drastically.

About half of a Jerusalem artichoke consists of inulin (see opposite). So if you eat a meal of just these tubers, your blood sugar level will remain virtually unchanged. The pancreas will not need to produce insulin to lower your blood sugar level as a result of the meal.

Another plus: Jerusalem artichokes contain only about 30 calories in a 3½-oz (100 g) serving. The same serving of potatoes contains nearly double the calories. Jerusalem artichokes are delicious fried, sautéed or baked in a gratin (see recipe, page 238). Try them in soups, fry slices into crispy chips or grate them raw into salads.

Polysaccharides: Inulin

Inulin, also known as alant starch, is another important example of how various sugars relate to blood sugar levels. It is a polysaccharide (a complex sugar) similar to starch, but it is not composed of multiple glucose molecules; it consists of many fructose molecules. Inulin contains only a single glucose unit at the end of a long chain of about 100 molecules. Many plants store this compound as an energy source for growth. Some examples are plants in the *Asteraceae* (or *Compositae)* genus, including Jerusalem artichokes, chicory, artichokes and salsify, and plants in the *Apiaceae* (or *Umbelliferae*) genus, including parsnips.

Because humans lack the corresponding cleaving enzyme called inulinase, inulin is not absorbed in the stomach or small intestine. Instead, inulin is broken down into short-chain fatty acids by bacteria in the rectum. Although it is a sugar composed of fructose units, inulin acts like dietary fiber in humans. We cannot digest this sugar, so the blood sugar level does not rise when we consume it. Plus, inulin is converted into valuable fatty acids in the colon.

Disaccharides: Sucrose, Maltose and Lactose

Disaccharides also play an essential role in today's diet. Depending on their composition, they behave very differently in terms of blood sugar levels. The most commonly used disaccharide is refined sugar, also known as industrial sugar or table sugar. Biochemically, it is referred to as sucrose. In addition to sucrose, there are other disaccharides that play a role in the human diet, including maltose (malt sugar) and lactose (milk sugar):

- **Sucrose** consists of equal parts glucose and fructose. Sucrose made from sugar beets is known as beet sugar (see box, page 76); sucrose made from sugar cane is called cane sugar. Beet sugar, cane sugar, granulated sugar, industrial sugar and household sugar are all synonyms for the same thing. Sucrose raises blood sugar levels rapidly.
- **Maltose** consists of two glucose units, and is broken down during digestion into two molecules of glucose, which are immediately absorbed into the blood, leading to a rapid, sharp rise in the blood sugar level.
- **Lactose** consists of one unit each of glucose and galactose. As it breaks down in the digestive tract, one molecule each

of glucose and galactose is released. Like fructose, galactose does not lead to an increase in blood sugar; galactose is taken up by cells that work independently of insulin, whereas fructose is slowly converted to glucose in the liver.

Isomaltulose: A Healthy Alternative

In nature, there also exist disaccharides that have some valuable properties. One of these is the little-known sugar isomaltulose, which is marketed under the brand name Palatinose. It was discovered in honey and sugar cane extract in 1957, and is becoming increasingly important due to its valuable biological properties.

Like sucrose, isomaltulose is composed of one molecule each of glucose and fructose. But while its structure is similar, it increases blood sugar to a much lesser degree than sucrose, because the glucose and fructose portions of isomaltulose are connected differently. This makes it harder for the body to break it down, and its glucose content is released more slowly.

The glycemic index (see box, page 78) of isomaltulose is just 32, so it has a very low impact on blood sugar. (In comparison, the glycemic index of white bread is 70 and that of glucose is 100.) Isomaltulose provides the body with energy more slowly, in a more sustained way. For the muscles and the brain, this means that energy is provided over a longer period, which curbs food cravings. But that's not all: isomaltulose also promotes fat burning and protects the teeth, because bacteria do not break it down in the mouth and cause tooth decay.

Unlike artificial sweeteners, isomaltulose is a naturally occurring sugar without side effects. It is a good substitute for household sugar in a low-carb diet. Unfortunately, its sweetening power is lower, but you can compensate for this by combining isomaltulose with sweeter sugars, such as tagatose or fructose, or by adding the natural sweetener stevia. For more on sugars and substituting them in recipes, see page 158.

Artificial Sweeteners, Sugar Substitutes and Fructose

Artificial sweeteners have much greater sweetening power than sugar; depending on the product, they are 10 to 3,000 times sweeter than granulated sugar. On the plus side,

Aspartame and Sucralose: Safe or Not?

When the body breaks down the sweetener aspartame, in addition to the amino acids aspartic acid and phenylalanine, the alcohol methanol also forms. However, the European Food Safety Authority has recently classified aspartame as safe, years after it was approved in North America. The sweetener sucralose (which was, coincidentally, discovered during the search for insect repellents) is a chlorinated carbohydrate. It was approved for use in food in the late 1990s in North America, but European authorities took more time to assess the pathways for its breakdown in the human body and its possible side effects. The European Union approved its use in food and beverages in 2000.

because they provide no food for decay-causing bacteria, they do not promote cavities in teeth. Another advantage is that these sweeteners have few or no calories. However, it is too early to assess the long-term risks of consuming them, because humans have used them for a relatively short time. Studies on possible adverse health effects have arrived at different results, so more research is needed.

Natural Sweeteners

It is a different story with stevioside, a natural sweetener made from the leaves of the South American stevia plant, which is 300 times sweeter than sucrose but does not lead to an increase in blood sugar. Stevia has been used for centuries by South American native communities to sweeten food and beverages; therefore, stevia is assumed not to pose any sort of health risk. In Japan, stevia has been used for decades to sweeten tea, soft drinks, toothpaste, cakes and candies. In recent years, it has been approved for use in North America and Europe, as well.

Sugar Alcohols

Polyols, also referred to as polyhydric alcohols or polyalcohols, are sugar substitutes and include isomalt, sorbitol and mannitol. They are produced by chemically manipulating sugar so that it provides the body with less energy than natural sugar. Since cavity-causing bacteria cannot (or can barely) break down these sugar substitutes, they are regarded as tooth friendly, just like artificial sweeteners.

The Glycemic Index

The glycemic index (GI) is a way to measure the effect of food on the blood sugar level. It indicates how strongly blood sugar is affected by the consumption of 50 grams of a particular carbohydrate food. The lower the increase, the lower the GI.

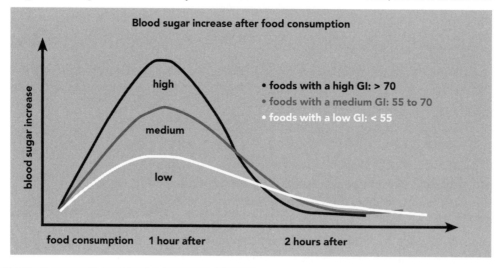

Sugar alcohols are especially useful for sweetening chewing gum and candies. Unlike artificial sweeteners, they do contain calories. And because they are largely broken down by intestinal bacteria, high doses can cause diarrhea and bloating. This is another reason why sugar alcohols are not generally seen as suitable replacements for sugar.

Fructose: Healthy Sweetness from Fruit?

Most people know that sugar is not necessarily part of a healthy diet. In contrast, when they rank the healthiest foods, fruit usually comes out on top. However, all fruit is not created equal, just like all sugars are not created equal. Some fruits are very healthy because they are rich in phytonutrients, vitamins and fiber. But some fruits require caution due to their high sugar content.

Although the term *fructose* suggests that it is the predominant sugar in fruit, most fruits contain a lot of glucose in addition to "healthy" fructose. Some modern apple varieties actually contain more glucose than fructose, and particularly sweet fruits, such as grapes, contain almost exclusively glucose. Remember: glucose is responsible for rapid rises in blood sugar and is, therefore, fuel for aggressive cancer cells (see page 37).

Sugar Trap: Dried Fruits

Dried fruits contain a lot of sugar, because they have been dehydrated. Raisins are particularly problematic, because grapes consist almost exclusively of glucose. In addition, most commercially available dried fruits are sulfurized (treated with sulfur as a preservative), and some are sweetened with sugar. This means you should eat dried fruits only from time to time and in moderation, and opt for fresh or frozen fruit more often.

Why You Need a Little Sugar

In order for the human body to work properly, most of the cells constantly take glucose from the blood and use it up. (One exception is heart cells, which live mainly on fatty acids, ketone bodies and lactic acid.) You should, therefore, not renounce sugar completely, but strive to balance your blood sugar level. By ingesting sugars other than glucose, such as tagatose, isomaltulose, trehalose and galactose, you can delay or even completely avoid blood sugar spikes. The other option is to significantly reduce your sugar consumption, adding tubers and roots that contain inulin, such as Jerusalem artichokes and parsnips, and avoiding starchy potatoes (see box, page 74).

Cooking Methods Count

A potato is a good example that shows clearly how processing or cooking can influence the amount of sugar that is released. If you mash boiled potatoes, the starch is more easily converted into glucose, because the potato pieces don't have to be digested in the stomach. Mashed potatoes, and the starch in them, are broken down quickly in the mouth and small intestine. Hence, their glucose is also more rapidly released.

One way to reduce this adverse effect is to let boiled potatoes cool after cooking (try them in a potato salad). As they cool, about 12% of the starch is converted into a starch paste, which cannot be broken down by enzymes in the body. You should, therefore, always let rice and potatoes cool completely before eating them — even if you reheat them again later.

Combining potatoes with fat reduces the speed of glucose uptake even more. French fries and sautéed potatoes make the blood sugar rise more slowly than boiled potatoes and, especially, mashed potatoes. Just make sure you use healthy, high-quality fat when frying. Hydrogenated vegetable fat, such as shortening, contains unhealthy trans-fatty acids.

DID YOU KNOW?

How Much Sugar the Body Needs

The normal glucose requirement of the human body is about 2 mg per 2.2 lbs (1 kg) of body weight per minute. So, per hour, an adult who weighs 165 lbs (75 kg) needs to consume seven to 10 g of sugar. If this adult ate 1 g of glucose once every 10 minutes, the consumption and use of sugar would be balanced, and the blood sugar level would not rise. Blood sugar increases are largely determined by the amount of sugar released over a specific period of time.

Research Study:
Carbohydrates and Cancer Recurrence

Carbohydrates also play an important role in cancer recurrence. Studies by U.S. researchers have shown that a carbohydrate-rich diet significantly increases the likelihood that cancer (such as colorectal cancer) will recur — and it causes more cancer-related deaths.

The role of carbohydrate consumption in cancer recurrence has also been demonstrated in breast cancer. Cancer researchers in California studied women with breast tumors and analyzed whether their tumors contained the IGF-1 receptor, which is closely related to carbohydrate consumption. After their tumors were surgically removed, women whose tumors had the IGF-1 receptor and who consumed as many or more carbohydrates than they did prior to the surgery had a 500% higher cancer recurrence rate than women who did not have the receptor. As a result, researchers have suggested dietary changes for patients who have tumors that are receptive to carbohydrates.

For deep- and pan-frying, saturated fatty acids are significantly better than unsaturated ones (see page 162). Unsaturated fatty acids are destroyed by frying and converted into less-healthy fatty acids. For cooking, frying or heating of any kind, choose fats and oils that contain a high amount of saturated fatty acids, such as butter, coconut oil, beef fat or lard.

Stabilizing Blood Sugar Values

Eliminating sugar from the diet — and the blood sugar spikes it causes — has a positive effect on more than just physical health. You'll also be emotionally and mentally more stable and balanced. It is believed that a diet low in glucose and starch has a liberating effect that can be attributed to the blockage of certain anxiety-inducing receptors. (These receptors are specialized cells that translate internal and external stimuli for the nervous system.) The reason: if sugar is no longer available in abundance, the local metabolism of the brain partially switches to metabolizing fat and using ketone bodies to create energy. Some of these ketone bodies occupy the receptors, preventing anxiety-creating compounds from coming in.

Anxiety reduction plays an important role in health, especially in patients with cancer, who are facing a life-threatening situation that causes great existential fears. Since a low-sugar diet not only makes life difficult for cancer cells, but also leads to emotional and mental stability, many patients are able to enjoy a noticeably more relaxed and stress-free life.

If you also exercise regularly, you'll empty the body's glycogen stores, ensuring that more ketone bodies are formed. Using special test strips from the pharmacy, you can easily check your urine to find out if your body has switched to fat burning and is forming sufficient ketone bodies. Simply dip the test strip briefly into a fresh urine sample; after a minute, you will be able to compare the color on the strip to a chart that will tell you how many ketone bodies are in your urine.

At a Glance: The Advantages of the Cancer-Fighting Diet

The harm caused to the body by high, constantly rising glucose levels is associated with much pain and suffering, and with enormous health care costs. And while insulin can reduce blood sugar, it cannot prevent the damage that excessive sugar consumption causes. Only a reduced-carbohydrate diet can do that. By reducing the amount of glucose in your diet, you achieve several important goals:

- Significantly reduce your risk of diabetes, Alzheimer's disease and heart attacks
- Harmonize your body and mind
- Supply your body with all the necessary and vital building blocks it needs
- Lose weight without difficulty
- Make it difficult for developing cancer cells to stay alive and to spread

A Real-World Analogy for Glucose Reduction

Imagine you have six vouchers for 10 g of glucose each day. You can use the vouchers throughout the day as you like — for example, two in the morning, three at lunchtime and one in the evening. You need to make sure, however, that you spread your vouchers over the whole day, more or less evenly, so that you do not take in too much glucose at one time. You should use more than four vouchers per meal only if you have been very active before eating or will be after your meal. In addition, you should always combine foods that are rich in sugar or starch with those that are rich in proteins and oils or fats. This will make the glucose they contain enter your bloodstream much more slowly.

Why Fasting Can Be a Miracle Cure

Many people fast to purge toxins and cleanse their bodies. During this time, they consume only liquids, such as water, unsweetened teas, vegetable stock, and/or heavily diluted fruit or vegetable juices. The strength and warmth these people need to live are drawn from their bodies' own energy deposits.

The Benefits of Fasting

The aim of fasting is to detoxify and cleanse the body, and to relearn the enjoyment of food in moderation. It also helps maintain your physical and mental abilities. Increasingly, fasting is also regarded as a preventive treatment for diet-related metabolic diseases. Medically or clinically supervised fasting is regarded as the most effective form of treatment. The positive effect is supplemented if you abstain from harmful social drugs, such as caffeine and nicotine; deliberately reject everyday stresses; and use regular enemas for bowel hygiene.

Cancer and Fasting

Fasting has a healing effect on cancer because it affects the fermentation metabolism of cancer cells. Intense fasting lowers blood sugar levels and reduces glycogen stores, so the body begins to burn its fat reserves. Glucose is allocated to only those cells that need it most to survive: the brain, nerves and retinas. But even the brain has to restrict its consumption and cover the majority of its energy needs by using ketone bodies. When the body is in this fat-burning mode, it is difficult for glucose-dependent, fermenting cancer cells to produce enough energy. This means that fasting forces fermenting cancer cells to alter their metabolism or, in the best-case scenario, even kills them off.

Who Can Fast?

Caution: fasting is useful only for patients who are not weakened by cachexia, or wasting of the body due to illness. There is a risk that the return to a normal glucose- and starch-rich diet after fasting could fuel the growth of cancer cells even more. To prevent this, a long-term change in the diet is required.

The Solution: Glucose Fasting

If you rigorously change your diet to include glucose fasting, you can achieve the same positive effect of fasting without suffering from hunger. Here's how:

- Reduce the amount of glucose you take in through food to 1 g per 2.2 lbs (1 kg) of your body weight per day.

- Support your diet by staying physically active and getting regular exercise.

- If you are overweight, cut your calorie intake. Even if you don't, you will likely lose 4½ to 6½ lbs (2 to 3 kg) at the beginning of glucose fasting. Why? Consuming fewer lectin- and gluten-containing foods curbs inflammation and water retention.

Fat: An Elixir of Health

For the body, fat is an essential nutrient. That's why, in recent years, nutritional scientists have increasingly distanced themselves from overall dietary fat reduction (in other words, low-fat diets). Instead, they have begun recommending that people consume a higher proportion of fats and oils.

In addition to quantity, the health-enhancing qualities of fats and oils are important. For example, some plant-based oils and some saltwater fish (such as salmon, herring and mackerel) contain valuable unsaturated fatty acids, which perform many important functions; chief among them is their role in human hormone metabolism, vitamin uptake and nervous system function (see page 84 for more information).

Fat is also valuable in controlling blood sugar levels. When carbohydrates are eaten with fat, the glucose level in the blood rises much more slowly. The body needs to digest fat or oil before it can use it, which significantly reduces the rate at which carbohydrates break down.

However, even if you can slow down rises in the blood sugar level this way, you can't take your eye off the ball: you still have to monitor the overall amount of glucose and starch you eat. As with fat, quantity counts for carbs. When you're eating out, by all means, enjoy a slice or two of white bread with oil, or a small portion of spaghetti with garlic and oil. But make sure you compensate for this by consuming fewer carbohydrates throughout the rest of the meal: avoid filling, carbohydrate-packed foods, such as a large main dish of pasta or a side dish of rice.

Essential Fatty Acids

Fats, which come in solid form (such as lard or coconut oil) or liquid form (such as oils), consist of several building blocks. The most important of these is fatty acids. The composition of a fat, the proportion of saturated to unsaturated fatty acids it contains and the type of unsaturated fatty acids it contains determine whether it is healthy or not. The most important thing is the right mixture of these different fats and oils.

Saturated fatty acids are an important energy source for the body. Thanks to their stable chemical properties, they are safe to consume; that is, they do not undergo unwanted and harmful reactions with other cell components, as is the case with sugar.

Monounsaturated and polyunsaturated fatty acids, however, are reactive and, therefore, unstable: they easily turn rancid. Because rancidity causes a significant change in their flavor, their shelf life is limited. This is one reason why these fats can be problematic for producers and sellers.

Just like vitamins, certain unsaturated fatty acids are absolutely essential for survival. This is why they are known as essential fatty acids; the body cannot make them itself but must absorb them through food. These essential fatty acids are the very popular omega-3 and omega-6 fatty acids. Flaxseed and hemp seed oils are particularly rich in omega-3s; walnut and rapeseed (canola) oils also contain valuable omega-3s. Safflower and soybean oils contain omega-6s. And while there are only minor differences between omega-3 and omega-6 fatty acids, the two have very different effects on the human body.

Omega-3 Fatty Acids: A Healthy Gift from Nature

Omega-3 fatty acids occur in plants only in the form of alpha-linolenic acid (ALA). The body must convert this into the usable omega-3 fatty acids docosahexaenoic acid (DHA) and eicosapentaenoic acid (EPA). The only way a sufficiently large quantity of these can be formed in the body is if you regularly eat plant-based oils that are rich in ALA, or a mix of leafy greens, sprouts, other vegetables, herbs, seeds and nuts.

The omega-3 fatty acids in meat and fish, on the other hand, exist in the forms that are right for our bodies: DHA and EPA. Game and grass-fed grazing animals (who do not eat an industrial grain-based diet) are also excellent sources of omega-3s. The same is true for cold-water fish, but you have to be careful because many are contaminated with heavy metals and toxins due to worsening pollution. A good alternative — especially for people who do not like fish — is omega-3 capsules derived from farmed algae, which are free from heavy metals and toxins. Just make absolutely sure your supplements are high quality; the oil they contain may not offer any health benefits if the fish has been taken from contaminated waters, or the oil has been heated during production.

DID YOU KNOW?

How to Slow Down Starch Digestion

Imagine you eat a slice of white bread. The starch compounds are split in a flash by digestive enzymes, and glucose is transported into the blood almost instantly. The result: your blood sugar rises very quickly. If, however, you dip your bread in olive oil before eating it, or spread it with butter, liverwurst or pâté, the carbohydrates are combined with oil. This slows down the splitting of the carbohydrates and the transportation of glucose into the bloodstream. It's a terrific little trick with great results. By the way, you can achieve the same effect by combining carbohydrates with proteins.

Seeds and nuts also contain valuable omega-3 fatty acids. In addition to walnuts and almonds, flax seeds and hemp seeds (or, to be botanically correct, hemp nuts), in particular, are rich in these essential fatty acids. Flax seeds and hemp seeds are also rich in proteins and fiber. They are well suited to use in many dishes, both hot and cold (you'll find lots of inspiring uses for them in the recipe section, starting on page 168).

The Right Dose

In the right amount, omega-3 fatty acids can protect you from cancer and cardiovascular disease, reduce blood pressure, stabilize the mind and improve intellectual development in children. In addition, they lead to a reduction in bleeding and reduce the danger of thrombosis, or blood clots that form in the circulatory system. Omega-3 fatty acids are also anti-angiogenic, which means they inhibit unwanted blood vessels from forming — a technique that is also employed by the most recent generation of anti-cancer drugs. Omega-3 fatty acids are a safe, cost-effective way to support cancer therapies.

Omega-3–Fatty Acid Content in Meat

Thanks to their diet and lifestyle, our ancestors naturally consumed a healthy mix of saturated and unsaturated fatty acids. Their diet was rich in proteins but low in glucose and starch. At the same time, their foods contained a high proportion of saturated animal fats and a moderate amount of unsaturated fatty acids from both animal and plant sources. The ratio of omega-3 to omega-6 fatty acids was also balanced, because the meat and fat of the plant-eating animals they hunted contained a rather large amount of omega-3 fatty acids.

Species-appropriate feeding directly affects the amount of these essential fatty acids in meat. This means that a cow that is allowed to graze on grass and eat hay will produce meat that is much richer in omega-3 fatty acids than an animal that is kept in a barn and fed grain. So treat yourself to something good: buy meat from animals that were kept and fed in a species-appropriate manner. The better taste and health benefits outweigh the higher price.

Meat: Healthy or Not?

Consumption of meat, especially red meat (that is, mainly beef and pork), is often suspected of carrying health risks. In studies that have examined this issue, the meat usually

DID YOU KNOW?

Omega-3s Protect Against Breast Cancer

Studies concerning fat uptake have been able to prove that the type of fat consumed has a significant effect on cancer risk. When your consumption of omega-3 fatty acids increases, you achieve a better ratio of omega-3 to omega-6 fatty acids in your diet, which lowers your risk of developing breast cancer.

DID YOU KNOW?

Omega-3s Require Caution, Too

Excessive amounts of healthy omega-3 fatty acids can lead to health risks. Too high a concentration may lead to a tendency to increased bleeding. Pay close attention to how much you're getting from your diet and supplements.

Salmon and Omega-3s

Freshly caught wild salmon, like other oily saltwater fish, is particularly rich in omega-3 fatty acids. If you're buying farmed salmon, however, make sure it is certified organic. Fish raised this way are significantly higher quality than those raised using conventional farming practices. The use of hormones, for example, is taboo in organic salmon.

Heritage Breeds and Omega-3s

You may be surprised to learn that grass-fed wild animals and some livestock raised today still contain a very high amount of omega-3 fatty acids. In some, their meat contains an even higher amount of omega-3 fatty acids than fish, which also ingest fatty acids in their food (such as plankton and algae). And it's not only the way an animal is kept and fed that affects the quality of its meat. The breeding of the animal can make a difference. Unlike many newer livestock breeds, heritage breeds are a better source of omega-3 fatty acids.

comes from animals that are not kept or fed in a species-appropriate way. It is, therefore, not surprising that the fatty acid composition of this meat is not particularly healthy. In addition, the meat may be contaminated with antibiotics and hormones (if processed meats are consumed, they are often chemically modified using nitrites, as well). Add to that the very real fact that red meat can also be prepared in an unhealthy manner. It may be cooked using the wrong type of fat or deep-fried in hydrogenated vegetable shortening, which contains harmful trans-fatty acids.

The question of whether to eat meat, both red and white, is not as crucial as the question of the quality of that meat. How can the white meat of a caged, industrially raised chicken be better than the red meat of a "happy" cow that grazes outside on grass? If red meat were unhealthy by its very nature, all of the big cat species — think lions, leopards and cheetahs — would have health problems. After all, they dine almost exclusively on red meat.

Unfortunately, the quality of the meat sold today is often terrible. Factory farming and species-inappropriate feeding lead to health issues, not only in the animals themselves but also in the humans who consume them. At the same time, milk and milk products made from animals raised using industrial farming techniques also show a negatively altered pattern of fatty acids, including too high a proportion of omega-6 fatty acids. The solution: always check the origin of the meat and dairy products you choose, and buy organic whenever you can.

Omega-6 Fatty Acids: Good in Smaller Amounts

We need to consume omega-3 fatty acids in our food, but we also need to get omega-6 fatty acids. In the Western world, however, we are likely to consume too much of these rather than too little. And this imbalance can have disastrous consequences: the body can chemically change some omega-6 fatty acids (also known as linoleic acid), via several intermediate steps, into a substance called arachidonic acid. From this four-way unsaturated fatty acid, the body can then form prostaglandins (tissue hormones), which promote inflammation.

The proper ratio of omega-6 fatty acids to omega-3 fatty acids in the body should not be more than 3:1. It's important to read nutrient labels and consume foods that contain these substances in the right proportions. In many foods, however, the ratio is clearly weighted in favor of omega-6 fatty acids; at times, the ratio can be as much as 50:1. The best way to create balance is to choose more foods that are rich in omega-3s while reducing your consumption of foods that are rich in omega-6s.

Just to be clear: omega-6 fatty acids are not bad for you. They are essential for survival. However, the amount you consume and the ratio of them to the omega-3 fatty acids in your diet are the important factors to prevent imbalance and inflammatory responses in the body.

Getting the Mix Right

Because the various types of unsaturated fatty acids have different effects — and because it can be hard to monitor their exact concentration and ratios in the body — even nutritional experts have a hard time determining which fatty acids are missing and which should be increased in a person's diet. So how are you supposed to decide for yourself whether you're in balance?

One way to determine this is to have a laboratory test a sample of your blood to find your fatty acid profile. From this data, you can discover whether you have any deficits or imbalances. Your insurance company or health care provider can tell you how much a test will cost and whether it is covered.

If your ratio of omega-6s to omega-3s is greater than 5:1, you should consume more omega-3 fatty acids from vegetable sources (which contain ALA) and/or animal sources (which contain DHA and EPA). Try special vegetable oil blends (see box, below), high-protein breads (see page 157) and grass-fed beef.

DID YOU KNOW?

Pork Can Be Healthy

It's not a meat most people associate with healthy eating, but pork can be good for you, too. Conventionally raised pigs are usually fattened with starchy food, so their meat is of comparatively poorer quality. However, some farms keep their pigs outside and let them feed in pastures, where they enrich their diet with green plants and acorns. Their meat not only tastes good but also contains many nutrients.

Special Oil Blends: A Secret Weapon

Special oil blends, including ones you mix yourself (see page 161), ensure a balanced supply of nutrients, with the proper ratio of omega-6 to omega-3 fatty acids. They also offer a beneficial proportion of unsaturated to saturated fatty acids, and of long- to medium-chain fatty acids, which are exactly adapted to the needs of the human body. In contrast, if you consume just one or two different vegetable oils, you won't get a blend of all the unsaturated and saturated fatty acids you need. No one oil is suitable as a sole source of fatty acids in humans.

Industrially Produced Oils

When oils and fats are industrially produced, they undergo some undesirable chemical changes. These fats and the foods made with them can cause serious health risks. One example of this is the hardening of unsaturated vegetable oils through a process called hydrogenation, which converts the fat's unsaturated carbon-carbon bonds (double bonds) into saturated carbon compounds. This chemical change creates a firmer, spreadable fat from liquid oil.

During the curing of these artificial fats, harmful trans-fatty acids can form. These compounds pose a number of health risks. In the United States and Canada, nutrition labels must list trans-fatty acid content. The state of California has gone so far as to ban the use of these fats in restaurants, and other local authorities in a number of states have also limited their legal use. A similar provision in the European Union is overdue. Beyond their trans-fatty acid content, industrially produced oils have a blend of fatty acids that can cause other health problems. The best advice is to avoid them when possible.

Use Caution When Heating Fat

Unsaturated fatty acids have one or more unsaturated carbon-carbon bonds. These so-called double bonds are very reactive; oxygen from the air is sufficient to get them going. No wonder, then, that unsaturated fatty acids easily turn rancid.

When heated, unsaturated fatty acids also tend to undergo a chemical reaction with oxygen or other unsaturated fatty acids. They are changed to such a degree that they can no longer perform their proper role in the metabolism. Moreover, at times, some dangerous chemical compounds are formed. Oils and plants with a high content of unsaturated fatty acids, such as flaxseed and hemp seed oils, are, therefore, not suitable for cooking or deep-frying, only for cold dishes. Saturated fatty acids, on the other hand, do not react with atmospheric oxygen and are stable when heated.

Use fats and oils with a high content of saturated fatty acids for cooking and deep-frying. Good options are coconut and palm oils, butter, beef fat and lard.

DID YOU KNOW?

There Are Multiple Types of Omega-6 Fatty Acids

To complicate matters, there are also large differences between the various types of omega-6 fatty acids. For example, gamma-linolenic acid, which is found in only a few plant oils (including those made from hemp seeds, borage, evening primrose and pomegranate seeds), has different properties and affects the body differently than linoleic acid. Gamma-linolenic acid, unlike linoleic acid, *positively* affects inflammatory processes in the body. Both of these fatty acids should be a regular part of your diet, in the proper amounts.

The Pillars of a Healthy Diet

Many patients with cancer repeatedly ask what they might have done "wrong." There simply is not an answer to that question, and even if cancer were your fault (which it definitely is not), no single answer would be applicable to everyone. The disease always occurs as a result of the unhappy combination of a number of different factors (see page 13).

This is why there cannot be any single recommendation for preventing cancer or choosing a treatment. One thing is certain, however: your health depends on a number of different factors. The more of these you take care of, the smaller your risk of developing cancer, and the greater the likelihood that you will be able to successfully fight the disease if it develops.

It's Time to Change Your Diet

If you are a patient with cancer, you know you should mostly give up unhealthy carbohydrates. This does not mean that you need to turn your entire diet upside-down. You simply

---

The Pillars of Personal Health Care

These are the basic factors you can control that will positively affect your health, reduce your risk of developing cancer and increase your chances of recovery if you do get cancer:

- Get regular preventive checkups, and have routine medical examinations and tests
- Eat a balanced diet that is low in carbohydrates and rich in protein and fiber, and contains a large amount of valuable oils and fats, and a sufficient supply of vitamins, minerals and phytochemicals
- Do aerobic exercise in the fresh air for 30 to 45 minutes at a time, at least three times a week, and include moderate weight training once a week
- Get regular and sufficiently long periods of sleep and rest
- Drink at least 8 to 12 cups (2 to 3 L) of still water throughout the day
- Do not smoke

More Pillars of Personal Health Care for Patients with Cancer

In addition to the strategies on page 89, patients with cancer have several other tools they can effectively use to battle the disease. Here are the most important ones:

- Get intensive medical care and use all available therapeutic options, maintaining strict control over your needs and progress. Make absolutely certain that the newest diagnostic procedures are used, including positron emission tomography (better known as PET) scans, which help reconstruct metabolic processes in the body (see box, opposite).

- Use the results from your diagnostic tests to select only those cancer treatments that promise the greatest chance of a cure *for your individual case*. Also take advantage of new testing methods to monitor the success of your treatment.

- Incorporate as many intense exercise sessions into your daily life as you can. Exercise empties the body's glucose reserves and deprives cancer of its food. When you exercise outdoors, thanks to the UV radiation from the sun, the body produces valuable vitamin D, which plays an important role in cell growth and can protect against cancer (see page 95). But be careful: always work out within your abilities and don't overdo it. Follow each exercise session with a period of rest and relaxation, which helps bring you inner peace.

- Make absolutely certain you stick to the low-carbohydrate foods of this cancer-fighting diet. It offers a high proportion of foods that contain lactic acid, phytochemicals, fiber, valuable plant-based oils and quality proteins.

have to replace high-glucose foods, such as pasta, bread and baked goods made from white flour, with alternatives that cause fewer blood sugar spikes — for example, high-protein bread and pasta, and baked goods made with flour milled from ancient grains are all smarter choices that provide the nutrients you need. This way, you can largely stick to your customary eating patterns, while gently and smartly fighting aggressive cancer cells.

At the same time, the cancer-fighting diet will help you slow down or stop the weight loss that often accompanies the disease. Statistically, cancer leads to complete cachexia (wasting and weakness) in 60% to 80% of people who have advanced-stage cancer, and one in five patients with cancer will die from this type of physical exhaustion. If you eat a diet rich in fats and proteins, you can supply the healthy cells in your body with energy while simultaneously "starving" aggressive cancer cells. You can eat your fill without making your blood sugar level shoot sky-high.

The most important thing is to take into account the quality of the food you eat. Your health should be worth the expense. You'll be pleasantly surprised by the great diversity of flavors you'll find in the recipe section starting on page 168.

Cancer Cells Demand Sugar

As long as cancer cells continuously remove glucose from the blood, the brain will always demand a new supply to keep the blood sugar level constant. This is why many patients with cancer experience cravings for sugary foods, such as bread, pastries, pasta and candy. To make matters worse, the body itself also produces sugar. If there is a lack of it, the liver can make glucose from the body's protein reserves to ensure an adequate supply. The result is that cancer then grows even more quickly at the expense of other tissues, such as the muscles. The liver desperately tries to cope and to continue supplying sugar, which, over time, depletes the body even more and leaves it emaciated. Serious weight loss may, therefore, be indicative of advanced-stage cancer.

Cancer also uses another evil strategy to feed itself: it releases the lactic acid generated during fermentation into body tissues. Because a fermenting cancer cell needs 20 to 30 times as much glucose as a healthy cell, the body has no choice but to transport the huge amount of lactic acid via the bloodstream to the liver. There, at the expense of considerable energy, it is once more converted to glucose, which speeds up the process of emaciation and renews the cancer cells' sugar supply.

Breaking the Vicious Circle

For patients with cancer, the consumption of glucose- and starch-rich foods has catastrophic consequences, because cancer cells make repeated and excessive use of blood glucose. As a result, the body increasingly resorts to using up its protein reserves; the patient can literally starve, even though he or she

DID YOU KNOW?

PET Scans Monitor Cancer Treatments
Positron emission tomography (PET) scans allow doctors to see glucose uptake by tumors, which can show early on how successful your chosen treatment is. For this scan, the doctor will inject you with a radioactively marked sugar called deoxyglucose. Aggressive tumors and metastases absorb this in the same way that they absorb glucose, which makes them show up when the body is examined in the PET tube. During a PET scan, the entire body is searched to find the location of the cancer, and to determine whether it has spread and how active it is. Ask your insurance provider if PET scans during cancer treatment are covered by your insurance; they are in some cases.

A Reminder

Remember: aggressive, fermenting cancer cells are dependent on glucose in the blood for their metabolism to work. If there is no new supply, the cells grow more slowly, which will eventually lead to disarmed tumor cells. In the best-case scenario, the cancer cells will simply die.

consumes plenty of calories. Patients too often try to cover their increasing energy needs by ingesting glucose-rich liquids or foods, which gives the cancer exactly what it needs to grow: simple sugar.

To break this vicious circle, you need to supply your body with more protein, valuable oils and fatty acids. And make sure your blood sugar level does not rise after meals. This way, you can slowly starve the predator in your body.

Limiting Unnecessary Sugar and Starch

I know what you're going to say: a consistent reduction of carbohydrates is difficult to achieve in real life. After all, in the Western world, foods with high glucose and starch contents traditionally rank high on the scale of importance. You'll be surprised, however, at how quickly you can get used to this change in your diet. After only two weeks, your desire for sweet, sugary or starchy foods will have lessened significantly. You will feel full of vitality and energy, and, generally, healthier.

The Three Types of Carbs

Foods that contain carbohydrates can be divided into three groups, depending on their effect on the blood sugar level:

- **Foods That Raise the Blood Sugar Level Quickly and Steeply.** Foods like bread, pasta, potatoes and sugary drinks contain a large amount of glucose and/or starch. They catapult the blood sugar to lofty levels, causing insulin to be released; all of this encourages cancer growth. The exception are breads and pastas that are low in glucose and starch (see page 157).

- **Foods That Raise the Blood Sugar Level Slowly and to a Limited Degree.** Foods in this category contain less glucose and starch, or other forms of sugar that are not converted into glucose until they reach the liver. This is why the blood sugar rises only a little and slowly after a meal; if consumed in moderation, these foods add variety to the diet. Berries, for example, contain valuable nutrients and a moderate amount of sugar. Just limit the quantity of these foods in your diet.

- **Foods That Raise the Blood Sugar Level Only a Little or Not At All.** Leafy greens, other vegetables, nuts, meat and fish contain a small amount of glucose and starch, so they hardly affect blood sugar at all. Healthy sugars, such as galactose, tagatose, isomaltulose and trehalose, also have little to no effect on blood sugar. When you eat these foods, cancer cells are unable to ferment properly and, in the best-case scenario, can even starve to death. Foods in this category should, therefore, make up the majority of your anti-cancer diet. You'll find a list of options on page 144.

And even if this change isn't so difficult for you, one question remains: how do you eat enough to be satisfied without the traditional fillers, such as bread, potatoes, pasta and rice? Don't worry. Even if you give up sugary and starchy foods altogether, your body will produce sufficient glucose, either from other sugar sources (such as fructose; galactose; and ribose, a sugar that forms part of our DNA) or from protein and glycerin (a component of fats). In addition, you will get plenty of glucose from fruit and vegetables, just in a much healthier form.

The body requires amino acids (the smallest protein building blocks), vitamins and some fatty acids, but glucose, starch and carbohydrates are, generally, not considered essential nutrients. Even if you do not supply your body with any carbohydrates over a long period of time and all your glucose stores are emptied, you won't suffer from a deficiency. The body will simply switch to making increased use of fats and proteins, and continue to maintain an uninterrupted energy supply. In emergency situations, the body is even able to produce its own glucose from protein and some fats. This way, it ensures that glucose-dependent tissues, such as the brain, the nerves and the retinas, will always be sufficiently provided for.

Lacto-Fermented Foods

In addition to low-carb foods, another important component of a healthy cancer-fighting diet is foods that have been preserved through lacto-fermentation (see box, page 94.) They are particularly low in sugar because the sugars that were originally present in them are converted to lactic acid.

Cancer cells cannot ferment the lactic acid in these foods a second time. This is quite unlike healthy cells (for example, in the heart muscle and other organs), which can easily use these foods to release energy.

Considering that fermenting cancer cells virtually flood the body with lactic acid, which stresses the metabolism, it seems hard to understand, at first glance, why we should feed the body additional lactic acid in food. The reason is that, as the liver breaks down lactic acid in food (the salt part of the lactic acid, called lactate, to be precise), this has a deacidifying effect on the body, which helps neutralize the lactic acid produced by cancer cells.

> **DID YOU KNOW?**
>
> **Magnesium Citrate**
> Magnesium citrate combines the deacidifying effect of citrate (or citric acid) and the cancer-protective properties of magnesium. Taking a high-quality supplement from your pharmacy can help you simultaneously reduce your body's acidity and supply sufficient amounts of the mineral. Different countries have different recommended daily allowances for this mineral, so check with your doctor or pharmacist to ensure you're getting the right dose for your age, sex and situation.

Common Lacto-Fermented Foods

Foods preserved using lacto-fermentation are old fashioned and have been consumed for centuries in a number of cultures. Some examples include

- Buttermilk and kefir
- Quark, a German fresh cheese similar to fromage frais
- Yogurt
- Cheeses (except mozzarella)
- Sauerkraut
- Sourdough bread (although this still contains plenty of starch)
- Pickled vegetables, such as kimchi or fermented dill pickles

This is an important point. Even more than in a healthy person, the body of a patient with cancer is prone to acidification due to lactic acid–fermenting cancer cells. It would be wrong to counter this simply by administering bases to neutralize the surplus acid. Adding bases would change the body's pH, making it even easier for cancer cells to release additional acid. Plus, adding bases would not eliminate the cause of increased acid production. That's why it is much more sensible to work on the underlying cause of increased lactic acid production. The solution is to reduce the supply of glucose and support the deacidification of the body with the salts of organic acids, such as lactic acid or citric acid (citrate).

Vitamins, Minerals and Other Micronutrients

Since biochemical reactions in the body are triggered by enzymes, which require vitamins and minerals in order to work properly, these micronutrients play an important role in the maintenance of bodily functions. Foods rich in glucose and starch often contain extremely low amounts of vitamins and minerals. If you consume foods that contain less sugar and starch, you will not only benefit from their natural cancer-inhibiting action, you'll also ensure that your diet is richer in vitamins and minerals.

Vitamin D: Cheap, Effective Protection from Cancer

Recent studies of breast, colon and prostate cancers have shown that a sufficiently high level of vitamin D in the blood is excellent protection from them. Vitamin D can reduce your risk of developing colon cancer by up to 50%.

The body can synthesize sufficient vitamin D in the skin only with the help of UV radiation, such as you get from the sun. The results of a follow-up in men with untreated prostate cancer showed that increases in prostate-specific antigen (PSA) levels in the blood (which signal tumor activity) during sunny months is lower than in the rest of the year. Further investigation showed that sun and UV exposure were directly related to prostate cancer occurrence and death from the disease. When subjects were exposed to UV radiation, their cancer risk decreased by 42%, and the number of deaths from the disease decreased by as much as 53%.

Our ancestors were exposed to solar radiation, at varying intensities, throughout the year. Modern humans, however, rarely spend that much time out in the open. Because window glass filters out sunlight, indoor light does not provide any amount of UV exposure. So make sure that you spend time in the fresh air as often as you can. Often, a long daily walk is sufficient to boost vitamin D levels. Just make sure your face and arms are exposed to the sun, without sunscreen, which blocks UV rays (but before you head outside, see the box below regarding the dangers of too much UV exposure). Even on cloudy days, enough UV radiation penetrates through the cloud cover to ensure good health.

DID YOU KNOW?

Two Reasons to Go Outside

Gentle aerobic exercise outdoors — for example, Nordic or regular walking — has a positive impact on your health in two ways. You empty your body's glycogen stores, and sunlight helps your body form enough vitamin D via the skin. Both help in the fight against cancer.

UV Light: A Blessing or a Curse?

Because UV light exposure is implicated in the occurrence of skin cancer (melanoma), more and more doctors quite rightly plead with their patients to protect themselves from UV radiation. But avoiding the sun completely is not a good idea, either. The trick is to learn how to deal with it responsibly. Go outside for about half an hour a day year-round. This way, you'll give your skin a chance to adapt to seasonal changes in sunlight and UV radiation with a corresponding change in pigmentation (and you'll help boost your vitamin D level). But don't stay in the sun too long, and put on appropriate sun protection during periods of increased UV radiation.

With increasing age, skin slowly loses its ability to produce vitamin D, even while the body's demand increases (for protection from conditions such as osteoporosis). Experts recommend that you take a vitamin D supplement to ensure you're getting enough; check with your doctor or pharmacist to ensure you're taking the right recommended daily allowance for your sex, age and situation. It's also smart to eat foods that are rich in vitamin D (see box, at left). Since the majority of the population suffers from vitamin D deficiency, the vitamin D levels of patients with cancer should be especially monitored and balanced with nutritional supplements, if necessary.

Coenzyme Q10 Keeps the Mitochondria Active

Everything that inhibits the activity of the mitochondria helps a tumor turn into cancer cells. In order for glucose combustion in the mitochondria to work at full throttle, it is necessary for energy-rich electrons (negatively charged particles) to be gradually transported to a lower energy level. Ubiquinone, also known as coenzyme Q10 or simply Q10, is a crucial element in this transport. If the level of ubiquinone in a cell is lowered, this can affect the activity of the mitochondria and, consequently, encourage fermentation. Studies in patients with cancer metastases have shown the role this substance plays in the disease: in these patients, a clear ubiquinone deficiency could be detected.

So how do you make sure you have a sufficiently high level of ubiquinone? There is a plentiful supply of the natural form of coenzyme Q10 in oily fish, liver and other offal; most nuts; and plant oils. Vegetables such as cabbages, onions, spinach, Brussels sprouts and broccoli also contain it. Coenzyme Q10 is heat sensitive, however, so it may be lost

Sources of Coenzyme Q10

Normally, you take in enough of this substance through food. The recommended daily dose is 10 to 30 milligrams. Particularly rich sources of coenzyme Q10 include

- Meat (3 to 4 mg per 3½-oz/100 g portion)
- Eggs and fish (6.5 mg per 3½-oz/100 g portion)
- Cold-pressed plant oils, such as olive oil (3 mg per 3½-oz/100 g portion)

Research Study: Is Vitamin C a Cancer Killer?

Until recently, giving patients with cancer vitamin C was not considered helpful. As a natural antioxidant, it was thought to protect healthy cells *and* cancer cells from radiation or chemotherapy. Now, however, studies have demonstrated that vitamin C causes cancer cells to die when it is administered intravenously and in high doses (about 500 times the normal recommended daily dose of 25 to 100 mg, depending on your age). Why? High-dosage vitamin C leads to the formation of cytotoxically active amounts of hydrogen peroxide in tumor cells, which inhibits cell growth.

Vitamin C intake also supports the positive effects of total-body hyperthermia, an established cancer-fighting procedure in which the patient's core temperature is raised to 107.2°F to 107.6°F (41.8°C to 42°C) for 60 minutes in an effort to kill cancer cells. The first successes with this combined therapy have been promising, especially because patients who responded to it had not responded to prior treatments using other therapies.

during cooking. The best idea is to use ubiquinone-containing plant oils to prepare cold dishes. Add these oils to salads and recipes made with fermented milk products.

Stress, disease, nicotine use, alcohol abuse and age-related reduction in receptivity can markedly lower the amount of coenzyme Q10 in the blood. Some cholesterol-reducing drugs (statins) also inhibit the body's production of ubiquinone and, therefore, have an unwanted cancer-promoting effect. In cases such as these, you should compensate by taking a supplement.

The Positive Effect of Selenium

The trace element selenium is considered *the* detoxifying substance par excellence. As an important component of antioxidant enzymes (the proteins that dispose of toxic free radicals in the body), it positively affects immune cell activity.

Unfortunately, soil depletion means that in many countries, there is a deficiency of this mineral in food. A connection exists between selenium deficiency and the appearance of lifestyle diseases, including diseases of the joints, internal organs, gastrointestinal system, nervous system and brain. Getting a sufficient supply of the mineral also plays an important role in cancer prevention.

Make sure, therefore, that the level of selenium in your body is high enough. Check with your doctor or pharmacist to ensure you're taking a supplement that contains the recommended daily allowance. And make sure to consume foods that are rich in selenium, such as offal (especially liver and kidneys) and nuts.

Zinc Activates the Immune System

Zinc is an essential mineral for all creatures. It is a component of important enzymes and proteins, which govern our genetic activity. In the body, this trace element fulfills a number of different functions: it plays a key role in sugar, fat and protein metabolism, and it is involved in the formation of genetic material and in cell growth. The immune system and many hormones also require zinc to function.

Just as for healthy people, it is important for patients with cancer to ensure they get sufficient zinc. Check with your doctor or pharmacist to see if you're getting the recommended daily allowance. Offal, beef, almonds, leafy greens and cabbage are all good suppliers of this mineral.

Drinks That Hydrate the Body

A healthy diet must also include an adequate amount of fluids. You should drink at least 8 cups (2 L) a day; if you do intense exercise, you should consume 12 cups (3 L) or more. But it's not just the amount that counts: which thirst-quenching drinks you opt for makes a big difference.

Water: The Source of Life

People often underestimate the importance of water to good health. It contains no calories so, in the strictest sense, it is not a food. But it is still the most important thing we consume. Water makes possible all the biochemical metabolic processes in the body, which are the foundations of life.

Two Types of Water

To stay healthy, we don't need pure distilled water, but rather water that contains a sufficient and healthy array of minerals and salts. Here are two options and some issues to consider:

- **Bottled (Mineral) Water.** With this type of water, there is no danger that you will burden your body with unwanted metals or halogens, such as chlorine or fluorine. However, mineral water has (as the name suggests) a high mineral content. If you don't exercise and/or perform heavy physical labor, you won't lose significant amounts of minerals through sweating. That means you should drink water with a lower mineral content, because it will more readily flush unwanted salts from the body. If you always drink mineral water (especially if it is high in sodium), you can stress your kidneys, which have to flush out the excess salts. This can lead to a rise in blood pressure.

- **Tap Water.** Water that comes directly out of the faucet can be good, but sometimes has drawbacks, too. Water often runs through pipes for many miles before it reaches your home. En route and as it stands, it can accumulate harmful metals. The best idea is to always let the water run for a while before you pour yourself a glass — especially if you haven't run the water through that faucet recently.

The Dangers of Fluoride

Fluoride, in the form of sodium fluoride, is added to tap water in parts of Canada, the United States and Switzerland. It inhibits the enolase enzyme, which is normally involved in sugar usage in the body, and promotes glucose fermentation, which can transform tumor cells into cancer. A study of American cities has shown that some types of cancer appear in greater numbers in areas that have fluoridated drinking water. In addition, sodium fluoride can trigger cancerous changes, chromosome damage and unplanned DNA syntheses. It's best to avoid fluoridated water and switch to a fluoride-free toothpaste.

Sugary Drinks

Energy-rich, sweet drinks will not quench your thirst. Generally, they contain between 12% and 15% sugar and act like a liquid turbocharger in the body. Let's take a bottle of lemonade as an example: in 4 cups (1 L), you will consume 120 to 150 grams of sugar. As a result of this blood sugar spike, your body's insulin release will be similarly strong.

What About Soy Milk?

More and more people have problems consuming cows' milk and switch to soy products. This is smart, because studies conducted around the world have repeatedly confirmed the health-promoting effects of the soybean. It encourages healthy digestion and lowers blood pressure. And thanks to its high protein content, it is an important basic food for vegetarians. You'll get an ideal daily dose in 10 oz (300 g) of tofu or 3⅓ cups (800 mL) of soy milk.

Like dairy, soy can also cause allergies and intolerances, so it is identified on food labels. A low-carb diet improves intestinal flora, which can, in many cases, make food intolerances recede or disappear. Like fermented milk products, special fermented soy drinks are also better tolerated than plain soy milk. This may be because proteins are present in a different form in a lacto-fermented environment, triggering fewer immune responses.

And it is not just artificially sweetened drinks that are dangerous to your metabolism and health. Depending on the variety, pure, unsweetened fruit juices may contain just as much sugar. But when compared with lemonade and similar sugary drinks, natural fruit juices do contain some valuable vitamins and phytochemicals. Fresh berries and vegetables, though, cover the body's requirements much better, without spiking blood sugar levels.

Milk

Unlike juices and sweet beverages that never occurred in the original human diet, there is one energy-rich drink that has always played a key role: milk. The lactose it contains is a disaccharide, composed of galactose and glucose (see page 75).

The ability of hunter-gatherers to break down and use lactose was limited: only babies and young toddlers had that capacity. In adolescents and adults, the body gradually stopped producing the lactase enzyme that is necessary to break down lactose. So when people in these age groups consumed milk, they experienced bloating and diarrhea. There is a simple reason for this: children had to be weaned so that milk would be available for the next child. Over millennia, genetic mutations took place in several populations and, slowly, adults also became able to break down lactose. From then on, the milk of cows, sheep and goats represented a high-quality food for these people.

If you get bloated and have diarrhea when you consume milk, that is a clear indication of lactose intolerance. (The symptoms cannot always be blamed on milk sugar, however, so it's worth consulting your doctor.) One solution to the problem may be switching to fermented milk products (see page 162). In these, bacteria convert most of the lactose into lactic acid, so people often do not have an adverse reaction to them.

Nature's Anti-Cancer Drugs

Natural, whole foods are filled to the brim with vitamins, minerals, trace elements and phytochemicals (see page 105). You simply cannot replace them, even with supplements that isolate beneficial nutrients or active ingredients. The door to Mother Nature's medicine cabinet is wide open — all you have to do is reach inside. The following foods taste wonderful, and they will greatly improve your health and well-being.

Cabbage and Broccoli: Vegetable Superstars

Cabbage, broccoli and other vegetables in the *Brassica* genus are packed with anti-cancer agents — for example, they contain glucosinolates, or sulfur compounds, that are released during the destruction of cell walls. These phytochemicals are able to protect human cells from damage by carcinogens and prevent tumor development. They detoxify carcinogenic substances and regulate estrogen levels. They are highly effective: just three or four servings of broccoli a week can significantly reduce your risk of breast or bladder cancer. In addition, like all members of the cabbage family, broccoli is a valuable source of vitamin C.

The active ingredients hibernate deep within these veggies, and only thorough chewing releases their anti-cancer action. Excessive heat reduces their effectiveness, so prepare broccoli and similar vegetables in a steamer, if possible, or heat them briefly in a skillet. Eat as much raw cabbage as you can and chew it well; every chomp increases its effectiveness.

Tomatoes: Healthy Red Giants

There is hardly a vegetable that lands on our plates as often as the tomato does — and for good reason. Nature wasn't stingy with taste or valuable compounds when it designed this fruit. Tomatoes ripened on the vine are jam packed with minerals, vitamins and phytochemicals. Lycopene is the compound responsible for the tomato's anti-cancer action. Lycopene is

DID YOU KNOW?

Dinosaur Kale
A delicious and easily digestible type of cabbage is dinosaur kale (also called black cabbage or cavolo nero). It is one of the oldest and most robust cabbage varieties.

DID YOU KNOW?

Wild Tomatoes
There are natural, wild forms of the tomato. If you can find them, use them. They have a much higher lycopene content than modern cultivars.

a type of carotenoid, or natural pigment, that gives tomatoes their appetizing, shiny red color. Unlike most phytochemicals, which are heat sensitive, lycopene actually *requires* heat in order to fully develop the effectiveness of its active substances. Concentrated tomato purée made from sun-ripened fruits and puréed cooked tomatoes contain the greatest proportion of lycopene.

Enjoying tomatoes in combination with high-quality oils increases the availability of lycopene. A puréed tomato soup made with garlic and olive oil, therefore, makes an ideal meal for preventing cancer. Try to include it in your diet at least twice a week.

Onions and Garlic: Fighting Cancer "Vampires"

Garlic and onions give so many dishes an appetizing flavor. But did you know that they are also highly effective weapons — entirely without side effects — in the fight against cancer?

The valuable active ingredients in these two mostly consist of strongly aromatic sulfur compounds, such as alliin, which converts into allicin when the cell walls are broken down and releases an unmistakable odor. Allicin is also responsible for the anti-cancerous effect of onions and garlic. To get the full benefit, you have to chop them into small pieces, and let them rest for about 10 minutes before use. A little oil further increases their efficacy. A word of caution: allicin is not stable when heated, so add garlic at the end of the cooking time and do not reheat the dish afterward.

Antibiotics: A Caution

The use of certain antibiotics can significantly threaten mitochondrial function. After all, mitochondria, the cell's "power plants," evolved from ancient bacteria (see page 26) and still have features typical of these microorganisms. This is exactly why some antibiotic treatments fight not only unwelcome, disease-causing bacteria, but also the mitochondria. When mitochondrial activity is reduced, the risk of glucose fermentation increases. You already know that this means a tumor can become aggressive and spread.

Use all available means to promote activity in your cellular power plants; the better they work, the harder it becomes for cancer cells to block them. With the right diet and regular aerobic exercise, you support their work. As you age, mitochondrial activity gradually decreases, so diet and exercise play an increasingly important role in keeping them healthy.

Onions also contain polyphenols, such as quercetin. These protect the body from cancer-causing agents, block the growth of cancer cells, activate glucose combustion and inhibit the fermentation metabolism. Eat them raw as often as you can — for example, in salads.

Citrus Fruits: More than Just Vitamin C

When you peel these colorful vitamin bombs, you can smell that there is so much more to them. The essential aromas they release belong to a group of compounds called terpenes. Citrus fruits also contain many highly active phytonutrients, especially in their zest, as well as great quantities of polyphenols, which, among other things, are potent anti-inflammatory agents. Citrus fruits' active substances seem to be able to intervene directly in the reproductive cycle of the cancer cell: they act as scavengers of free radicals and help detoxify the body. Citrus fruits also increase the absorption and effectiveness of other plant substances. Plus, they activate and strengthen the immune system.

You can take advantage of citrus power in so many ways. Season your salads with a spoonful of lemon juice to increase your body's absorption of vitamins, minerals and phytochemicals. Lemon juice will also protect the oil in the salad from oxidation. Other tasty options are to use bitter orange marmalade (just pay attention to the sugar content), and add grated lemon zest to desserts and sauces.

Dark Chocolate: A Healthy Snack

Chocolate is a gourmet food with great potential, and not only for the taste buds. Like blueberries and grapeseed flour, cocoa is one of the most effective suppliers of the plant component proanthocyanidin, a flavonoid that neutralizes free radicals and protects the cell before mutations can occur. This compound also interferes in the energy generation of cancer cells by promoting combustion and inhibiting fermentation. Additionally, cocoa contains a large amount of polyphenols.

A daily snack of just a few squares of regular dark chocolate (made with more than 70% cocoa) or chocolate sweetened with healthy sugars, such as galactose, tagatose or trehalose, will provide you with a great quantity of these nutrients without raising your blood glucose level.

DID YOU KNOW?

A Smart Combination

A simple rule: the darker the chocolate, the higher the cocoa content and the more effective the antioxidative action. But the combination of chocolate and healthy sugar is a very good alternative. Bars of chocolate made with a higher percentage of cocoa (more than 70%) that are sweetened with healthy sugars are especially valuable.

Fresh Berries: Gourmet Health Food

Raspberries, blackberries, blueberries, black currants and strawberries: just the thought of them makes your mouth water, and that's a good thing. Almost no other type of fruit provides such highly effective phytochemicals. Berries contain large quantities of polyphenols, which inhibit cancer by blocking the formation of blood vessels (also called angiogenesis) and speeding up the programmed suicide of cancer cells. In addition, polyphenols are strongly antioxidant, so they trap free radicals, which can lead to premature aging and the destruction of healthy cells.

Include berries in your diet as often as you can, blueberries especially. You can safely use frozen berries; the active ingredients will survive the cold. Just keep an eye on the amount you eat, so you don't exceed the recommended daily amount of sugar.

Turmeric: Spice and Medicine

Turmeric is an intensely yellow-orange, light-sensitive spice made from the rhizome of the turmeric plant (*Curcuma longa*). Traditionally, this powdered spice is an essential component of curry powder. Thanks to its intense color, turmeric is also used in the food industry as a natural coloring agent — for example, in margarine, packaged rice dishes, baked goods, mustard and candy.

Turmeric does much more than just stimulate the taste buds. It contains curcumin, which counters the development of chemotherapy resistance, hampers the invasion and metastasis of cancer cells, and reduces angiogenesis. At the same time, it promotes the death of cancer cells. This is why turmeric is one of the most effective natural anti-cancer foods.

Like all phytochemicals, curcumin is very sensitive to light, heat and oxygen. Make sure the spices and extracts you buy are carefully processed, transported and stored so that they do not lose their biological effectiveness.

Green Tea: A Potent Elixir

Today, green tea has an established place in cancer prevention. Its special value lies in its gentle processing. Unlike black tea, green tea is unfermented, which preserves the valuable, cancer-preventing polyphenols (called catechins) in the tea leaves. Catechins prevent the formation of blood vessels that supply cancer cells.

DID YOU KNOW?

Pepper and Turmeric Are a Great Team

Curcumin, the cancer-fighting compound in turmeric, degrades fairly rapidly in the liver and the intestinal mucosa, which limits its availability to the body. You can counteract this by seasoning turmeric-infused food with black pepper. The piperine it contains inhibits the degradation of curcumin.

Just 3 cups (750 mL) of green tea a day significantly inhibits cancer growth. The catechins are optimally released when you let the tea steep for eight to 10 minutes, so set a timer and relax while you wait. The Japanese varieties gyokuro or sencha uchiyama are the best choices, because they have the highest polyphenol content.

Phytochemicals

In addition to vitamins and minerals, fruits and vegetables supply countless phytochemicals. A number of them are responsible for the cancer-preventive effects of food. They capture free radicals, inhibit growth in cancer cells and neutralize cancer-causing substances.

Phytochemicals That Fight Cancer

Here are three good reasons to eat more fruits and veggies. The following phytochemicals have been shown to inhibit cancer growth:

- **Resveratrol.** In animal experiments, resveratrol had a demonstrated life-prolonging effect. It also reduced weight gain associated with diets that were particularly rich in fats. At the same time, it significantly increased physical endurance. Resveratrol encourages cancer cell death, because it inhibits a protein (called nuclear factor-kappa B) that is essential to their survival. This means that apoptosis, or programmed cell death, can be turned back on in these cells.

- **Quercetin.** This phytochemical, from the class of polyphenols, has a direct effect on cancer cell metabolism. In 2008, Dutch scientists were able to demonstrate that it promotes combustion and inhibits fermentation in these cells.

- **Salvestrols.** These compounds protect plants from invasive pathogens, such as fungi. In humans, they attack tumor cells without affecting healthy cells. Why? The CYP1B1 enzyme, which is active only in tumor cells, ensures that salvestrols are converted into substances that trigger a number of different processes, including apoptosis. Modern foods contain only small amounts of salvestrols, thanks to pesticide use and breeding to remove them and their bitter taste. Opt for heirloom fruits and vegetables whenever you can. Cooking methods can also decrease the amount of salvestrols. Cooking vegetables in lots of water can remove them; steam, stir-fry or roast veggies to preserve salvestrols' anti-tumor benefits.

Cancer Is Not a Punishment

Chance plays a critical role in the development of cancer. Knowing this reassures many patients who blame themselves for their illness. Never forget that the formation of tumor cells can be triggered by random mutations that occur while DNA is being duplicated. Cancer is never your fault.

You can, however, positively influence the progress and treatment of your condition. Make use of the strength that comes from eating the right diet, exercising regularly and keeping your mind healthy. Try with all your might to think positively and to live for the future.

Inhibitors Require Caution

Many phytochemicals inhibit the formation of new blood vessels around a tumor; this process is called anti-angiogenesis. This makes it difficult for the tumor to gain access to the blood vessels; due to lack of access to oxygen and nutrients, it cannot grow and will die. This process becomes dangerous only when tumors receive further nutrients in the form of excessive glucose. They are then virtually forced to switch to an oxygen-free energy supply: fermentation via the TKTL1 enzyme.

Unfortunately, cancer drugs that specifically inhibit blood vessel formation by tumors often have adverse effects. Invasive tumors may be formed and spread. That's why you should always follow a low-carbohydrate diet if you use either artificial or natural inhibitors. Omega-3 fatty acids (see page 84) are an example of a natural inhibitor.

Günter G. on How Changing His Diet Affected His Prostate Cancer

Q: When a prostate tumor was discovered in your body, how did you react? What did your doctors recommend?

A: Because I had an elevated PSA [prostate-specific antigen] value, a tissue sample was taken and a prostate tumor was detected. For me, the diagnosis was as surprising as it was devastating. I had always believed that nothing like that could ever happen to me because I led a very healthy life.

Q: What did your doctors advise you to do?

A: My doctors informed me that, because of the test results, I urgently had to undergo either radiation or immediate surgical removal of the entire prostate to eliminate the cancer. This is not an easy undertaking; after all, the nerves that lie close to the prostate must not be damaged, because that could lead to impotence and incontinence. Despite the risks, however, I opted for surgery; my prostate was completely removed. And the operation seemed to have gone well. According to the surgeons, I was healed. I was overjoyed when I heard the good news.

Q: So you were considered completely healthy?

A: Yes. But after two years, my PSA value rose again. Since the increase was minimal, I did not let it worry me at first. Then, my doctor told me that in men who have had their prostates removed, PSA could have been formed by prostate cells and released into the blood only if metastases had already formed before the operation. And my increase in PSA was a clear alarm signal. Now I knew that the cancer was still there, after all. That whole time, I had thought I was cured. My shock was even greater when I was once again diagnosed with cancer. I was aware that my prospects for recovery were much worse this time. After all, the cancer cells had already spread. Then I accidentally came across an article about the discovery of the TKTL1 gene by Dr. Coy.

Q: What did you do with that information?

A: I studied Dr. Coy's diet plan, and realized that this way of feeding myself seemed absolutely feasible. I was immediately ready to change my diet so that I could be actively doing something to fight the disease. It was initially strange to purge familiar foods from my diet, such as pasta, potatoes, cakes and bread. But since I started, special breads and pastas have been developed that I can eat in moderation. I managed to change my diet without feeling like I had to abstain from everything. I also learned to appreciate many foods that I had previously shunned because of their high calorie content.

Q: Did you have any problems with the transition?

A: Yes, but they had nothing to do with the "new" foods. They mainly came from the fact that I was always asked about my diet at parties or events. Many people only smiled benignly at me because I believed in the importance of diet in the battle against cancer — which, by the way, I still do today.

Q: Did you stick with the diet despite all the criticism?

A: Yes, and for several reasons. First, I could easily follow it and didn't feel that my pleasure in eating was diminished. Second, it was very motivating to notice that I was feeling better in general. I have been trying to eat no more than 60 grams of carbohydrates a day. If I don't exceed this maximum, I can afford to occasionally eat a slice of normal bread or a roll. So even today, I don't have to punish myself in any way.

Q: Did following Dr. Coy's diet affect your PSA value?

A: My PSA level was low, but it increased slowly and steadily. A subsequent PET scan confirmed the PSA test results, and showed a lymph node metastasis in my abdomen. My doctor advised me not to opt for radiation, but instead to try anti-hormone therapy. In addition, I adhered more strictly to the principles of the cancer-fighting diet and visited a naturopath, who treated me with complementary remedies, including vitamin C, mineral salts and deacidifying powder. I then started the anti-hormone therapy recommended by my urologist. Within 20 days, my PSA value dropped from 1.66 to 0.22, a clear indication of the positive results of the treatment. I continued to eat according to Dr. Coy's principles and to take my naturopath's preparations. Recently, my PSA value dropped again, to the magnificent, almost negligible level of 0.05.

Q: Are you concerned that your PSA value may rise again?

A: Of course I am. But regular PSA and EDIM-TKTL1 tests will help me discover early on whether new cancer cells are growing in my body. Should this be the case, I will fight them in a very targeted way again. I now see the whole experience much more calmly. Because I understand the strategy pursued by the cancer cells in my body, I can actively defend myself against them.

Q: How are you now?

A: I am very glad that I changed my diet according to Dr. Coy's plan when my prostate cancer metastases were detected. At that time, conventional medicine thought my case was incurable, but by changing my diet, I have been able to survive for five years after the diagnosis of metastasis. The patients with prostate cancer who I met nine years ago when we were initially diagnosed did not believe in the importance of diet and laughed at me when I began making changes. Unfortunately, they have all since died. I still eat the same diet today, and it has stimulated my physical and mental performance, allowing me (at 75 years of age) to expand the company I run.

How the Mind Helps You Heal

There aren't many topics that are as hotly debated as the importance of the mind in the occurrence and treatment of cancer. The fact is that there is no scientific evidence that psychological factors encourage or even trigger the formation of tumor cells. But while there's no proof from studies, there is a definite connection between the development of tumors and the mind. After all, the latter has a remarkable influence on the immune system.

If the immune system is sufficiently strong, it will locate and destroy tumor cells, which are constantly developing in the body. If the immune system is weak, the rate of new mutant cell formation will gradually become higher than the rate of destruction, and a tumor will develop. Emotional factors — such as fear, stress, helplessness and social isolation — suppress the immune system, weakening its ability to fight this constant onslaught.

When you are relaxed and unstressed, and feel safe and happy in your circle of family and friends, you strengthen your immune system. Seen from this point of view, a stable psyche can contribute significantly toward building good health.

DID YOU KNOW?

Relearning Old Habits

Humans are optimally adapted to alternating phases of stress and relaxation. We've simply unlearned how to deal with stress and instead remain tense for too long. Try, therefore, to actively address stressful situations, then consciously relax when they are done.

What Does Relaxing Mean to You?

Relaxing doesn't always mean doing nothing. Quite the opposite! If you lounge around on the couch for hours, you'll feel tired, not relaxed. Moderate activity that focuses on something specific is the best way to switch off stress. Some people relax best while gardening, others when they go for a long walk, still others when they piece together a jigsaw puzzle.

There are many structured relaxation techniques, too, such as autogenic training (see page 120), progressive muscle relaxation (see page 120) and qigong (see page 122). All these activities have you focus on something else, liberating the mind from the negative thoughts that revolve around cancer, and get you back in touch with life. Fill your leisure hours with as many of these positive activities as you can. They will improve your well-being and mental balance, and you'll find the strength and courage to face your illness.

A Stressful Diagnosis

A cancer diagnosis can throw even the strongest personalities off track. There's hardly any other news that will affect your mind as seriously as the fact that a malicious growth has taken root in your body. Cancer causes fear — in everyone.

The ways in which people deal with the diagnosis, however, vary greatly. Some will ask themselves what they did wrong, or ask why they had to be the ones to get cancer. Others will blame themselves for the disease because they always did what they were supposed to do, always wanted to please everyone and always just swallowed everything anyone said to them. But there is no point in pondering, in blaming yourself or in wasting your energy analyzing the past. The key is to think only of the future.

New Hope

The new findings about the importance of fermentation in cancer cells, presented for the first time in this book, are meant to encourage you — and to demonstrate ways that you can actively fight your cancer. It is difficult to defeat fermenting cancer cells with just the established therapies. However, when you combine them with a change in diet, regular physical activity and techniques that strengthen the mind, you can create synergies that significantly increase your chances of beating cancer.

The findings in this book will help you understand how the enemy in your body works and how you can fight it. They will enable you to take effective countermeasures. The most important thing: do not slide into a passive, fearful role. Cancer is not a fate that you have to blindly accept. On the contrary, with the right nutrition and a conscious lifestyle, you can actively engage in the battle.

Learning to Control Stress

One very important aspect of treatment is keeping your immune system active, or reactivating it if it is weak. And stress can cause it harm.

Don't forget how important it is to your health to alternate periods of tension and relaxation. In the long term, you can perform at your peak only if you give your body time to regenerate after it has been stressed. This doesn't mean avoiding stress at all costs or relaxing all the time. Quite the contrary! Learning to cope with unavoidable stress is the key. Plus, some types of stress can also have a positive effect: the term *eustress*, which literally means "good stress," promotes efficiency and improves concentration.

Stress Can Help You Survive

Our bodies' reaction to fear and stress still works the same way as it did for our prehistoric ancestors. In order to react optimally to a life-threatening situation, the body responds with a number of metabolic processes. For example, when a Neanderthal man stood facing a saber-toothed tiger, the situation triggered stress signals that prepared him for an immediate fight-or-flight reaction (see box, below). In the subsequent fight or during the flight, his pent-up stress hormones and the released sugars were broken down. If the hunter survived, the life-threatening situation was followed by a phase of relaxation and regeneration. Used-up reserves were replenished, wounds healed and the hunter recovered.

For most of human development, this emergency program worked beautifully. It is only in our modern, hectic times that problems have emerged. Many people today are in a state of permanent stress — due to noise, overcrowding, financial worries, pressures at work, media overload and much more — with all its negative consequences for their metabolism, immune system, physical regeneration and mental health. And this is all because they can no longer sufficiently work off their stress hormones through physical activity.

What Happens During Fight or Flight?

When the body prepares for fight or flight, it increases the release of hormones, which crucially influence blood circulation and blood sugar metabolism. Glucose is released, which raises the blood sugar level. The heart, skeletal muscles and lungs are optimally supplied with nutrients and oxygen, while the outer blood vessels and inner organs are narrowed and cut off from the energy supply. With this adaptation, the body is perfectly prepared for the upcoming, strenuous muscle activity it anticipates.

But Stress Also Encourages Cancer

If no physical activity follows a stressful situation, the stress hormones and sugar that have been released break down very slowly. In addition, restricted blood flow reduces the body's supply of oxygen. All this promotes fermentation in cancer cells.

It is particularly important for patients with cancer to break down stress hormones and sugar through exercise. They must also improve tissue oxygenation with the help of enhanced respiration (ideally, in the fresh air). This helps cancer cells switch back to combustion from fermentation. Moreover, relaxing periods of rest activate self-healing and the body's own regenerative powers.

The Pillars of a Strong Mind

- Eating a balanced, low-carbohydrate cancer-fighting diet
- Getting physical activity in the fresh air at least three times a week for about 30 minutes at a time
- Enjoying a healthy emotional balance, alternating between periods of stress and periods of relaxation
- Getting sufficient regenerative sleep
- Maintaining a positive attitude toward life
- Actively participating in the healing process

Promoting the Powers of Self-Healing

O. Carl Simonton, an American oncologist and radiology specialist, is considered to be the pioneer of psycho-oncology (see opposite). For more than 30 years, he has successfully supported patients with cancer, and strengthened their self-healing powers, markedly improving their quality of life.

Of particular note in his process is visualization, a method of imagining and finding a person's inner source of strength. The patient works out goals that affirm that life is worth living. The technique can develop self-healing resources and reduce chronic stress. As patients realize that they can influence the conditions of their lives — and, accordingly, no longer feel helpless — their stress levels decrease. The feeling of mastery over the situation can even help reduce the need for painkillers and shorten postoperative recovery periods.

Activity Helps

Three things you can do right away to help your treatment are to get active, accept your situation and stop fighting your fate. Staying active in your leisure time and getting sufficient exercise will bring mental harmony and increase your will to live and enjoy life.

Endorphins, hormones that make you feel good, are released during physical activity. They act like little bursts of happiness, boosting your mood. At the same time, stress hormones, such as cortisol and adrenaline, are reduced by exercise, which strengthens your immune system. Physical activity, in combination with a low-carbohydrate diet, also promotes the formation of ketone bodies (see page 43), which inhibit anxiety-triggering mechanisms in the brain. And, as you've learned, a protective lactic acid shield forms around cancer cells; but these lifestyle changes interrupt that, allowing the immune system and conventional cancer therapies to work on the once-resistant cells.

Strengthening Your Mind

Besides exercise, there is a whole range of measures you can employ to boost your mental and physical well-being at the same time. Psycho-oncology, or psychosocial oncology, deals with the mental side effects of cancer, and working with practitioners in this field can positively influence your mood. Complementary therapies — such as homeopathy, acupuncture, reflexology, aromatherapy and sound therapy — can also help you achieve physical and mental balance.

No single method works for every person. Every patient has to discover what does work for him- or herself. The best idea is to try something new and make a decision based on your gut feeling; rely on your intuition. Your body will give you clear signals about what feels right.

Psycho-Oncology: Professional Support During Treatment

Psycho-oncology, or psychosocial oncology, is a fairly new branch of psychotherapy. It deals with the connections between cancer and its psychological consequences for the patient. As early as the 1970s, scientists began searching for factors that might contribute to the formation of tumor cells in introverted "cancer personalities." They soon found that

DID YOU KNOW?

Homeopathic Remedies

Homeopathic remedies are not · administered in their full-strength form but rather diluted. This process is called potentiation. Remedies are usually given in the form of milk sugar beads called globules. Although one might assume that dilution would weaken the medicine's efficacy, the exact opposite happens: the power, or potency, of the remedy is increased.

DID YOU KNOW?

One Size Doesn't Fit All

For optimal homeopathic results, a practitioner should perform a diagnostic assessment and take a detailed medical history before treatment. Each homeopathic remedy must be individually adapted to the patient, his or her complaints, and his or her physical and mental condition.

psychological problems do not directly cause the formation of tumor cells. However, they discovered that long-term stressful situations, such as the death of a close relative or job loss, can inhibit and damage the immune system to such a degree that existing tumor cells can multiply more easily, and turn into cancer cells and cancerous growths.

The Mind-Body Connection

The close interaction between the brain and the immune system makes it clear that positive mental reinforcement directly builds and strengthens immunity. And this provides powerful support in the fight against cancer. Think positive — even if it is hard to do some days.

It's vital to make use of all the resources available to you to regain inner balance and free yourself from the vicious circle of fear and immune system suppression. Don't be afraid to ask a psychologist for support. Psycho-oncologists are specially trained to help patients resolve past stressful events. They can also teach you strategies to actively deal with any ongoing challenges.

Complementary Healing Methods

Western, or conventional, medicine is very much focused on the body. Disease is considered to be a measurable change in bodily function, caused by one or more breakdowns in normal physical, chemical or biological mechanisms. And these changes do need to be addressed to ensure healing.

Since the middle of the 20th century, however, growing numbers of complementary therapies have become increasingly important tools for treatment. For example, homeopathy, phytotherapy, aromatherapy and traditional Chinese medicine are used to care for not only the body but also the emotions, to encourage healing. A bonus: many of the methods mentioned on the following pages are largely free from side effects.

Homeopathy

The gentle healing method of homeopathy comes from the teachings of Samuel Hahnemann (1755–1843), a German doctor and chemist. Following the Latin principle of "Similia similibus curentur" ("Like cures like"), Hahnemann asserted that a substance that causes the symptoms of disease in a healthy person may also be able to heal that person if he or she actually develops this particular disease.

Plant-Based Cancer Remedies

The following are just some of the plant remedies used in cancer treatment.

Compound	Effect
Mistletoe extract (see box, page 116)	Stimulates the immune system
Fermented wheat germ extract	Acts as an anti-inflammatory, antimetastatic and antioxidant agent; stimulates the immune system
Fermented hot-water extract of rice hemicellulose B	Stimulates natural killer cells, and cytotoxic T-cells and B-cells
Indian incense	Fights cancer cell proliferation in glioblastoma (the most common malignant brain tumor in adults)
Willow bark extract	Inhibits angiogenesis around tumors
Medicinal mushroom extracts	Stimulate the immune system

Homeopathy does not differentiate between physical, general and mental symptoms. Instead, a practitioner always takes all three into account when making a diagnosis and selecting a suitable remedy. Once the right remedy has been found, improvement usually occurs very quickly. Physical symptoms subside, and general well-being and energy increase. In the mental area, too, an impact is perceptible — patients are, for example, less frightened and find new courage. As an accompaniment to cancer therapy, homeopathy can be used to regulate the immune system and psychological balance.

Phytotherapy: Healing with Plants

Phytotherapy, or herbal medicine, prevents and treats diseases using a variety of plants, plant parts and preparations made from these. Some of these natural healing substances are used to make cancer treatments, as well; for example, a class of chemotherapy drugs called taxanes are derived from a type of yew. They have a strong growth-inhibiting effect. However, like some other herbal ingredients, paclitaxel (one of the taxanes) is highly toxic to not only cancer cells but also healthy cells.

DID YOU KNOW?

Future Therapies
Anti-TKTL1 agents are in clinical development but are not currently approved for use. Scientists are testing an altered form of vitamin B1 (thiamine), which appears to inhibit the TKTL1 metabolism in cancer cells, thereby increasing the efficacy of radiation and chemotherapy. For more on treatment options, see page 122.

Caution: Mistletoe Preparations

Among the best-known plant remedies used in cancer treatment are mistletoe preparations. In addition to other benefits, they modulate or stimulate the immune system.

In contrast with naturally increasing immune system performance through exercise and diet, artificially increasing it using immunostimulating preparations can have a downside. Sometimes these remedies can activate cells (called suppressor cells, regulatory T-cells or Tregs) that suppress immune response. Serious stress or physical exertion can also trigger immune suppression. So if, during a period of overload — called an "open window" in sports medicine — you use immunostimulatory agents, they may further suppress and weaken the immune system.

To prevent this, always have your doctor do an immune status blood test before starting immunostimulatory therapies. This will tell you whether these compounds will boost or suppress your body's defenses. If you get the all clear from your doctor, mistletoe preparations are well suited to promote immune system function.

Essential Oils for Cancer Treatment

The scent of aromatic oils can help lift patients with cancer out of a low mood, or even relieve pain gently and effectively. Below are some essential oils to try for different effects. Make sure you buy organic oils; look for them at health food stores and pharmacies. They may be a little more expensive, but they are pure and effective. Cheaper scents are often synthetic and have no therapeutic effect.

Effect	Essential Oils
Stimulating	Bergamot, geranium, jasmine, cardamom, orange and tea tree
Mood lifting	Mandarin, lemon balm and orange
Analgesic (especially for headaches)	Chamomile, lavender, peppermint and rosewood
Calming	Chamomile, lavender, patchouli and rosewood
Relaxing	Clary sage, black spruce, fir, ylang-ylang and cedar

Try a Sound and Breathing Exercise

Sit comfortably on a chair or a cushion on the floor. If you can, cross your legs or move into the lotus position. Close your eyes and breathe calmly and evenly for a while. Then, take a deep breath. As you breathe out, loudly and powerfully say, "Om." Hold the tone as long as you can, then inhale deeply through your nose. Repeat the exercise three times.

The calming sound of the "Om" puts your upper body into a soothing vibration, which is extremely relaxing. In addition, you will unconsciously be "forced" to exhale long and hard. This helps the body dispose of metabolic toxins and regenerate more easily. The deep inhalations improve blood oxygenation and strengthen you in your fight against cancer.

The aim of phytotherapy is to identify herbal substances that inhibit the growth of cancer cells without adversely affecting healthy cells at the same time. Studies have been able to identify a variety of plant constituents that function this way, especially the phytochemicals resveratrol, quercetin and salvestrols (see page 105).

Aromatherapy

Aromatherapy is a special branch of herbal medicine. You may think the use of carefully dosed aromas is just a spa treatment with pleasant psychological effects, but the origins of this effective therapy date back to Ancient Egypt. Modern, international research studies have confirmed, time and time again, that essential oils not only create feelings of well-being, but also have measurable therapeutic effects on body and soul when compared with pharmaceuticals. Experts today regard aromatherapy as a safe, reliable form of natural complementary medicine.

Essential oils influence our sense of smell, awakening pleasant memories and feelings via the limbic system, which is the seat of our emotions. Essential oils also undergo various metabolic reactions in the body. The scents can have a calming, relaxing or stimulating effect, but they can also bring about medical outcomes. Because the inhaled vapors pass via the nasal mucosa into the bloodstream, they move, via the blood, directly to various organs and the central nervous system, where they have their full therapeutic effect.

DID YOU KNOW?

Aromatherapy Applications

Aromatherapy treatments are administered in a variety of ways. Oils and essences can be absorbed directly through the skin — for example, in an aroma oil massage or an aroma oil bath. (Stir the essential oil into a little cream or jojoba oil before adding it to warm bathwater.) They may also be taken orally via a steamy inhalation.

Music or Sound Therapy

Music therapy is considered one of the oldest treatment methods in holistic medicine. Tiny vibrations transmitted through echoes work like a kind of micro-massage for the entire body, which can lead to deep relaxation, stress reduction and activation of lymphatic flow. Toxins are, thereby, flushed out more quickly, which promotes healing. Current research in the field of psychoneuroimmunology also confirms that high sound frequencies stimulate the cerebral cortex and the limbic system. They also increase the release of the body's own pain-inhibiting substances.

Singing can also improve health. It strengthens the muscles in the respiratory system; this can be extremely beneficial to patients with lung cancer. As you sing, your improved oxygen uptake helps boost the immune system. Last but not least — and this may go without saying — singing instantly improves your mood.

Acupuncture

Like the other holistic methods already mentioned, traditional Chinese medicine also considers humans in their entirety. It is an important complement to Western, technology-based

DID YOU KNOW?

Instruments for Music Therapy

A variety of musical instruments, including gongs, singing bowls, rain sticks, drums, chimes and monochord instruments, are used to improve mental, physical and spiritual health. The process usually involves passively listening to music and sensing its vibrations. Singing bowls are sometimes placed on the skin to transmit the vibrations directly to the body. The sound waves help your body swing back into natural harmony.

How Does Acupuncture Work?

Acupuncture involves puncturing the skin at precisely defined points with tiny, sterile needles. The treatment affects neurotransmitters, which bring pain relief.

Around 400 points are known, distributed along the meridians in the body; meridians are channels through which qi, or life energy, flows. Qi is composed of yin and yang; as long as these two forces are in balance, a person is healthy. When the relationship is out of kilter — for example, if a blockage prevents the qi from flowing — or there is a chronic imbalance, the person gets ill.

Acupuncture points are linked to specific organs; stimulating a point with a needle balances the qi flow in and around that organ. Because meridians run through the whole body, acupuncture points that are far removed from the site of pain may play an important role in its treatment. Often, the entire functional circuit must be energetically stabilized for the treatment to be successful.

Acupuncture offers proven, successful, side effect–free pain management for patients with cancer. And now, in addition to the traditional method of acupuncture, which calls for needles, there is a newer method, which uses pain-free laser impulses and, therefore, makes treatments much more comfortable for pain-sensitive patients.

Do Your Own Reflexology Treatment

The following foot massage helps combat stress, and you can do it just about anywhere. An important note: take your time, and spend about five minutes performing each step.

1. **Gently Activate the Spinal Zone.** Massage the area that runs in a gentle S-shaped curve along the inside edge of the foot. This curve starts at the first joint of the big toe, runs through the metatarsophalangeal joint (just below the big toe) to the navicular bone (just in front of the ankle) and about 1 inch (2.5 cm) below the ankle up to the Achilles tendon.

2. **Massage the Solar Plexus Point.** Using your thumb and making small circles, rub the area in the center of the sole of your foot, directly below the ball. Increase the pressure as you inhale, and decrease it when you exhale.

3. **Activate the Lymph Zones of the Pelvic and Abdominal Cavities.** Grasp the middle of the lower leg with both hands and stroke toward the heel without applying pressure. Then push both hands toward the tip of the foot; as you do so, your index and middle fingers will slide along above the ankle, your ring fingers and pinkies below. To finish, gently stroke your foot.

medicine. The best-known and most widely recognized therapeutic method in traditional Chinese medicine today is acupuncture. Scientific studies have repeatedly proven its effectiveness, and conventional medicine recognizes its benefits. Many health benefit programs actually pay for acupuncture treatments these days.

Reflexology

The selective activation of certain reflex points on the foot increases general well-being. It also has a balancing, and even a healing, effect on individual organs and body parts.

So how does it work? Therapists have found that specific areas on the sole of the foot have solid connections (called reflex paths) that run to other regions of the body. When a specific reflex zone is massaged, energy flow is stimulated and blockages are removed.

Unfortunately, attempts to scientifically prove the effectiveness of reflexology have failed so far. Anecdotally, however, it is known that the gentle touch of a therapist during the massage, and the subsequent soothing relaxation that occurs, represent a very significant benefit in the healing process.

DID YOU KNOW?

Specific Points Help Specific Problems
Acupuncture points on the ear have been found to be especially effective against cancer pain. Stimulation of a point called P6, which is located on the inside of the forearm, helps decrease nausea and vomiting during chemotherapy. And stimulation of a point called LV2, which is located between the big toe and the second toe, is a soothing, side effect–free treatment for insomnia and headaches.

Active Relaxation

There are a number of relaxation techniques that you can use on your own after instruction by an experienced teacher. Using them, you can take a break whenever you want or need to.

If you have trouble falling asleep or sleeping through the night, try doing a short relaxation program in the evening. Do a few yoga poses, 15 minutes of qigong (see page 122) or progressive muscle relaxation (see below) before going to bed. You'll fall into a restful, deep slumber without needing sleeping pills.

Autogenic Training

This relaxation technique not only helps combat stress and sleeping problems, but also tackles fear, restlessness and depression. It was developed by Johannes Heinrich Schultz (1884–1970), a German physician, in the years between the First and Second World Wars. The underlying principle is quite simple: the more you focus on the weight and warmth of your relaxing body, the more external stimuli lose importance. As a result, you feel calm and relaxed. Incorporating special, individual formulas into your exercises can help you address specific personal problems.

Autogenic training is a proven strategy for pain management, so it is valuable in the case of cancer. Patients can focus their thoughts on a self-selected point to make the pain — like other external stimuli — recede into the background. Plus, relaxing the muscles lowers the patient's degree of alertness. This information is transferred to specific brain regions, in which, it is assumed, lie the sites of pain perception, pain awareness and pain processing. There, the sensation and localization of the pain is diffused. The result is that, while the patient can still feel the pain, it no longer hurts as much.

Progressive Muscle Relaxation

Progressive muscle relaxation (PMR) is another relaxation technique, created by physician Dr. Edmund Jacobson in the early 20th century. During PMR, each individual muscle group of the body is first deliberately tensed, then completely relaxed.

As you learn to focus on each feeling, you'll become increasingly sensitive to the degree of tension you carry in your muscles. With regular practice, you'll soon be in a position to detect and release tense muscles using brief contractions. Pros in this technique can react immediately to critical situations when tension builds, and can even prevent the harmful tensing of muscles from the start.

PMR is so effective that more and more community colleges and public health agencies offer courses in the technique. If you prefer to learn and practice on your own, there are some excellent books and interactive CDs that will help you learn the process.

Try a PMR Routine

Many of us carry muscle tension around all day and get no break from it. This routine will help release those muscles and bring on a feeling of relaxation.

1. Lie down on your bed or an exercise mat. Relax your muscles.

2. Direct your full attention to your right foot. Tense the muscles in that foot, pointing the toes, then lift that foot slightly off the ground. Hold the tension for about five seconds.

3. Curl your right toes up toward your body. Release the tension once more.

4. For about 30 seconds, observe closely the small but important difference between how your right foot and your left foot feel.

5. Now tense the muscles in your lower right leg. Briefly hold the contraction before relaxing.

6. Focus on the relaxed feeling afterward, and compare the difference between the right and left legs.

7. Repeat this exercise using all the muscles in the right half of your body, one group at a time, from the thigh and bottom to the hand and arm to the shoulder, back and neck.

8. Scrunch up your face as if you'd bitten into a lemon, then relax your face.

9. Repeat the same path in reverse, this time down the left side of the body. Start at the neck and move down to the shoulder and back to the arm and hand to the leg and foot. Tense each muscle group firmly, then relax again.

10. To complete the exercise, lie calmly on the bed or mat for a moment. Can you feel the refreshing state of relaxation, right down to your toes?

Your Options: Cancer Therapies

There are many ever-evolving conventional treatments available to fight cancer. Here's an overview of the major categories:

- **Surgery.** Surgical removal of a tumor is still one of the most successful cancer therapies available. If all of the tumor tissue can be removed, you have the best chance for a complete cure. This is why it is vital to identify tumors through screening tests as early as possible. It is also extremely important to have well-controlled, frequent follow-ups to detect recurrences as early as possible. If a tumor cannot be removed completely, or if there is a danger that it has already metastasized, chemotherapy and radiation are available.

- **Chemotherapy.** Chemotherapeutic agents are made from a variety of substances. One important class uses phytonutrients (see page 115) that inhibit and/or stop tumor cell growth; examples are taxanes, made from the yew shrub, and vinorelbine, made from periwinkle. Another class of drugs administers modified building blocks of the cell, such as 5-fluorouracil, which inhibit the growth and division of cancer cells. Metal compounds, such as cisplatin, are also common because they damage DNA and inhibit tumor growth. Some other forms of chemotherapy use altered vitamins; methotrexate, for example, is an altered form of vitamin B9 (folic acid), which inhibits a tumor cell's metabolism and its growth.

- **Radiation.** Another important form of treatment is radiation. During this treatment, free radicals are produced in the cells by high-energy radiation (X-rays) in order to damage and kill cancer cells.

Qigong

Qigong is a traditional form of meditation, concentration and movement developed in Ancient China. It is said to strengthen the body and mind in a holistic way. A technique of traditional Chinese medicine, qigong also increases and harmonizes qi, or the life force, in the body.

Qigong combines breathing, body awareness, movement and concentration exercises. It strengthens the muscles and the mind, and sets countless metabolic reactions in motion. That means it's ideal for rehabilitation after major surgery, for conditioning prior to returning to exercise after a long absence and for overweight people. After just one training session, you'll start to feel the energy that the exercises release within the body.

How Does the Cancer-Fighting Diet Help Other Therapies?

Studies have demonstrated that resistance to chemotherapy drugs (for example, paclitaxel and cisplatin) and radiation is based on a cancer cell's switch to the sugar fermentation metabolism. The discovery of the TKTL1 metabolism explains why this resistance happens, and gives us the tools to fight it. By following the cancer-fighting diet, you'll make your conventional treatments more effective, and you'll be able to tolerate them more easily.

By adhering to a strict ketogenic diet for three days before beginning chemo or radiation, you can force TKTL1-positive cells to go into sugar withdrawal and switch their metabolisms back to normal combustion. This restarts the mitochondria, which makes cancer cells susceptible to free radicals and vulnerable to processes that encourage programmed cell death (apoptosis). The result: cancer cells that are once more sensitive to radiation and chemotherapy, and, thus, can be killed more easily.

Studies show that inhibition of the TKTL1 metabolism, which can also be achieved by fasting, lowers the risk of cancer recurrence and metastasis formation by up to 75%. Fasting, however, can be hazardous for patients with cancer, especially in the advanced stages of the disease, when they may already be struggling with malnutrition, weight loss and emaciation (cachexia).

For this reason, specialist organizations (such as the German Society for Nutritional Medicine) recommend that the diets of patients with cancer include more fats and proteins. Furthermore, a sufficiently high proportion of omega-3 fatty acids and natural vitamin E in the form of gamma- and delta-tocotrienol should be ingested to combat the inflammatory processes that often occur during cachexia. Gamma- and delta-tocotrienol also directly inhibit the growth of cancer cells, and eliminate them by triggering cell death. At the same time, they protect healthy tissue from radiation damage.

In clinical settings, these new findings are being put into practice. There now exist liquid supplements (called sip feeds) that are rich in fat and protein; contain sufficient omega-3 fatty acids and anti-inflammatory gamma- and delta-tocotrienol; are sugar free and low in carbohydrates; and ensure an optimal supply of vitamins, minerals and trace elements. They are ideal for generating a ketogenic metabolism, and increasing the effectiveness of radiation and chemotherapy. Ketogenic sip feeds can easily be taken in place of meals during a hospital stay, or to enrich the ketogenic metabolism.

After successful cancer therapy, it is sensible to maintain the changes you've made by following the cancer-fighting diet, in order to prevent recurrence of the disease. This includes keeping your blood sugar level steady through moderate consumption of low-GI sugars and carbohydrates (see page 158), healthy fats and oils (see page 161) and phytochemicals (see page 105). The only thing you don't have to compromise on is taste, as you'll see in the recipe section that starts on page 168.

Exercise Helps Cancer Treatment

Not that long ago, bed rest and quiet were recommended for patients with cancer. Today, we know better. Moderate to intense activity not only helps prevent cancer, but is also useful once the disease has occurred. A series of studies have proven the hypothesis that consistent exercise is one of the most effective means of fighting cancer. When patients exercise regularly, the death rates for some of the most common types of cancer, such as colon and breast cancer, may be reduced by up to 40%. That's why getting active is an ideal complement to conventional cancer treatments.

Of course, sports cannot — and should not — replace medical interventions for cancer. But they are an ideal way to support such interventions. If you get active, you can, in a manner of speaking, simply run away from your disease. Take advantage of the good feeling you get from taking a major part of your recovery into your own hands.

Exercise: More Effective than Some Drugs

The benefits of regular activity and exercise in the fight against cancer are still massively underestimated, just like the role of diet. Yet our bodies are veritable power machines and extremely versatile ones at that. Whereas animals mostly focus on a single type of movement, humans can perform a whole series of highly complex sequences. Thanks to our flexibility, we can adapt to a variety of external conditions: humans can run, climb, jump and much more. In prehistoric days, this brought us an immense advantage in the daily struggle to survive.

As a consequence of this ability to adapt to nearly all environmental conditions, we have also (seemingly) adapted to our modern, civilized and comfortable lifestyle. We are almost at a complete standstill. Over millions of years, our ancestors were constantly on the move and had to work hard physically to survive. Accordingly, their energy consumption was very high. Today, however, we hardly move at all, but

Hormones: How Do They Work?

Hormones trigger a variety of reactions in the cells and organs. They are responsible for many important metabolic processes in the body.

- **Insulin.** This is the main metabolic hormone. It provides cells with nutrients and disposes of excess nutrients (sugars and fats) by storing them in fatty tissue. Like growth hormone (see below), insulin has an anabolic, or building, effect; this is why it is also referred to as the "fattening hormone."

- **Adrenaline.** Also known as epinephrine, adrenaline is the antagonist of insulin. It gives the signal that tells the body to open sugar stores in the cells and release glucose. If too much adrenaline circulates in the body (such as in times of stress), it will weaken the immune system. The best way to break down surplus adrenaline is to exercise regularly and intensely.

- **Growth Hormone.** Also known by its abbreviation, GH, this is an important hormone for reproduction, growth and regeneration. Enhanced insulin secretion caused by elevated blood sugar levels reduces production and distribution of healthy growth hormone. In this way, insulin acts as GH's opponent and weakens the body's regenerative processes.

- **Melatonin.** This hormone makes the body feel tired and eases it into sleep. It also protects against damage by free radicals, activates major regeneration processes, strengthens the immune system and protects against cancer. Melatonin is formed only when you are exposed to darkness; that's why you should always sleep in a darkened room.

every day we still consume plenty of energy in the form of carbohydrates and fats. No wonder, then, that an imbalance has arisen, which can lead to illness over the long term. It's time to help your body regain its balance between energy intake and energy use.

Adrenaline Protects Against Cancer

For our ancestors, movement revolved mostly around fighting, fleeing and searching for food. To make rapid, sudden use of glycogen-based energy reserves in fight-or-flight situations, the body releases the hormone adrenaline, the antagonist of insulin. Adrenaline ensures that the glycogen stores in the cells (especially in the liver) break down quickly.

A large amount of glucose, the body's "turbo fuel," is released in the process, which ensures that the muscles are supplied with sufficient energy to fight or flee. Without an adrenaline rush, stored glucose cannot be broken down. If this spike in glucose is not used up through activity, it remains available for fermentation, promoting the growth of cancer cells.

Because our muscles aren't being used to escape or fight like our ancestors' were, our bodies do not use up the excess glucose that floods our systems when we're under stress. Intense exercise is the solution to this problem. Performing just three 30-minute sessions of aerobic exercise per week cuts your cancer risk in half. For patients who have already undergone cancer surgery, chemotherapy or radiation, 45 minutes of aerobic activity a day are recommended to stimulate the metabolism and empty the glucose stores.

Runner's High

Movement represents a loss of energy for the body. When you run, before your body taps its energy reserves, it tries to dissuade you from wasting them: your legs begin to feel heavy, breathing becomes difficult and your muscles start to burn. If this doesn't work, the body changes strategy and releases adrenaline, which signals "flight." The results? Your glycogen stores open up and release glucose. The blood vessels that supply the organs and muscles needed for fight or flight expand, while those that feed the digestive tract contract. The outer blood vessels in the skin also narrow to prevent blood loss in case of injury.

In the brain, adrenaline also triggers emotions that motivate you to push yourself to the limit. The consequences are evident: your legs seem to run of their own accord, and you feel euphoric and carefree. In runners, this mechanism is known as runner's high. When it happens, you feel like you're running weightlessly.

DID YOU KNOW?

Adrenaline's Other Functions

In addition to facilitating energy procurement, adrenaline has another role in fight-or-flight situations. It causes the peripheral, or outer, blood vessels to narrow, which minimizes blood loss in the case of an injury. Simultaneously, adrenaline expands the inner blood vessels, so that enough oxygen and glucose can enter the muscles.

Target Heart Rate

To train effectively, you first need to know your maximum heart rate. As a general rule, this is

- For women: 226 minus your age

- For men: 220 minus your age

Beginners work out initially at 60% to 70% of their maximum heart rate; when they are more advanced, they will increase to 65% to 75% of their maximum heart rate. If you suffer from another medical condition or want to know more about your heart health, consult your doctor or a sports medicine specialist before you start training. He or she can offer advice and determine your status using a stress test.

The only way to attain this moment of happiness is to exercise in the aerobic zone, where you're breathing heavily and your heart is pumping toward the higher end of your capacity (see box, opposite). This gives your body sufficient oxygen to burn up the glucose in your bloodstream, then draw extra energy from your fat stores.

Sports Stimulate the Mind, Too

Sure, regular exercise gives you immediate physical results, but it also has a positive effect on the mind. During aerobic exercise especially, a large number of endorphins, the body's happiness hormones, are released.

Social contact also plays a major role in mental wellness. Patients with cancer frequently suffer from social isolation, as friends turn away in confusion over what to say or do. Some patients also initially feel alienated from their own bodies, which they now have to share with a malicious "roommate." Alone, they have to face difficult questions: am I allowed to exercise? Should I take it easy and save my strength?

Once you get active, you'll notice a rapid improvement in your mood. You'll gain self-confidence, and, most of all, you'll feel in control of your situation. Many self-help groups offer exercise programs. Go — and use the opportunity to speak with other patients about your fears and joins forces with them to fight cancer.

DID YOU KNOW?

Movement Activates the Mitochondria

Intense physical activity releases more than just adrenaline. Oxygen is the basis for combustion in the mitochondria (see page 26), so the right sort of exercise will also boost the activity of these tiny cellular power plants, making life difficult for cancer cells.

Getting Started with Exercise

Through moderate aerobic exercise, you can effectively strengthen your body and improve your health. Start by setting a tough but measurable challenge for yourself. A muscle can grow only if it works hard, whether it's your biceps or your heart.

Systematic Training

Endurance training increases your overall vitality — provided you exercise regularly and systematically. Do not go right up to your limits, but rather pay close attention to your body. Make sure it is supplied with sufficient oxygen while you exercise in the aerobic zone, so that your muscles can get their energy by burning both glucose and fat.

The easiest way to determine the intensity of your activity is to wear a heart-rate monitor; it will check your heart rate continuously and accurately while you exercise, and you can increase or decrease your exercise intensity according to the readout. In a pinch, you can also use the less-precise "talk test": as long as you can talk and breathe without difficulty while exercising, you are in the aerobic zone. If you are out of breath and can no longer talk fluently, the intensity is too great and you should shift down a gear.

Exercise is even more effective if you combine endurance training with moderate weight training or a gentle stretching program once a week. Gradually increase the intensity, so you don't overdo it. Perform each exercise slowly and with your full concentration.

Should You Exercise Immediately After Cancer Treatment?

Recent studies directed by Dr. Freerk Baumann at German Sport University in Cologne, Germany, confirm that it is sensible and healthy to begin light workouts while still in the hospital after cancer treatment. The old assumption that this is dangerous has been refuted by these studies. It's prudent to initially avoid sports that use jerky, uncontrolled movements, such as raquet sports or soccer, so that healing can take place without complications. Suitable sports for patients with cancer are

- Water therapy, water aerobics and swimming (only after wounds have healed)
- Cycling
- Walking, Nordic walking and jogging
- Cross-country skiing
- Inline skating (though there can be a higher risk of injury associated with this activity)
- Dancing
- Working out on an elliptical trainer

Get Moving, Without Joining a Health Club

Many people want to move more, but are reluctant to sign up at a gym or sports club. Here are some simple ways to get moving without doing that:

- Pick up the newspaper each morning, by bike or on foot, instead of having it delivered.

- Avoid escalators and elevators as often as possible, and walk or climb stairs instead.

- Spend time moving in the fresh air for at least one hour a day, whatever the weather. The UV exposure from the sun will stimulate your vitamin D production, free of charge (see page 95).

- Arrange to meet friends for a walk instead of inviting them for coffee. You can have just as inspiring a conversation, and you'll also be spending time outside.

When Exercise Isn't a Good Idea

If you are suffering from certain physical problems, it is better not to do any exercise until you have healed. Rest and avoid exercise if you are suffering from severe pain or have a fever, which can be a sign of infection. Likewise, skip training if your blood platelets (thrombocytes) are below 10,000 as a result of chemotherapy. If your platelets are below 20,000, you should train only under medical supervision.

Pick Yourself Up

Exercise is an essential part of our biology; all our bodily processes are adapted to it. But in modern life, our bodies are more and more at rest. To return to a life where you are in harmony with your body, you have to break through the vicious cycle of lethargy and poor nutrition. With each activity session, you'll feel a little healthier and happier.

Sports and exercise are not much different from diet: most people think of them only in terms of staying slim. But they are worth so much more to your health. A nice figure and tight skin are merely the external, although highly motivating, signs of the positive changes that exercise makes to your body on the molecular and biochemical levels.

Make a Gentle Introduction

If you are physically restricted and should not (yet) engage in sports, moderate exercise on a mini-trampoline or using a special vibrating exercise device will help prevent muscle wasting. You can also use either apparatus to gently but effectively prepare your body for the resumption of sporting activities.

The mechanical vibration and shaking motion created by a vibrating exercise device produces 25 to 50 muscle contractions per second in the body. You can use it while standing or lying down, so it can get the muscles working without much moving around. On a mini-trampoline, you determine the pace of your movements. Keep it slow, and don't worry about jumping high, as you would on a normal

10 Reasons Why Patients with Cancer Should Exercise

1. You will enhance the efficiency of your body's immune system.

2. You will actively reduce your stress-induced adrenaline level and empty glucose stores.

3. You will improve microcirculation in the spine, the intervertebral discs and the bones, counteracting back pain and osteoporosis.

4. You will activate your metabolism and speed up the removal of metabolic waste materials.

5. You will improve your coordination, reducing the risk of falls.

6. Your pancreas will secrete insulin in a more constant way, and your cells will increase the formation of insulin receptors.

7. Your blood vessels will become more elastic, and will adjust better as a result. You will also grow more red blood cells, ensuring increased oxygen transport.

8. Your brain will enjoy better blood circulation, increasing the growth of new nerve cells and keeping you feeling young. At the same time, your nerve cells will release more endorphins, the body's happiness hormones, which improve mood.

9. You will improve your stamina and strengthen your cardiovascular system. Your heart will beat more regularly and strongly. Your blood pressure will also remain constant, because your heart can powerfully pump oxygen into even the smallest capillaries.

10. Your lung volume will expand, a benefit of the utmost importance for health, especially in patients with lung cancer.

trampoline. Simply stand on the surface, and slowly start to bob to train your muscles in a gentle way. You'll improve your balance at the same time.

Have a Checkup Before You Start

Even if you meet all the health criteria for exercise, it's best to have a thorough medical exam before you begin any exercise program. This is true for everyone over 35 years of age, and is particularly important for patients with cancer.

Get checked regularly, paying special attention to your heart. You can have appropriate fitness and function tests done as part of a routine physical with your family doctor, or you can make an appointment with a sports medicine specialist. The exam should include a blood pressure check; a resting and an exercise electrocardiogram (ECG or EKG); and a thorough ultrasound examination of the heart muscle, heart valves, coronary arteries and neck arteries.

Off You Go!

According to the results of a 2009 Nestlé dietary study on the topic of healthy lifestyles, the majority of people surveyed said they would like to exercise more. However, in practice, people rarely do. The reasons they usually give are lack of time and motivation.

To make sure this won't happen to you and that you're full of vim and vigor, check out the box opposite. The reasons presented there should help chase your inner couch potato off its warm, cozy seat. Remember: the joy of activity is innate in every human being. Sometimes you just have to find it again. The best part is that once you start down your new path, you'll feel so good you'll want to stay active.

The Right Exercise for Your Cancer

If you saw an orthopedic surgeon about your back pain, you'd probably be very surprised if all he or she recommended were warmth and rest. You would probably argue, and rightly so, that this treatment, as pleasant and helpful as it may be, did not seem particularly well targeted to solve the problem.

It's exactly the same with exercise and cancer. We take for granted that any kind of movement is an improvement over total immobility. And while that's true, there are certain

DID YOU KNOW?

Exercise for People with Chronic Pain

If you suffer from musculoskeletal problems, such as back or joint pain, you should also consult an orthopedic surgeon about any restrictions. In most cases, he or she will still recommend moderate exercise, such as walking, hiking or cycling. Continuous rest and relaxation are never the right solution.

The Best Motivational Tips

- **Start Slowly.** Integrate small activity units into your everyday life, such as walking to the bookstore or cycling to work.

- **Train with a Good Friend.** If there are two of you, it's easier to get motivated — and more difficult to find an excuse if you don't feel like going.

- **Make It a Fixed Date.** Schedule exercise in your appointment book. Don't put off training; it is important and should not be cancelled.

- **Set Realistic Goals.** If you start jogging, don't set your sights on the New York City Marathon right away (though, in the long term, you can probably achieve this goal). There are few age restrictions on these races; at the Berlin Marathon, for example, more runners in their 70s cross the finish line every year.

- **Reward Yourself.** Celebrate the small victories by treating yourself to new exercise gear, booking a spa appointment or making room for a leisurely day of pampering at home.

- **Enjoy Your New Diet.** When you are physically active, eating healthily is much easier. After an exercise session in the fresh air, you will automatically prefer fruit over a burger.

- **Enjoy Feeling Good.** Exercise has a balancing and stimulating effect, immediately improving your mood. You will feel like a new person in your body.

exercises that will help you improve your particular situation in a more targeted way. On the following pages, you'll find out which types of activity offer the greatest success in treating the three most frequent types of cancer: colon, breast and lung cancer. If yours is not on this list, pay close attention to your individual needs, and speak with your doctor about effective training strategies for your situation.

Colon Cancer

Because the abdomen is opened during surgery, patients with colon cancer undergo a major medical intervention. In some cases, patients must be fitted with a colostomy bag to remove waste. The stoma, or the opening into the intestines, that the bag fits over presents an obstacle and restricts patients' ability to exercise.

The most important things are to avoid heavy lifting and intense physical work. Due to the possibility of infection and/or injury to the wounds, dangers lurk in everyday life. Gardening and carrying heavy boxes are taboo. Once the interior surgical wounds have healed, there's nothing to stop you from pursuing your favorite sports, especially if you don't have a colostomy. You can increase the intensity of your exercises if you do so gradually.

Activities for Patients with Colon Cancer

Moderate aerobic activities, such as cycling, swimming, walking and Nordic walking (see box, page 134), are particularly suitable. Because they require trunk rotation and involve uncoordinated, sudden stopping movements, tennis, golf and other ball-centered games are not recommended.

An elliptical cross-trainer machine is excellent for strengthening your cardiovascular system and muscles without straining your spine or joints. Another advantage of this machine is that you can train at home or in a fitness studio, and you can stop at any point to visit the toilet. This aspect of colon cancer recovery can play a major role in outdoor sports. Many patients suffer from diarrhea or frequent bowel movements, so making sure there is a toilet nearby helps relieve stress. Drinking plenty of water, evenly spaced throughout the day, is a particularly important thing that all patients with colon cancer should do.

In addition to aerobic exercise, you should carefully strengthen your abdominal and back muscles. Before beginning a program, have your overall fitness and strength checked by a sports medicine expert, a physiotherapist or a qualified fitness professional to find out what and how much you can do. He or she will provide you with a personal training plan that's right for you. Start gently and avoid stretching the healing tissue too much. Avoid all jerky, pulling movements so that there is no strain on the scars. Slowly increase intervals and weights, and control your breathing: exhale while tensing muscles, and inhale as you relax.

DID YOU KNOW?

Patients with Colon Cancer Can Enjoy Swimming
If you like to swim, you can! Just empty your colostomy bag right before you get into the water. If you don't want to encourage unwanted curiosity from others, you can buy a special belt that will cover the area. Women can easily conceal their abdominal area with a shirred swimsuit.

Breast Cancer

There is some very good news. Women who have had breast cancer surgery that removed only the so-called guardian lymph nodes can resume almost any type of exercise immediately after a complication-free recovery. Getting fit helps many women quickly feel healthy and attractive again.

In the hospital, you can actively speed up healing. Special physiotherapy can help prevent the occurrence of lymphedema, a condition that often occurs after breast cancer surgery. Physiotherapy can also rapidly heal existing edema.

With increased muscle work, the lymph channels are pressed so that lymph flows more easily (this is called the lymphatic pump) and swelling disappears.

Activities for Patients with Breast Cancer

Self-help groups for patients with breast cancer are often especially well organized. Get in touch with a group; almost all of them offer exercise-focused activities. When you work out with other people who understand your situation, you'll soon start to feel stronger.

In principle, the following applies generally to all patients with breast cancer. Avoid all uncoordinated and quick movements. Instead, choose exercises that can be done in a flowing, controlled manner, and make sure to include arm movements in your training (see box, below). Ideal sports are swimming, cross-country skiing, Nordic walking and regular walking. If you are in great shape, you can also go jogging.

Swimming is excellent because water automatically prevents any jerky movements and provides plenty of resistance for an effective workout. In addition, it lightly massages tissues, promoting lymph flow. One important note: make sure you swim in water that is between 75°F and 86°F (24°C and 30°C); anything warmer can strain your circulation.

Almost as important as endurance sports in breast cancer treatment are flowing relaxation methods, such as yoga, qigong and tai chi. They improve body awareness and inner balance, and give you back the self-confidence and feeling of physical well-being that many patients lose after diagnosis and therapy.

Arm Movements Are a Must

When exercising after recovering from breast cancer surgery, always allow your arms to swing far back and forth. This helps you achieve optimal upper body rotation, which is transmitted to other muscles. If you go Nordic walking immediately after healing, use your poles more gently than usual. Let your arms swing loosely to prevent any lymphedema from worsening.

Pay special attention to your handwork: when you swing your arm back, open your fist; when you swing it forward, close your fist. This way, you'll activate the lymphatic pump even more. Once you've healed well, you can start walking as energetically as you did before surgery. To apply pressure to the muscles and activate the lymphatic pump, stretch your hands upward several times a day, energetically opening and closing your fists several times.

Lung Cancer

The majority of patients with lung cancer are or were heavy smokers, and most did little or no exercise before their illness. For this patient group, activity is especially important to strengthen the respiratory muscles and rebuild lung function. While these aspects improve, patients will also improve their general physical condition and well-being.

Activities for Patients with Lung Cancer

For these patients, even gentle endurance sports, such as Nordic walking or cycling, will likely be difficult at first, especially if part of the lung has been removed. Slow, gentle training can, however, quickly improve physical fitness. Start by setting small goals, because even a little progress is a big step on the way back to good health. Initially, cover only short distances, then rest up properly after exertion.

Once your surgical wounds have completely healed, swimming is excellent for building endurance and strong core muscles. Until you're ready for this, cautiously do moderate weight training to strengthen the entire upper body, back and abdominal muscles. Strong core muscles will help you sit and stand more easily, and breathe more freely.

For safety's sake, start your exercise program under the guidance of an experienced physiotherapist. He or she can show you how to restore flexibility to scar tissue using special stretching exercises; this can help loosen even the smallest adhesions, and improve the blood supply to those tissues. This speeds up healing, so you'll be able to breathe better and participate in everyday life. Once you learn the movements, you can continue to perform them on your own at home.

A qualified physiotherapist can also teach you special breathing techniques that will facilitate respiration and make your lung muscles strong. This improves both physical well-being and mental health, which can positively influence the healing process.

DID YOU KNOW?

Fresh Air Is Important
For patients with lung cancer, getting exercise in the fresh air is especially important, because it helps strengthen the lungs and improve breathing.

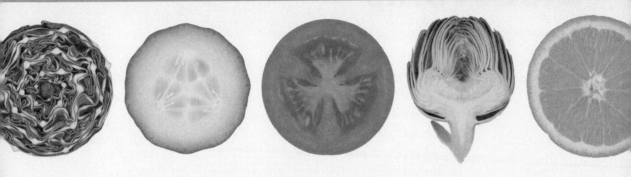

PART 3

The Healthy Cancer-Fighting Kitchen

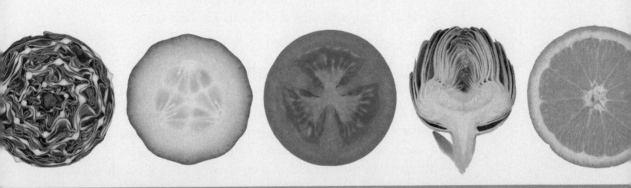

How the Cancer-Fighting Diet Works

A typical Western daily menu might look a little like this: an English muffin, fruit-on-the-bottom yogurt and some cereal for breakfast; a simple sandwich made with your favorite bread, lean cold cuts and a slice of cheese for lunch; a serving of spaghetti and some veggies for dinner; and a few snacks of sweet, juicy fresh fruit in between. Sounds like a healthy, balanced diet that provides a reasonable number of calories and amount of energy, right? But it deserves a closer look.

Today, "healthy," slim people are developing cancer at an early age — simply because they are feeding their bodies too many carbohydrates, and too few nutritious oils and fats. To be fair, we have been told for decades that carbohydrates are healthy and that fat is unhealthy. But it's actually sugar and starch, two forms of carbohydrates, that are making us ill.

It doesn't have to be like that, though. It's actually easy to revamp your eating patterns, and combine the pleasure of eating with healthy nutrition. The diet outlined in this book is the practical response to what has only recently been understood: the fermentation metabolism in cancer cells (see page 29). The discovery of the TKTL1 enzyme and the process of glucose breakdown connected with it have revealed entirely new connections between diet and various illnesses, especially cancer. And they have enabled everyone to take a new, more effective approach to fighting cancer: combining a rigorous change in diet with physical activity to enhance traditional medical treatments, such as chemotherapy and radiation.

Eat Yourself Healthy

First off, the cancer-fighting diet is not actually a diet. It is a consistent, nutritious eating plan that will help you maintain a healthy body and mind, and protect you from lifestyle diseases. For patients with cancer, it ensures that the body is supplied with energy that will give maximum advantage to healthy cells while inhibiting the growth and proliferation of cancer cells. By following this plan, you can ensure you have adequate energy and counter the risk of cachexia (emaciation), which can weaken you dangerously (see box, at right).

The Basics

The cancer-fighting diet contains large amounts of protein, fat and dietary fiber, and very small amounts of carbohydrates. When you eat this way, your blood sugar level should not increase significantly after meals, and insulin secretion should be minimal.

The quality of the ingredients you choose is important. Opt as often as possible for organic products, which are not contaminated with pesticides, herbicides, chemicals, radioactive compounds, antibiotics or heavy metals. Also avoid ready-made foods whenever possible, because important biologically active compounds are often destroyed during manufacturing and packaging. (The health-enhancing effects of phytochemicals, in particular, play an extremely important role in the cancer-fighting diet, so choose fresh whole foods whenever possible.) When selecting meat and dairy products, animal welfare and species-appropriate feeding are also of great importance, since these have a direct impact on the biological value of the food (see page 85).

Limits Aren't a Disadvantage

You can easily do without prepared foods and sugary candies if necessary. But you might wonder how your daily diet will work without bread, potatoes, pasta and rice. After all, your body still needs some carbohydrates. Recent studies have determined that the key for patients with cancer — and anyone looking to prevent cancer in the first place — is to avoid starchy foods that lead to a diet that's extremely high in sugar.

Changing your diet is not as hard as you might think. You can still enjoy food and benefit from reducing your carbohydrate intake. There are still plenty of delicious ingredients to choose from, and some newly developed products that deliver the low-carb, high-protein calories you need. Even a moderate change in your diet — including eating healthy sugars with a low GI, such as galactose, isomaltulose, tagatose and trehalose — can help you fight cancer. And along the way, you will also be protecting yourself from other lifestyle diseases, such as diabetes, heart disease and Alzheimer's disease. Plus, you'll more easily control your weight, which always feels good.

How to Build Your Cancer-Fighting Diet

- **Lay the Foundation.** The first step toward better health is to turn off the sugar supply. Slash your carbohydrate intake to the bone: eat no more than 1 g of carbohydrates per 2.2 lbs (1 kg) of body weight each day (for a 132-lb/60 kg person, this is 60 g carbohydrates per day). Make sure to spread your carb intake throughout the day to avoid blood sugar spikes, which feed cancer cells.

- **Add Pillar 1: The Right Fats.** Supplying your body with sufficient, good-quality fat is almost as important as reducing your sugar intake. You can add fats by making and consuming your own special oil mixture (see page 161). You need to eat 1/8 tsp (0.5 mL) of the special oil mixture per 2.2 lbs (1 kg) of body weight each day (for a 132-lb/60 kg person, that's just 2 tbsp/30 mL per day). By doing this, you will avoid blood sugar spikes and stimulate combustion in the mitochondria. At the same time, you'll inhibit inflammation, which can weaken the immune system.

- **Add Pillar 2: Protein, Fiber and Phytochemicals.** High-quality protein gives the body energy and essential amino acids without triggering a sharp rise in blood sugar. Dietary fiber also prevents blood sugar spikes, so substituting specific whole-grain flours and protein-rich fiber powder (see page 155) for white flour in baking and cooking is an important component of the cancer-fighting diet. Low-carbohydrate vegetables, fruits, nuts, oily seeds and whole-grain flours are not only rich in vitamins and minerals, but also contain many phytochemicals that are important for maintaining body functions and inhibiting cancer cell growth. Substitute these foods for the carbohydrates you're eliminating.

- **Add Pillar 3: Gentle Deacidification.** To counteract the over-acidification of the body that arises from cancer cells' increased lactic acid production, you should regularly eat deacidifying foods. In particular, you should consume plenty of lactic acid–fermented foods, such as buttermilk, cheese, yogurt, sauerkraut and lactate drinks (see page 162). These are all very low in sugar, and cancer cells cannot use the lactic acid in them for fermentation or energy release. You can also deacidify with the help of citrate; for example, you can take a magnesium citrate supplement (see box, page 93).

The Structure of the Cancer-Fighting Diet

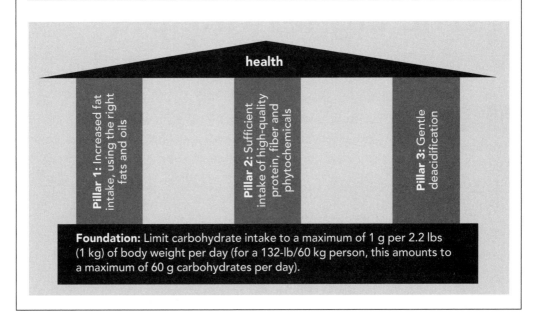

health

Pillar 1: Increased fat intake, using the right fats and oils

Pillar 2: Sufficient intake of high-quality protein, fiber and phytochemicals

Pillar 3: Gentle deacidification

Foundation: Limit carbohydrate intake to a maximum of 1 g per 2.2 lbs (1 kg) of body weight per day (for a 132-lb/60 kg person, this amounts to a maximum of 60 g carbohydrates per day).

Vitamins Are Key, Too

Simply by restricting your intake of sugar- and starch-rich foods, which are usually nutrient poor, you will be eating a diet much richer in vitamins and minerals. If you consult your doctor and find out you have a specific deficiency, you can add an appropriate dietary supplement. But be careful: excessive doses of vitamin supplements can sometimes have the opposite of the desired effect. For example, too much vitamin A taken in the form of supplements leads to an increased rate of lung cancer in smokers.

As well, vitamin C, which is a type of fermentable sugar, can weaken the effectiveness of chemotherapy — if you take a daily supplement that contains more than 1,000 mg. On the other hand, very high doses of vitamin C given intravenously seem to be beneficial to the health of patients with cancer (see box, page 97).

Eat According to the Traffic Light Principle

The tables on the following pages show how different foods will affect your blood sugar level. Following the traffic light principle will help you avoid heavy-duty carbohydrates from the start, and customize your diet so that it works for you (and tastes great). The foods are identified by the colors of a traffic light: green means "go"; yellow means "proceed with caution"; and red means "stop."

- **Green-Light Foods.** You can safely consume normal-size portions of these foods and drinks because they will not (or will hardly) raise your blood sugar. In the recipes starting on page 168, you can substitute any green-light food for another (assuming it will taste good with the other ingredients!).
- **Yellow-Light Foods.** The foods and drinks on this list are healthy, but should be eaten only in limited amounts on the cancer-fighting diet. They are relatively higher in sugar than Green-Light Foods.
- **Red-Light Foods.** These are the foods and drinks that you should avoid or consume only in minute quantities on the cancer-fighting diet. The prepared foods on this list (such as bread and pasta) are the "traditional" recipes, which contain ingredients that raise blood sugar quickly and steeply (such as table sugar or all-purpose wheat flour). Today, there are many different types of bread, pasta, pizza, cakes, chocolate and even ice cream that will raise your blood sugar level slightly or not at all.

Become a Label Reader

Carefully study the detailed information on food and drink packaging before you buy. Use the traffic light lists and the information on these pages to help you decide whether a food is a good bet. If you decide to have a snack from the Red-Light Foods list, you'll be able to see at a glance how many carbohydrates it contains, whether low-GI sugars are used in it and how much you can eat without exceeding your carb quota for the day.

Decoding Nutrition Labels

So what do all those terms on packages mean? And how do you figure out what's good and what's not? Here are some hints to help you decode food labels. Keep in mind that different countries have different laws governing labeling. Check your local regulations so you know what you're getting:

- **Ingredients.** These are always listed in the order of relative weight. So, for example, if sucrose (table sugar) is second or third on the ingredient list, the product is very sugary.

- **Carbohydrates.** Included in this number are a number of different types of carbs, including polysaccharides (such as starch), oligosaccharides, monosaccharides and disaccharides. Other substances may also affect the calculation of this number. The proportion of carbohydrates is usually determined after subtracting protein, fat, fiber, ash and water content.

- **Sugar.** This number indicates the quantity of monosaccharides and disaccharides, such as glucose and sucrose, in the food. Check the ingredient list to see whether healthy, low-GI sugars were used.

- **"No Added Sugar."** No monosaccharides, disaccharides or other sugary sweetening ingredients, such as maple syrup or honey, were added to these foods. If the ingredients that go into the product contain natural sugars (which is often the case), this may be indicated on the label with the words "Contains naturally occurring sugars." Not all manufacturers add this label, though.

- **"Lower in Sugar" or "Reduced Sugar."** Foods that are marked with this statement must contain 25% less sugar than the normal version. They must contain at least 5 g less sugar in the standard reference amount (usually 3.5 oz/100 g).

- **"Sugar-Free."** This claim can be placed only on food that contains less than 0.5 g of sugar per serving of the standard reference amount.

Green-Light Foods

The following foods are best suited to the cancer-fighting diet; you can eat these to your heart's content, and fill yourself up in a healthy way. Use them in recipes, or eat them as snacks between meals.

Fruits

- Lemons

Leafy Greens

- Arugula
- Belgian endive
- Cress
- Curly endive (chicory)
- Dandelion greens
- Lettuce (such as Batavia, green or red leaf, iceberg, lollo rosso, oakleaf and romaine)
- Mâche (lamb's lettuce)
- Mesclun mix
- Purslane
- Radicchio (regular and Treviso)
- Sorrel
- Spinach
- Watercress

Mushrooms

- Birch boletes (orange and regular)
- Cèpes (porcini)
- Chanterelle
- Hen of the woods
- Ling zhi (reishi)
- Morel (dried and fresh)
- Oyster
- Portobello
- Saffron milk cap
- Shiitake
- Slippery Jack
- Truffles (dried and fresh)

Other Vegetables

- Artichokes
- Asparagus
- Avocados
- Bamboo shoots
- Bean sprouts
- Beans, green
- Bell peppers (any color)
- Bok choy
- Broccoli
- Brussels sprouts
- Cabbage (such as Chinese, green, pointed, red, savoy and white)
- Cauliflower
- Celeriac
- Celery
- Chard (such as rainbow and Swiss)
- Cucumbers
- Eggplants
- Garlic
- Jerusalem artichokes
- Kale (such as curly and dinosaur)
- Kohlrabi
- Lactic acid–fermented vegetables (such as beets and sauerkraut)
- Leeks
- Lotus roots, fresh
- Nettles
- Okra
- Olives
- Onions (such as cooking, green and Spanish)
- Parsnips
- Radishes (such as daikon and red)
- Ramps
- Romanesco
- Salsify
- Seaweed
- Sprouts (such as alfalfa; avoid chickpea and soy sprouts)
- Tomatoes
- Turnips
- Zucchini

Herbs and Spices

- Basil
- Borage
- Capers
- Caraway seeds
- Chervil
- Chile peppers
- Chives
- Cilantro
- Cumin
- Curry powder
- Dill
- Galangal
- Garden cress
- Hyssop
- Lemon balm
- Lovage
- Marjoram
- Nutmeg
- Oregano
- Paprika
- Parsley
- Pepper, ground (black and white)
- Peppercorns (green and black)
- Peppermint
- Rosemary
- Sage
- Salad burnet
- Savory
- Tarragon
- Thyme
- Turmeric

Meats

- Beef (filet mignon, ground, loin, prime rib roasts, stewing cubes and tenderloin)
- Charcuterie (such as bacon, bresaola, ham, prosciutto, salamis and speck)[1]
- Lamb (chops, fillet, legs, loin, medallions and tenderloin)
- Liver pâté (such as liverwurst)[1]
- Offal (such as bone marrow, brains, kidneys, liver, lungs, oxtails and tongue)
- Pork (belly, chops, cutlets, fatback, fillet, ground, knuckles, loin, neck and stewing cubes)
- Rabbit
- Sausages (such as bratwursts, frankfurters, Polish sausages and veal sausages)[1]
- Veal (breasts, cutlets, fillet, leg and stewing cubes)

Poultry

- Chicken (breasts, legs, poussin, thighs and whole)
- Duck
- Goose
- Turkey (breasts and legs)

Game

- Antelope (such as chamois)
- Buffalo (bison and water buffalo)
- Hare
- Ostrich
- Partridge
- Pheasant
- Pigeon
- Quail
- Venison
- Wild boar

[1] Organic, if possible; containing no added sugar or nitrites

Fish

- Anchovies
- Bream
- Carp
- Catfish
- Caviar and other fish roe
- Cod
- Eel, freshwater
- Eel, smoked saltwater[2]
- Flounder
- Haddock (fresh and smoked)
- Hake
- Halibut
- Herring (fresh, kippered, pickled and salted)[2]
- Mackerel (fresh and smoked)[2]
- Perch
- Pike
- Plaice
- Red mullet
- Redfish (ocean perch)
- Salmon (fresh wild, and smoked)[2]
- Sardines (canned and packed in oil, and fresh)[2]
- Sole (such as Dover and lemon)
- Sprat[2]
- Surimi (imitation crabmeat)
- Swordfish (dorado)
- Trout (such as brown and speckled river)
- Tuna[2]
- Turbot
- Whitefish

Seafood

- Crab (canned and fresh)
- Crayfish
- Langoustines (Dublin bay prawns or Norway lobsters)
- Lobster
- Mussels
- Oysters
- Scallops
- Shrimp
- Squid (fresh)

Dairy Products and Eggs

- Buttermilk, regular
- Cream, whipping (35%)
- Crème fraîche
- Eggs, chicken
- Sour cream

Cheeses[3]

- Appenzeller
- Blue cheeses (such as Bavarian Blue, Bleu d'Auvergne, Bleu de Bresse, Gorgonzola and Roquefort)
- Brie
- Camembert
- Cottage cheese
- Cream cheese
- Danbo
- Edam
- Emmental
- Feta
- Fresh cheeses (such as fromage frais, paneer and quark)
- Goat cheese
- Gouda
- Gruyère
- Limburger
- Mascarpone
- Mozzarella
- Parmesan
- Provolone
- Raclette
- Ricotta
- Sheep cheeses
- Swiss cheeses (such as Tête de Moine)
- Tilsit

Fats and Oils

- Almond oil
- Avocado oil
- Butter (clarified, ghee and organic)
- Canola oil[2]
- Coconut oil
- Drippings, beef
- Flaxseed oil[2]
- Goose fat
- Grapeseed oil
- Hemp seed oil[2]
- Lard
- Margarine (nonhydrogenated)
- Olive oil
- Palm oil
- Peanut oil
- Pomegranate seed oil
- Pumpkin seed oil
- Sesame oil
- Walnut oil

Sweeteners

- Stevia (see page 77)

Thickeners

- Agar-agar
- Gelatin
- Guar gum
- Locust bean gum (carob bean gum)

Drinks

- Chicory coffee
- Coffee, unsweetened (brewed and espresso)
- Lemon juice
- Tea, unsweetened (black and green)
- Water (mineral and tap)

Miscellaneous

- Broth cubes and granules (beef, chicken and vegetable)
- Flax seeds and flaxseed flour
- Mustard, hot
- Sambal oelek
- Soy sauce (watch out for sugar content)
- Tofu
- Vinegar (all types)
- Worcestershire sauce

[2] High in omega-3 fatty acids

[3] Do not consume cheese rinds, especially if the cheese is made from unpasteurized milk. Avoid blue cheeses, such as Roquefort, if your immune system is impaired, because they increase the risk of infection.

Yellow-Light Foods

You may enjoy these foods without feeling guilty, but in limited quantities. Make sure that the foods you choose are unsweetened and not highly processed. Each of the very exact portions below contains 5 g of carbohydrates; an accurate digital kitchen scale is a terrific tool for measuring these foods, especially very small amounts.

Fruits

- Apples (1.4 oz/40 g)
- Apricots (1.9 oz/55 g)
- Bananas (1.4 oz/40 g)
- Black currants (1.75 oz/50 g)
- Blackberries (2.8 oz/80 g)
- Blueberries, cultivated (0.9 oz/25 g)
- Blueberries, wild (1.9 oz/55 g)
- Cherimoyas (1.4 oz/40 g)
- Cherries, sour (1.75 oz/50 g)
- Cherries, wild (1.4 oz/40 g)
- Cranberries (2.8 oz/80 g)
- Elderberries (2.6 oz/75 g)[1]
- Figs, fresh (1.4 oz/40 g)
- Gooseberries (2.1 oz/60 g)
- Grapefruits (2.1 oz/60 g)
- Guava (2.6 oz/75 g)
- Kiwifruits (1.6 oz/45 g)
- Kumquats (1.2 oz/35 g)
- Limes (9.7 oz/275 g)
- Lychees (1 oz/30 g)
- Mandarin oranges (1.6 oz/45 g)
- Mangos (1.2 oz/35 g)
- Melons, honeydew (2.8 oz/80 g)
- Nectarines (1.4 oz/40 g)
- Oranges (1.75 oz/50 g)
- Papayas (7 oz/200 g)
- Passion fruit (1.4 oz/40 g)
- Peaches (1.9 oz/55 g)
- Pears (1.4 oz/40 g)
- Persimmons (1 oz/30 g)
- Plums (1.6 oz/45 g)
- Pomegranates (1 oz/30 g)
- Pomelos (1 oz/30 g)
- Prickly pears (2.5 oz/70 g)
- Quinces (2.5 oz/70 g)
- Raspberries (3.2 oz/90 g)
- Red currants (2.3 oz/65 g)
- Rhubarb (12.3 oz/350 g)
- Rose hips (1 oz/30 g)
- Star fruit (5 oz/143 g)
- Strawberries, cultivated (2.8 oz/80 g)
- Strawberries, wild (3.2 oz/90 g)
- Watermelons (2.1 oz/60 g)
- White currants (1.9 oz/55 g)

Vegetables and Legumes

- Beets, cooked (3 oz/85 g)
- Carrots, raw (3 oz/85 g)
- Chickpeas, cooked (0.4 oz/12 g)
- Hearts of palm, canned (4.2 oz/120 g)
- Lentils, cooked (1 oz/30 g)
- Pickled gherkins, sour (14.1 oz/400 g)
- Potatoes, waxy pan-fried (1.2 oz/35 g)
- Pumpkins (3.5 oz/100 g)

Grains and Flours[2]

- Almond flour (2.5 oz/70 g)[3]
- Amaranth, whole raw (0.31 oz/9 g)[3]
- Barley, pot (0.28 oz/8 g)
- Buckwheat flour (0.25 oz/7 g)[3]
- Coconut flour (0.8 oz/23 g)[3]
- Einkorn flour (0.31 oz/9 g)
- Emmer flour (0.31 oz/9 g)
- Grapeseed flour (1 oz/30 g)[3]
- Millet (0.28 oz/8 g)[3]
- Oat bran flour, low-carb (0.4 oz/12 g)
- Oats, rolled (0.28 oz/8 g)
- Pumpkin seed flour (1.2 oz/35 g)[3]
- Quinoa (0.28 oz/8 g)[3]
- Rye flour (0.28 oz/8 g)
- Spelt flour (0.28 oz/8 g)

[1] Do not eat raw
[2] For reference; use full quantities given in recipes

Nuts and Seeds

- Almonds (4.2 oz/120 g)
- Brazil nuts (4.9 oz/140 g)
- Chestnuts, cooked (0.5 oz/14 g)
- Coconut, fresh (3.5 oz/100 g)
- Coconut, shredded dried unsweetened (2.8 oz/80 g)
- Hazelnuts (1.6 oz/45 g)
- Hemp seeds, shelled (2.3 oz/65 g)
- Macadamia nuts (1.2 oz/35 g)
- Peanuts (1.75 oz/50 g)
- Pecans (3.9 oz/110 g)
- Pine nuts (2.1 oz/60 g)
- Pistachios (1 oz/30 g)
- Poppy seeds (4.2 oz/120 g)
- Pumpkin seeds (1.2 oz/35 g)
- Sesame seeds (1.75 oz/50 g)
- Sunflower seeds, shelled (1.4 oz/40 g)
- Walnuts (1.6 oz/45 g)

Dairy Products

- Ayran ($\frac{2}{3}$ cup/150 mL)
- Buttermilk, full-fat ($\frac{1}{2}$ cup/125 mL)
- Kefir ($\frac{1}{2}$ cup/125 mL)
- Milk, 1% or 2% (7 tbsp/100 mL)
- Milk, raw unpasteurized (7 tbsp/100 mL)
- Milk, skim (6 tbsp/90 mL)
- Milk, whole (7 tbsp/100 mL)
- Whey (7 tbsp + 2 tsp/110 mL)
- Yogurt, plain unsweetened ($\frac{1}{2}$ cup/125 mL)

Sweeteners[4]

- Agave syrup (1 tsp/5 mL)
- Fructose, powdered (1 tsp/5 mL)
- Maple syrup (1 tsp/5 mL)

Beverages, Nonalcoholic[5]

- Beer, alcohol-free ($\frac{2}{3}$ cup/150 mL)
- Berry juice from berries on Yellow-Light Foods list, unsweetened (scant 1 cup to 1$\frac{2}{3}$ cups/200 to 400 mL)
- Café au lait, unsweetened (7 tbsp/100 mL)
- Cappuccino, unsweetened (7 tbsp/100 mL)
- Coffee, brewed unsweetened with milk (7 tbsp/100 mL)
- Red wine, dry alcohol-free (scant 1 cup to 1$\frac{2}{3}$ cups/200 to 400 mL)
- Soy milk, unsweetened ($\frac{2}{3}$ cup/150 mL)
- Sparkling wine, brut alcohol-free (scant 1 cup/200 mL)
- Vegetable juice from vegetables on Green-Light Foods list, unsweetened (scant 1 cup/200 mL)
- Vegetable juice from vegetables on Yellow-Light Foods list, unsweetened (7 tbsp/100 mL)
- White wine, dry alcohol-free (scant 1 cup to 1$\frac{2}{3}$ cups/200 to 400 mL)

[3] Naturally gluten free

[4] You may also enjoy low-GI sugars in limited quantities. Your body will use only 30% of the energy in tagatose, so you can consume about three times more than other healthy sugars. Other good options are galactose (a protective sugar for the brain and neurons that cannot be used by cancer cells), trehalose (a sugar that slowly and steadily releases glucose during digestion) and isomaltulose (a sugar that slowly and steadily releases glucose and fructose during digestion). For more information, see pages 158 and 159.

[5] You can also enjoy in limited quantities any beverages made with low-GI sugars.

Beverages, Alcoholic

- Beer, Pilsner and wheat (2/3 cup/150 mL)
- Beer, reduced calorie and light (2 cups/500 mL)
- Champagne, brut (scant 1 cup/200 mL)
- Cider, hard (scant 1 cup/200 mL)
- Red wine, dry (scant 1 cup to 1 2/3 cups/200 to 400 mL)
- Rosé wine, dry (scant 1 cup to 1 2/3 cups/200 to 400 mL)
- Sherry, dry (scant 1 cup/200 mL)
- Sparkling wine, brut (scant 1 cup/200 mL)
- White wine, dry (scant 1 cup to 1 2/3 cups/200 to 400 mL)
- White wine spritzer, dry sour (1 2/3 cups/400 mL)

Miscellaneous[6]

- Amaranth, puffed (0.31 oz/9 g)
- Gingerroot (1.6 oz/45 g)[7]
- Peanut butter, natural unsweetened (1.75 oz/50 g)
- Peanut butter, sweetened (1 oz/30 g)
- Tahini (1.75 oz/50 g)

[6] You can also eat in limited quantities chocolate made with low-GI sugars.
[7] An effective remedy for nausea during chemotherapy

Red-Light Foods

Red means "stop," so these are the foods you should avoid completely (or consume only in minute quantities, very infrequently) when you're following the cancer-fighting diet. They contain too many carbohydrates.

Fruits

- Banana chips
- Dried fruit (such as apple rings, apricots, dates, figs, prunes and raisins)
- Grapes

Vegetables

- Corn, fresh
- Kidney beans, red and white
- Peas

Potatoes

- Potato dishes (such as dumplings, gnocchi, pancakes and soup)
- Potato starch
- Potatoes, baked
- Potatoes, boiled (peeled and unpeeled)
- Potatoes, deep-fried
- Potatoes, mashed and puréed

Nuts

- Cashews
- Mixed nuts (may contain cashews)
- Trail mix (contains dried fruit)

Grains and Cereals

- Barley, pearl
- Bread crumbs
- Bulgur
- Cereals, cold, ready-to-eat (such as corn flakes, muesli, multigrain cereals and puffed wheat)
- Corn, dried (cornmeal)
- Cornstarch
- Couscous
- Polenta
- Semolina
- Wheat berries
- Wheat bran
- Wheat flour (such as cake, high-gluten, white and whole-grain wheat flours)
- Wheat germ
- Wheat starch

Baked Goods[1]

- Breads (such as baguettes, and multigrain, pumpernickel, rye, sourdough, white and whole-grain wheat breads)
- Buns, hamburger and hot dog
- Cakes
- Cookies
- Crackers and crisp breads
- Pitas
- Pizza
- Pretzels
- Rolls (white and whole wheat)
- Tortillas (corn and flour)
- Waffles, ready-made

Pasta and Rice[2]

- Pasta (such as egg noodles, and durum wheat, white and whole-grain pasta)
- Rice (such as basmati, brown, quick-cooking/instant, white and wild)
- Rice noodles
- Rice pudding
- Rice starch
- Spaetzle, ready-made

Dairy Products and Cheese

- Buttermilk, flavored
- Cheese, processed slices
- Quark (flavored and sweetened)
- Sweetened condensed milk
- Yogurt (flavored and sweetened)

Snacks

- Chips (corn and potato)
- Popcorn
- Pretzels
- Puffed rice
- Rice crackers

Sweeteners

- Dextrose (glucose)
- Fructose syrup
- Honey
- Invert sugar
- Jam, ready-made fruit
- Jelly, ready-made fruit
- Lactose
- Maltodextrin
- Maltose
- Molasses
- Sugar (such as brown, granulated and table)

[1] Made with "traditional," high-carbohydrate, refined ingredients
[2] You can enjoy high-protein pasta in limited amounts (see page 157).

Beverages, Nonalcoholic

- Barley malt drinks
- Carrot juice
- Coffee, sweetened
- Cola drinks, sweetened
- Fruit juice, undiluted
- Fruit nectar
- Hot chocolate
- Iced coffee and tea, ready-made sweetened
- Lemonade
- Oat drinks
- Rice milk
- Soy milk, sweetened
- Sports drinks (isotonic drinks), sweetened
- Tea, sweetened
- Vitamin-infused water, sweetened

Beverages, Alcoholic

- Beer (such as beer mixed with lemonade or flavorings, and dark or strong wheat beer)
- Bitters
- Liqueurs (herbal liqueurs are better than sweet liqueurs)
- Malt beverages
- Sparkling wine, sweet
- Spirits (such as gin, schnapps, vodka and whisky)
- Wine (such as dessert, light, mulled, semi-dry and young)

Miscellaneous

- Convenience foods (in general)
- Ketchup
- Mustard, sweetened
- Salad dressing, ready-made sweetened
- Sauces and gravies thickened with flour or starch
- Seitan (wheat protein meat substitute)
- Soups thickened with flour or starch
- Tapioca

Sweets

- Candy
- Chocolate, less than 70% cocoa
- Ice cream
- Pudding

Ingredients: Content Matters

The recipes in this book call for a variety of regular ingredients, and some that are a little different or special. To make the dishes in this book as low in carbohydrates as possible, you'll need to read labels and choose some ingredients that meet specific requirements. Here are some to watch for.

Grains and Grain Products

"Normal" wheat flour (white and whole grain) is harmful, and not recommended in the cancer-fighting diet. The gluten in wheat also triggers strong intolerance reactions in some people (see page 61). But it's easy to replace in recipes, so you won't have to go without your favorite foods.

The ancient grain einkorn contains less starch and more protein than wheat and other grains, such as spelt, oats or rye, so it is a top choice. Flours made from oats, barley and rye are much healthier than wheat flour, too. Ancient grain flours are also highly recommended, and are suitable for making cakes, biscuits, cookies, waffles and pasta, and for using as a partial replacement for potatoes in dumplings.

For low-carbohydrate baking and cooking, the following flours have also proved successful:

- Oat bran flour (with low sugar and starch content)
- Almond flour
- Coconut flour
- Flour made from oily seeds, such as pumpkin seeds and flax seeds (see box, opposite)
- Flour made from fruit seeds and kernels, such as grapeseed and pomegranate seed flour

In some cases, these flours have a strong taste; for example, if you use only coconut flour to make a cake, it will taste like coconut. Mixing different flours, such as oat bran, coconut and almond, with protein-rich fiber powder (see opposite) creates an even, fairly neutral taste. Fiber powder also improves the texture of baked goods by binding together the dough, so it won't crumble. You can supplement low-carb flour mixtures with some relatively starchy flours made from ancient cereals, oats, rye or barley, and make a wide variety of cakes, waffles, pastas and baked goods.

Protein-Rich Fiber Powder

Dietary fiber is widely available in powder form. Initially, it was meant only to supply the fiber necessary to keep the intestines and digestion moving along, and to lower the energy density of foods. But then it was found to reduce or delay rises in blood sugar, because fiber slows down the release of glucose — and it became an ideal supplement for people with diabetes.

This powder contains both protein and dietary fiber from different plant seeds or husks, so it is especially effective at making you feel full (unlike sugar). The fiber it contains reduces the amount of usable energy in it, which means you can eat more of it, and take in fewer calories, at the same time. In addition, protein-rich fiber powder hardly increases blood sugar and insulin levels. As a matter of fact, if you cook or bake with it (or dissolve some of it in berry juice and

What About Flaxseed Flour?

Still largely unknown, flaxseed flour can be made from cakes of pressed flax seeds left over after cold pressing (oil mills sometimes sell these cakes). The pressed cakes are sold whole, so you'll have to grind them at home; an electric coffee grinder is a good tool. Flaxseed meal is particularly high in fiber and saturated with healthy flaxseed oil. Another valuable flour is made from cakes of pressed pumpkin seeds. It contains less fiber than flaxseed flour, but it offers a large amount of valuable protein.

Flours made from these oily pressed seeds are very good for you. They do not absorb the valuable components of other foods, unlike other types of isolated dietary fiber (for example, cellulose). And they will not make you gain weight, despite their rich oil content. In contrast to "normal" sugar- and starch-rich flours, which are truly fattening, they will not raise your blood sugar or insulin levels. Plus, they help keep you feeling full for a long time.

Oily seed flours are best in blends, because they are dark and have a strong flavor. Flour made from oat bran is similarly low in glucose and starch, and is better on its own in baking.

mineral water, and drink it before a meal), your blood sugar and insulin levels will rise more slowly after your meal. At the same time, the high amount of protein it contains supplies the body with valuable amino acids, which are cell building blocks and energy suppliers.

Adding protein-rich dietary fiber powder is good for everyone's diet, but patients with cancer get an extra benefit: the energy it provides does not stoke fermentation in cancer cells, even though it offers a steady energy supply. Use these powders, including plain ground psyllium husks or ground flax seeds, as wheat flour substitutes in baking and cooking. They are terrific for breading meat or fish, and will thicken sauces. Very finely ground (instant dissolving) protein-rich fiber powders have an additional benefit: they can be easily dissolved in beverages and won't make your mouth feel gritty.

Make a Blueberry Fiber Spritzer

Protein-rich fiber powder is good for mixing into drinks, such as fruit juice spritzers. The consistency of the beverage becomes creamier and the taste fuller. Stir 1 tsp (5 mL) of protein-rich dietary fiber powder into a glass of blueberry spritzer (nine parts water mixed with one part pure, unfiltered, unsweetened blueberry juice) and mix well. Refrigerate the drink for 5 minutes or until thickened. Stir again before drinking.

Choosing a Healthy Mix

When you're choosing a high-protein fiber powder, look for one that contains both soluble and insoluble fiber. This ensures healthy intestinal flora will receive a good food supply, which strengthens your immune system and protects you from intestinal inflammation (see page 64).

Today, there are dietary fiber powders that have a good mix of soluble and insoluble fiber, as well as a high proportion of protein. They are excellent for baking; dough enriched with them will bind well even without gluten. It's best to choose a product that contains less than 5% biologically available carbohydrates, such as oat bran, ground flax seeds, ground psyllium husks or pumpkin seed flour. (When using oat bran, make sure that the proportion of usable starch is less than 5%.)

Always cast a critical eye over ingredient lists before buying. (That's a good idea no matter what ingredient you are purchasing.) Many commercially available oat brans contain a large amount of starch, and are not suited to the cancer-fighting diet; like "normal" flour, they will spike blood sugar and insulin levels.

High-Protein Bread

Around the world, bread is one of the top staples in most households. And no matter whether the bread is white, rye or whole wheat, it supplies vast amounts of carbohydrates that boost blood sugar.

Today, there are some newer, special breads that contain less than 20% carbohydrates. They contain more protein (at least 12%) and sufficient dietary fiber (more than 10%), so they still make you feel full. Many include oil seeds, so they are rich in healthy fats, especially omega-3 fatty acids (at least 2%). If you opt for these breads, you won't need to stop eating sandwiches. You can also find high-protein, oil-rich breads that are made entirely from gluten-free grains. This way, you can combine a low-carbohydrate diet with a gluten-free one.

But you still need to be cautious. Read labels or if you're buying artisanal breads, ask your baker. Some high-protein breads still supply large amounts of carbohydrates. If you can't find any low-carbohydrate bread, simply bake your own: there are tasty recipes on pages 205, 206 and 208.

DID YOU KNOW?

Wheat Bran
Never use wheat bran when you're on the cancer-fighting diet. It is extremely rich in gluten, just like wheat flour, and may cause immune or inflammatory responses.

High-Protein Pasta

Pasta can be another option you don't have to give up entirely. Choose varieties that have a minimum protein content of 50% and a maximum carbohydrate content of 20%. Those with a high proportion of dietary fiber are also beneficial; they will fill you up with fewer calories.

Buyer Beware: "No Added Sugar"

Some products are advertised with the promise of "no added sugar" (see box, page 143). This may mean a couple of different things, which you need to keep in mind. Don't let packaging claims lead you astray:

- **In Candy and Chewing Gum:** If the label says "no added sugar," a sugar substitute, such as isomalt, may have been used instead. Isomalt is a sugar alcohol (see page 77), which is broken down slowly; your body uses only about 50% of the energy it contains. Isomalt should, therefore, really be classed as dietary fiber, which helps create a sweet flavor without noticeably raising blood sugar and insulin levels. When consumed in large quantities, however, isomalt can cause bloating and diarrhea. Look for products made with the low-GI sugars tagatose, galactose, trehalose and isomaltulose, which do not cause bloating and diarrhea, especially when you combine them. A mix of these sugars is the best choice.

- **In Products That Contain Starch:** The "no added sugar" label does not guarantee that the product will cause your blood sugar and insulin levels to rise slowly. These products, generally, contain plenty of starch, often in the form of white flour. Remember that white flour will spike your blood sugar faster than granulated sugar will (see page 73).

Pasta made from ancient grain flours is also recommended. These varieties are particularly delicious and healthy when, besides sufficient fiber, they also contain herbs and vegetables. These may be commonly used garden herbs and vegetables, such as basil and tomatoes, but more and more organic and health food stores also sell pasta made with traditional medicinal herbs, which offer additional benefits.

Healthy Sugars and Sugar Substitutes

There are many different healthy sugars and sugar replacements, which act like a form of dietary fiber and are metabolized slowly or not at all by the body. Their names resemble one another, making them hard for the layperson to tell apart. Isomalt is a carbohydrate almost indigestible to humans; it is a type of dietary fiber that is similar to inulin (see page 75) that is broken down by bacteria in the colon. Isomaltulose, on the other hand, is an easily digestible, healthy disaccharide with a low GI (see page 76). Tagatose, trehalose

DID YOU KNOW?

Liquid Sweeteners
Many healthy sugars and sweeteners come in powdered form, but some also come in liquid form, which is better for use in beverages and liquidy dishes.

and galactose are sugars with low-GI values that create a long-lasting energy supply for your body without increasing your blood sugar level.

Dextrose, maltose, maltitol, malt syrup, mannitol, fructose syrup, sorbitol, xylitol: with so many similar names, what are you supposed to do? Buy foods only if you know what type of sugar was added to them and how they affect your body (for a list of synonyms for glucose, see box, page 160).

Isomaltulose and Fructose

As you read on page 76, isomaltulose is a healthy form of sugar that is marketed under the brand name Palatinose. This disaccharide is a particularly suitable dietary choice, because it offers a good compromise between pleasure and health.

Isomaltulose breaks down slowly in the body, ensuring a slow rise in blood sugar. This helps prevent dangerous blood sugar spikes and insulin-induced hypoglycemia. It is a very good alternative to granulated sugar; it has the same baking properties and does not absorb moisture. It has a little less sweetening power, however.

Three Other Healthy Sugars

These sugars are not in wide circulation for consumer use in North America, but some health food and therapeutic-product websites sell them and will ship them to you:

- **Trehalose.** This is an excellent sweetener, because it offers uniform, prolonged glucose release. It also inhibits tooth decay and promotes fat burning. It is relatively new to the market in Europe and North America, so it might be harder to find for consumers.

- **Galactose.** This option is especially good for supplying the brain with the sugar it requires, even in people who experience insulin resistance, which inhibits glucose uptake in the brain. Recent studies have concluded that galactose protects against neuronal damage, and a study from the United States has also shown that it induces fat burning in obese women. Galactose protects teeth, unlike table sugar, which causes decay.

- **Tagatose.** Another very healthy option, tagatose is as sweet as table sugar, but it contains only one-third of the calories. It slows down the uptake of other sugars in a meal, which helps stabilize your blood sugar level and increases fat burning. It also helps remove dental plaque, inhibits tooth decay, and promotes the growth of beneficial, protective bacteria in the colon.

The Names Glucose Hides Under

On package labels, glucose can wear a lot of disguises. Watch carefully for these terms as you read ingredient lists:

- Agave nectar
- Amylopectin
- Amylose
- Apple nectar
- Beet sugar
- Brown sugar
- Cane sugar
- Caramel
- Corn syrup
- Dextrin
- Dextrose

- Fondant
- Glucose syrup
- Granulated sugar
- Honey
- Icing sugar
- Invert sugar syrup
- Isoglucose
- Lactose (milk sugar)
- Malt syrup
- Maltodextrin
- Maltose (malt sugar)

- Maple syrup
- Pear juice concentrate
- Pearl sugar
- Preserving sugar
- Refined sugar
- Starch
- Sucrose
- Table sugar
- Vanilla sugar
- Whole cane sugar

DID YOU KNOW?

Jam and Hidden Sugar

It's best to eat jam that contains at least 55% fruit. Make sure it is sweetened with sugar substitutes or with sugars that have a low GI (see page 158). Organic and health food stores offer a wide range of seemingly healthy fruit spreads, but many are made with agave or apple nectar, which both also contain plenty of fructose and glucose.

Fructose affects the blood sugar level even less than isomaltulose does, but you shouldn't use large amounts of it. Excessive consumption can cause fatty liver disease and can sometimes increase uric acid levels in the blood.

Make Your Own Sweetening Mix

You can combine a number of different healthy sugars that have low-GI values, such as galactose, trehalose, isomaltulose and tagatose (see box, page 159). This combination is particularly good at ensuring that healthy cells maintain their protective sugar metabolism. Trehalose, tagatose, isomaltulose and galactose prevent the rise of insulin and insulin-like growth factor 1 (IGF-1) in the blood, which can be associated with growth signals in cancer cells. They also induce fat burning, prevent tooth decay, and supply a steady, secure source of energy to the brain.

These healthy sugars are a very powerful tool that can help you enjoy a little sweetness in the cancer-fighting diet. If you want, you can add other sweeteners, such as stevia or aspartame, to increase your mix's sweetening power. Don't use them without low-GI sugars, though — your brain will be tricked into thinking you're taking in enough glucose for its needs, but no glucose will be delivered.

Special Oil Mixture

There is no single vegetable oil that covers all the nutritional needs of the human body, so your best bet is to use a combination of oils. Doing so will add nutrients, healthy fats and great flavors to your recipes.

The ideal blend should contain a high proportion of natural vitamin E, with more of the tocotrienol form of the vitamin than the more-familiar tocopherol form. Oils that contain a large amount of gamma-tocotrienol are especially recommended. It should also contain between 20% and 30% omega-3 fatty acids, and the ratio of omega-3 to omega-6 fatty acids should be between 1:1 and 2:1. Including a source of gamma-linolenic acid (GLA) is also desirable, and 20% to 30% of the mixture should consist of medium-chain fatty acids (also known as medium-chain triglycerides, or MCTs). In addition to having a positive effect on blood sugar levels, this blend will inhibit inflammation and activate glucose combustion in the mitochondria.

Sounds complicated, right? It doesn't have to be. Just read oil labels to make sure they contain what you need, and make sure you get a wide variety of them to ensure good nutrition. Blend mixtures according to your taste; for example, start with a mixture of flaxseed, walnut, argan and hemp seed oils, and then add some palm kernel oil and MCT oil (a ready-made blend that contains a high proportion of medium-chain trigylcerides). Use an immersion blender and a tall cup to mix your favorite oils, or simply shake everything vigorously by hand in an airtight jar. To keep the mixture from going rancid, store it inside the fridge, but not in the door, which gets too warm and moves too much when you open and shut it.

Quality Comes at a Price

High-quality cold-pressed vegetable oils are the best choice, but they are expensive. Cold pressing extracts the oil slowly so that the temperature does not exceed 107°F (42°C), because heat damages the beneficial compounds within. Be careful, though: the words *cold pressed* on the label are not absolute proof of quality. They indicate only that no external heat was applied to the oil during manufacturing. Some oil seeds are pressed so fast that they heat up through mechanical compression and friction. Choosing and buying reliable vegetable oils is a matter of trust, so research different brands.

Hemp Seeds

The seeds of the hemp plant, also called hemp nuts, contain about 50% nutritious hemp seed oil, and are excellent sprinkled over salads, muesli or yogurt. They offer essential amino acids and lots of omega-3 fatty acids, so they're a nutritious addition to your diet.

You can eat hemp nuts unshelled; however, the shell cracks when you chew it (that's why many people prefer them shelled). To give hemp nuts a wonderful aroma reminiscent of sesame or sunflower seeds, toast them in a dry nonstick skillet. Walnuts, pumpkin seeds and almonds are similarly rich in oil and protein (see page 149 for a guide to serving sizes). So are flax seeds, which you can eat freely.

Fats for Frying

DID YOU KNOW?

Browned Butter
To make this delicious, simple sauce, simply melt butter in a skillet and cook over medium heat until browned and fragrant. Drizzle it over dishes for a healthy, sophisticated touch.

Cold-pressed vegetable oils should not be heated. They're too valuable, and their health benefits are destroyed by cooking. Use them in cold dishes, such as spreads or salad dressings, or for drizzling over dishes. For frying and deep-frying, coconut oil is the best choice; it does not create any toxic by-products when heated. If you don't like its coconut flavor, butter, lard and beef fat are smart, tasty alternatives. Canola oil and olive oil do not have a very high proportion of unsaturated fatty acids, so they can be another option, if you prefer them.

Lactate Drinks

Lactate drinks are beverages that contain a blend of healthy vegetable oil and lactic acid–fermented milk or soy milk. Lactic acid–fermented milks are relatively high in protein and extremely low in carbohydrates; when mixed with valuable vegetable oils, they have an extremely positive effect on the metabolism. Food manufacturers in Germany combine these two components into ready-made products (and are moving their products into North American markets soon), but you can mix the components to taste in your kitchen. If you buy a commercial version, make sure it contains less than 2% carbohydrates and has a high proportion of unsaturated fatty acids.

Fermented milk or soy milk is ideal for mixing with berry juices (try two parts fermented milk to one part pure, unsweetened blueberry or raspberry juice). You can vary the flavor and keep making new combinations, which add variety and fresh nutrients to your diet. By adding some of your special oil mixture (see page 161), you'll increase the content of valuable fatty acids and secondary nutrients even further. You can vary the drink by adding a bit of protein powder, fresh fruit or low-sugar jam.

Buttermilk and Other Lactic Acid–Fermented Foods

Lactic acid fermentation significantly reduces the amount of sugar and starch in foods and drinks. Unfermented foods make blood sugar and insulin levels rise quickly, whereas fermented foods don't. They also have a deacidifying effect on the body. They give you energy without benefiting fermenting cancer cells.

Buttermilk is versatile. You can use it in baking and even marinate meat in it to make it more easily digestible. Sour cream, which also contains lactic acid, is excellent for baking, cooking and adding to salad dressings. And don't forget about lactic acid–fermented vegetables, such as sauerkraut and kimchi, which are also extremely healthy.

Diet Know-How

The recipes starting on page 168 were specially developed by home economists for patients with cancer. The recipes are, however, equally good for healthy people, and can help prevent cancer and other lifestyle diseases, such as diabetes, cardiovascular disease and Alzheimer's disease.

Try to stick to the diet as consistently as possible. In just a couple of months, it will be second nature to you. In some people, a regression in cancerous tumors, metastases and tumor markers can be noticed after only two weeks. The positive effect on body and mind usually becomes obvious after only three to five days, which helps you stay motivated.

Keep Your Diet Exciting

The ingredients you invite into your cancer-fighting kitchen should provide as much variety as possible while fulfilling the criteria of the diet. They should contain minimal carbohydrates; emphasize proteins, and healthy fats or oils; and contain a variety of bioactive substances, phytochemicals and sufficient dietary fiber. Let the lists of Green- and Yellow-Light Foods (pages 144 to 150) be your shopping guides.

Tips for Eating Well on the Road

Once you get the hang of this new diet, you will find it easy to eat healthily without sacrificing enjoyment or avoiding social situations — even when you're not in your own kitchen. It's true that there are very few ready-made foods that fit the diet (never mind what's on offer in restaurants). But with the following tips, you can make wise choices even when you're out and about:

- Always combine meat or fish with salad or vegetables (but not with potatoes, beans, peas or chickpeas).
- Watch for hidden sugar in salad dressings. If you're in doubt, ask for oil and vinegar, and mix your own dressing at the table.

DID YOU KNOW?

You Can Cheat Wisely

There will be days when you want to take time out from everyday healthy eating. If you don't follow the cancer-fighting diet 100% of the time, you can still reap the benefits — if you learn a simple trick. If you know that you are going to eat out or go to a party, empty your glycogen stores by consuming very little glucose or doing intense exercise before going out. The missing glycogen will be replenished first from the food you eat, so your blood sugar will rise more slowly, and your body won't be negatively affected by the sinful food.

- Avoid filling side dishes, such as pasta, rice, potatoes and bread, and choose vegetables or salad instead. You can eat a lot more of these without having to think about their carb content.
- Craving a hot dog or sausage? No problem. Just skip the bun and the ketchup; opt for mustard instead (avoid sweet or honey mustard, which contains plenty of sugar).
- Feel free to indulge in crisp sautéed potatoes (or even fries) once in a while. Both release less glucose than boiled or mashed potatoes, and release it more slowly.
- If you want to eat a carbohydrate-rich main course, have a salad, vegetables or high-fat soup as a starter. This will slow down carbohydrate metabolism.
- Skip soups that contain pasta or noodles. Instead, choose soups that contain vegetables or legumes on the Green-Light Foods list (see page 144). Plain chicken soup and oxtail soup are ideal choices.
- Request substitutions at restaurants; many will be happy to oblige. Ask them to hold the high-carb sides and serve meat or fish with vegetables or a salad.
- If you want to indulge in a slice or two of baguette or other white bread, spread them with a little butter or drizzle them with olive oil. Make sure the other components of your meal contain small amounts of glucose and starch.
- For dessert, have a simple dish of berries with cream, or a high-fat custard, such as panna cotta. Don't worry about the calories. It's better to have extra cream, because it slows down the rise in blood sugar.

Snacks to Take with You

Some days you may find your stomach growling between meals. Here are some good-for-you snacks that can satisfy hunger pangs:

- **Nuts and Seeds.** Almonds, walnuts and pumpkin seeds are ideal.
- **Special (Chocolate-Based) Energy Bars.** Look for those made with protein-rich ingredients, low-GI sugars, good fats and fiber. Watch ingredient lists for unhealthy sugars; regular energy bars contain an awful lot of glucose.
- **Dried Meat.** If you like cold cuts, dried beef (also called bresaola) will help you master energy lows. Skip meat jerky made with nitrates and added sugar.
- **High-Protein Bread.** If you can't live without bread, take along a slice or two of high-protein bread. Loaves that have been pasteurized keep longer at room temperature.

- For another sweet dessert option, choose plain cheesecake; just don't eat the carb-rich crust.
- Drink mainly water, unsweetened tea and decaffeinated coffee. You can also enjoy spritzers made with nine parts of mineral water to one part of pure, unsweetened, unfiltered berry juices (see page 163), such as raspberry, strawberry and elderberry. Or choose beverages containing small amounts of low-GI sugars (which may be combined with other sweeteners, such as stevia or aspartame).
- Opt for diluted vegetable juices, but watch their sugar content. Choose those made from veggies on the Green-Light Foods list (see page 144).
- Feel free to indulge in beer from time to time. Opt for bitter barley beers, such as Pilsner, which often contain fewer carbohydrates than wheat beers (which also contain gluten).
- Treat yourself to a glass of red wine; the phytochemicals it contains render it a healthy option.

Test Your Results

Adhere strictly to the cancer-fighting diet before you begin a course of chemotherapy or radiation. In the first weeks of following the cancer-fighting diet, you should check the effect it has on your metabolism. You can do this by finding out if your sugar reserves have been used up, and your body has started burning fat to make energy. If so, your urine will contain ketone bodies (see page 43), which can be detected using a simple test strip. For more accurate results, you can test your blood with a different type of test strip. Both are available at pharmacies.

If you are following the cancer-fighting diet in a more moderate way, for cancer prevention or to prevent recurrence, ketone bodies will not be present in your urine. And while ketone bodies won't show up on a test, the low-GI character of the diet will still hinder the growth of aggressive cancer cells.

If you don't find a moderate approach to the diet is working, follow it strictly, especially if you're preparing for a new round of chemotherapy or radiation. In this case, you need to see that the ketone bodies are present in your urine, to ensure that the diet will help your therapies be more effective.

The Five Steps You Can Take to Fight Cancer

Don't accept cancer as an unalterable fate. Look ahead, full of confidence that you can change your life. The following five strategies will support you in your undertaking:

1. **Follow the Cancer-Fighting Diet.** The discovery of the TKTL1 metabolism shows that aggressive cancer cells differ significantly from healthy cells. In order to obtain energy, they rely on the constant supply of glucose. This is why you can significantly improve your chances of a cure by simply changing what you eat. See the box on page 140 for more on the pillars of this diet.

2. **Get Moving.** Exercise is the most effective way to empty your body's glycogen stores. At the same time, the oxygen supply to the tissue improves, thereby facilitating the switch from fermentation to combustion in cancer cells. Last but not least, exercise increases self-confidence, helping you feel better about your body. This has a positive effect on your state of mind. Set aside three 30-minute periods each week for intense endurance exercise. An extra session is also recommended if you know that you are going to "sin" shortly thereafter, perhaps because you are invited to a big party with excellent food. To increase muscle tone, you should also do gentle weight training once a week. And remember to always consult your family doctor, a physiotherapist or a sports medicine specialist before you start, so you know what your limits are.

3. **Get Professional Help.** The most important thing you need to know after a cancer diagnosis is that you are not to blame for the disease. You also need to know that you are not alone; a large team of professionals can assist you in all matters. Make use of this professional help. If you suffer from depression and anxiety, a psycho-oncologist can help you come to terms with the past, resolve problems and open your eyes to the possibilities of the future.

4. **Try Complementary Medicine.** In contrast to conventional Western medicine, complementary healing methods treat the symptoms of a disease while considering the entire person. Methods such as homeopathy, aromatherapy and music therapy are not meant to replace conventional cancer treatments, but to support them in a gentle manner by strengthening the immune system and the mind. Acupuncture (see page 118) also helps patients cope with pain and nausea (for example, during chemotherapy).

5. **Relax the Right Way.** There are many relaxation methods that can help you consciously unwind, building the proper balance between tension and relaxation, which is so important for health. Autogenic training (see page 120), PMR (see page 120) and qigong (see page 122) can easily be done at home after a short introduction by an experienced teacher. You'll only need to set aside a little time — and make the decision to do something good for your own well-being.

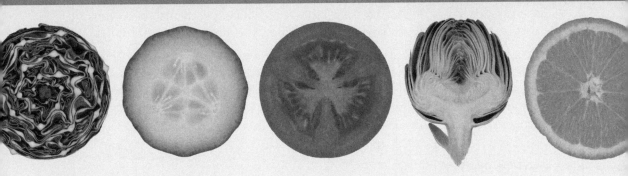

PART 4

Recipes

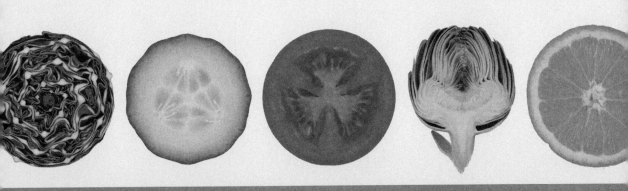

Recipe Basics

- Most of the recipes in this book serve one person (with the exception of baked goods, cakes and desserts). If you want to share a particular meal with family or guests at a dinner party, simply multiply the ingredients accordingly.

- At the bottom of each recipe, you'll see the nutrient values per serving. This helps you keep an eye on the calories — and especially the carbohydrates — that you're taking in each day. Make sure you don't exceed your maximum daily intake of carbohydrates (see box, below). Distribute this amount as evenly as possible throughout the day.

- Make sure you eat enough of your special oil mixture to ensure good health (see box, page 161).

- If you are hungry between meals, help yourself to Green-Light Foods (page 144).

Health Begins in the Kitchen

In your own home, the everyday implementation of the cancer-fighting diet is very easy. The recipes in this section of the book clearly show you how varied this type of diet can be. Even desserts, cake and savory snacks are allowed, provided you do not exceed the maximum daily amount of carbohydrates (1 g carbohydrate per 2.2 lbs/1 kg body weight per day). This is where using healthy, low-GI sugars can really help.

When planning your menu, make sure you do not use in a single day several recipes that have relatively higher carbohydrate contents. On the other hand, if the amount of carbohydrates you eat is lower that your maximum daily limit, that's no problem. Your body can also make glucose from protein and meet its energy needs (see page 91).

Breakfasts and Beverages

Spinach Omelet

**Prep time:
20 minutes**

*Well seasoned and
packed with healthy
spinach, this omelet is a
satisfying way to start
the day. It fills you up
and keeps you full.*

Tip

Before you wash and
prep spinach, always
pick through and
discard any wilted or
yellow leaves.

5 oz	fresh spinach (see tip, at left)	150 g
1 tsp	butter	5 mL
	Vegetable broth granules	
	Turmeric	
1	tomato	1
2	eggs, separated	2
½ tsp	heavy or whipping (35%) cream	2 mL
	Salt and freshly ground black pepper	
	Grated nutmeg	
1½ tbsp	coconut oil	22 mL

1. Pick over and thoroughly wash spinach; drain. In a saucepan, melt butter over medium-high heat. Add spinach with water clinging to leaves; sauté for 5 minutes or until wilted. Season to taste with vegetable broth granules and turmeric. Set aside.

2. Core and cut tomato into wedges. In a bowl, whisk egg yolks with cream; season with salt, pepper and nutmeg. In another bowl, beat egg whites until stiff peaks form. Gently fold egg whites into yolk mixture.

3. In a nonstick skillet, heat coconut oil over medium heat. Pour in egg mixture; cook for 3 minutes or until golden on bottom and almost dry on top. Arrange spinach over one half of omelet; fold over uncovered half.

4. Transfer omelet to a plate; garnish with tomato wedges.

Prep Tip

It's a good idea to wash all produce thoroughly to remove any surface dirt or grit. Use plenty of cold water and rub or swish gently to prevent bruising, especially when preparing delicate greens or tender vegetables.

Nutrients per serving	
Calories	280
Fat	26 g
Carbohydrates	3 g
Protein	12 g

Fried Eggs and Bacon

Makes 1 serving

**Prep time:
10 minutes**

This isn't just a Sunday favorite; it's also a high-protein breakfast that's easy to prepare on weekday mornings.

Tip

This breakfast is especially delicious when big, beautiful garden tomatoes are in season. They're so juicy and fresh alongside the eggs and crispy bacon.

2	slices bacon (about 1½ oz/45 g), see tip, below	2
1	tomato (see tip, at left)	1
1 tsp	butter	5 mL
2	eggs	2
	Salt and freshly ground black pepper	

1. Chop bacon. Core and cut tomato into wedges. Set aside.

2. In a nonstick skillet, melt butter over medium heat. Add bacon; fry, stirring often, for 5 minutes or until crisp and browned. Break eggs into skillet; fry just until set or until desired doneness.

3. Transfer bacon and eggs to a plate. Season to taste with salt and pepper. Garnish with tomato wedges.

Substitution Tip

Sodium-reduced bacon also works well in this dish if you prefer a less-salty result.

Nutrients per serving	
Calories	340
Fat	30 g
Carbohydrates	2 g
Protein	16 g

Herby Scrambled Eggs

*Fresh herbs give simple
scrambled eggs an
attractive and delicious
makeover. The bacon
adds a smoky note that's
very satisfying.*

Tips

Eating eggs for breakfast
gives you plenty of
energy and keeps you
feeling full all morning.
They're an excellent low-
carbohydrate option.

You can add up to 2 tbsp
(30 mL) chopped fresh
herbs if you like more
of their fresh flavor in
your eggs.

2	eggs	2
1 tsp	heavy or whipping (35%) cream	5 mL
1 tbsp	chopped fresh herbs (see tips, at left)	15 mL
	Salt and freshly ground black pepper	
1 tbsp	finely chopped bacon	15 mL

1. In a bowl, whisk eggs with cream. Stir in herbs. Season with salt and pepper.

2. In a dry skillet over medium heat, fry bacon, stirring often, for 3 minutes or until crisp and browned. Pour in egg mixture. Cook, stirring, for 2 minutes or until set.

Shopping Tip

You can vary the herbs according to your preferences and what's available. Try fresh chives, basil or tarragon, or experiment with other herbs to find your favorite.

Nutrients per serving	
Calories	265
Fat	20 g
Carbohydrates	4 g
Protein	21 g

Cheese and Bacon Waffles

Makes 6 servings

**Prep time:
30 minutes**

*Bacon is always tasty
with waffles, but it's even
better inside them. The
waffles are excellent
served hot or cold.*

Tip

Einkorn is an ancient
form of wheat that's very
nutritious. If you can't
find it at the supermarket
or a health food store,
whole-grain spelt flour
is a good alternative.

- **Waffle iron**

4	eggs	4
1 cup + 2 tbsp	grated Parmesan cheese	280 mL
¾ cup + 2 tbsp	butter, melted	200 mL
½ cup	sour cream	125 mL
5	slices bacon, finely chopped	5
⅔ cup	whole-grain einkorn flour (see tip, at left)	150 mL
¼ cup	finely ground oat bran (see tip, below)	60 mL
1 tsp	baking powder	5 mL
1 tsp	dried thyme	5 mL
	Salt	
1 tsp	coconut oil	5 mL

1. In a bowl, beat eggs. Whisk in Parmesan cheese, butter, sour cream and bacon.

2. In another bowl, whisk together flour, oat bran, baking powder and thyme. Stir into egg mixture until almost smooth. Season with salt.

3. Heat waffle iron according to manufacturer's instructions. Brush coconut oil over hot waffle iron. Spoon some of the batter onto iron, spreading almost to edges. Bake until crisp and golden. Repeat with remaining batter to make 6 waffles.

Shopping Tip

Oat bran may be coarsely or finely ground. The finely ground version may be labeled as a hot cereal or as oat bran powder; either will work in this recipe.

Nutrients per serving	
Calories	480
Fat	42 g
Carbohydrates	9 g
Protein	18 g

Mini-Pancakes with Apple and Cinnamon Cream

Now you can make pancakes just for yourself. These nutty delights are the perfect guilt-free morning meal.

Tip

To incorporate the apple directly into the pancakes, coarsely grate it instead of slicing. Drizzle with lemon juice as directed; fold into batter. Cook pancakes as directed.

2 tbsp	whole-grain spelt flour	30 mL
1 tbsp	coarsely ground almonds	15 mL
½ tsp	cream of tartar	2 mL
1	egg	1
⅓ cup	buttermilk	75 mL
1 tsp	raw cane sugar	5 mL
Pinch	salt	Pinch
2 tsp	butter	10 mL
¼	Granny Smith apple (about 1½ oz/45 g), peeled and cored	¼
1 tsp	lemon juice	5 mL
2 tbsp	crème fraîche	30 mL
	Ground cinnamon	

1. In a bowl, whisk together flour, almonds and cream of tartar. In another bowl, stir together egg, buttermilk, sugar and salt. Stir in flour mixture until almost smooth.

2. In a large nonstick skillet, melt butter over medium heat. Using 1 tbsp (15 mL) for each, spoon batter into skillet to make 6 pancakes; cook for 2 minutes or until bottoms are golden. Turn and cook for 2 to 3 minutes or until golden all over and center is cooked through.

3. Meanwhile, cut apple into thin wedges; immediately drizzle with lemon juice to keep from browning.

4. Arrange pancakes on a plate; garnish with apple wedges and crème fraîche. Season to taste with cinnamon.

Nutrients per serving

Calories	457
Fat	31 g
Carbohydrates	32 g
Protein	13 g

Jam Sandwiches with Papaya

Makes 1 serving

**Prep time:
5 minutes**

Who says you have to wait until lunch for a sandwich? This one is naturally sweet rather than savory — perfect for the morning.

Tip

Berry jams are especially tasty in this open-faced sandwich. Try raspberry (with or without seeds), strawberry or mixed berry.

1	slice high-protein bread (see page 157), about 1½ oz (45 g)	1
1 tsp	butter	5 mL
1 tsp	jam (see tip, at left)	5 mL
1	piece fresh papaya (4 oz/125 g) (see tip, below)	1
	Lemon juice	

1. If desired, toast bread. Spread butter, then jam over bread.
2. Peel and seed papaya; cut into thin slices. Season to taste with lemon juice.
3. Arrange papaya slices over jam.

Storage Tip

The remaining papaya will keep well in the crisper drawer of the refrigerator for another breakfast (like Papaya with Cottage Cheese, page 181). Cover the papaya tightly with plastic wrap to keep it fresh.

Nutrients per serving

Calories	172
Fat	9 g
Carbohydrates	11 g
Protein	7 g

Nut and Fruit Yogurt

Makes 1 serving

**Prep time:
10 minutes**

*A mix of crunchy, fresh
and creamy tastes, this
bowl of goodness is the
perfect way to wake up.*

Tips

Kefir is a fermented
milk drink that's packed
with beneficial bacteria
that aids digestion.
You'll find it in health
food stores and most
supermarkets. You can
also buy cultures to make
your own at home.

Use full-fat yogurt for
this recipe. It's creamy
and has the healthy
fat your body needs to
fight cancer.

¼ cup	fresh blueberries (see tip, below)	60 mL
¼ cup	kefir (see tips, at left)	60 mL
3 tbsp	plain yogurt (see tips, at left)	45 mL
2 tsp	special oil mixture (see page 161)	10 mL
	Sweetener (see page 158)	
	Ground cinnamon	
1 tbsp	ground hazelnuts	15 mL

1. Wash and pick through blueberries, discarding any that are wrinkled or bruised. Set aside a few for garnish.

2. In a bowl, stir together kefir, yogurt and special oil mixture. Season to taste with sweetener and cinnamon. Stir in hazelnuts.

3. Spoon blueberries into a small bowl; pour yogurt mixture over top. Refrigerate for 30 minutes or until chilled. Garnish with reserved blueberries.

Substitution Tip

Instead of fresh blueberries, you can substitute 2 tsp (10 mL) mixed berry jam, stirring it into the yogurt mixture until blended.

Nutrients per serving	
Calories	220
Fat	19 g
Carbohydrates	6 g
Protein	4 g

Tofu and Raspberry Breakfast Pudding

Makes 1 serving

Prep time: 10 minutes

Silken tofu is a great alternative to dairy in smoothies and breakfast dishes like this. It has a delicate taste, so it takes on the flavors around it.

Tip

Vanilla powder is a concentrated flavoring made by grinding vanilla beans. Look for bottles that don't contain added sugar or starch.

• **Blender**

2 oz	silken tofu, drained (see tip, below)	60 g
½ tsp	almond butter	2 mL
½ tsp	special oil mixture (see page 161)	2 mL
¼ cup	fresh raspberries	60 mL
Pinch	vanilla powder (see tip, at left)	Pinch
	Sweetener (see page 158)	

1. In a blender, purée together silken tofu, almond butter and special oil mixture until smooth. Pour into a small bowl.

2. Set aside a few raspberries for garnish. In another small bowl, and using a fork, mash remaining raspberries. Stir into tofu mixture.

3. Stir in vanilla powder. Season to taste with sweetener; garnish with reserved raspberries.

Storage Tip

To keep leftover tofu fresh, drain it daily and cover with fresh filtered water to keep it moist. Cover tightly and use up in a couple of days.

Nutrients per serving	
Calories	150
Fat	11 g
Carbohydrates	6 g
Protein	7 g

Strawberry Quark with Flaxseed Crunchies

A layered parfait like this is as pretty as it is delicious. The flaxseed crunchies are really addictive — they might be your favorite part of breakfast.

Tips

Unless a recipe calls for the low-fat version specifically, always choose the full-fat varieties of quark and sour cream when you're on the cancer-fighting diet. Your body needs the fat they contain to make energy.

In summer, you can make this dish with other berries, such as fresh blackberries or raspberries. Or, for a different taste, try it with diced honeydew melon.

2 tsp	raw cane sugar	10 mL
2 tbsp	coarsely chopped flax seeds	30 mL
½ cup	fresh strawberries, hulled	125 mL
⅔ cup	quark (see tip, below)	150 mL
2 tbsp	sour cream (see tips, at left)	30 mL
2 tsp	lemon juice	10 mL

1. In a small nonstick skillet, melt sugar over medium heat until caramel-colored and syrupy. Stir flax seeds into caramel. Remove from heat; let cool.

2. Halve or quarter strawberries, depending on size. Set a few pieces aside for garnish.

3. In a bowl, stir together quark, sour cream and lemon juice until smooth. Stir in half of the flaxseed crunchies. Alternately spoon quark mixture and strawberries into a cereal bowl. Garnish with reserved strawberries. Sprinkle with remaining flaxseed crunchies.

Substitution Tip

Quark is a German fresh cheese that is similar to a French fresh cheese called fromage frais. If you can't find either, you can drain plain yogurt to make yogurt cheese and use that instead.

Nutrients per serving

Calories	479
Fat	33 g
Carbohydrates	20 g
Protein	23 g

Papaya with Cottage Cheese

Makes 1 serving

**Prep time:
15 minutes**

This mix of tropical fruit, mild cheese and nuts is packed with nutrients. The cocoa powder is a decadent topping, but you can omit it if you prefer.

Tip

The remaining papaya will keep well in the crisper drawer of the refrigerator for another breakfast (like Jam Sandwiches with Papaya, page 177). Cover tightly with plastic wrap to keep it fresh.

1 tbsp	raw cashews	15 mL
½	ripe papaya (about 7 oz/210 g), see tip, at left	½
1 tbsp	lime juice	15 mL
¾ cup + 2 tbsp	cottage cheese	200 mL
2 tsp	walnut oil (see tip, below)	10 mL
Pinch	grated organic lime zest	Pinch
	Liquid sweetener (see page 158)	
	Unsweetened cocoa powder	

1. Chop cashews. In a dry nonstick skillet over medium heat, toast cashews, shaking pan often, for 5 minutes or until golden brown. Remove from heat; set aside.

2. Peel and seed papaya; cut into wedges lengthwise. Arrange on a plate. Drizzle with lime juice.

3. In a bowl, stir together cottage cheese, walnut oil and lime zest until creamy. Season to taste with sweetener.

4. Spoon cottage cheese mixture over center of papaya slices. Sprinkle with cashews. Season to taste with cocoa powder.

Storage Tip

Walnut oil is highly perishable. Keep it in the refrigerator to prevent it from going rancid.

Nutrients per serving	
Calories	514
Fat	32 g
Carbohydrates	14 g
Protein	31 g

Berry Sour Cream with Honeyed Almonds

The combination of sour cream and crème fraîche makes for a very tangy dish. It would also be good made with plain yogurt instead of sour cream.

Tips

This fruity and fresh berry cream also tastes delicious as a dessert after a low-carb meal.

If you use frozen berries, it's best to let them thaw overnight in the refrigerator.

1 tbsp	sliced almonds	15 mL
1 tsp	liquid honey	5 mL
7 tbsp	sour cream	100 mL
2 tbsp	crème fraîche	30 mL
Pinch	vanilla paste (see tip, below)	Pinch
	Liquid sweetener (see page 158)	
1/3 cup	fresh or thawed frozen raspberries (see tips, at left)	75 mL
1/4 cup	fresh or thawed frozen blackberries	60 mL

1. In a small dry nonstick skillet over medium heat, toast almonds, shaking pan often, for 5 minutes or until golden brown. Remove from heat. Stir in honey until combined. Let cool.

2. In a bowl, stir together sour cream, crème fraîche and vanilla paste. Add sweetener to taste. Top with raspberries and blackberries.

3. Garnish with cooled honeyed almonds.

Shopping Tip

Look for pure vanilla paste in health food and gourmet stores. It's a potent, alcohol- and sugar-free way to add flavor to recipes. It can be pricey, but a little goes a long way.

Nutrients per serving	
Calories	474
Fat	42 g
Carbohydrates	17 g
Protein	6 g

Kiwi with Ginger Ricotta

Ricotta is a mildly acidic fresh cheese made from whey rather than whole milk. It is a delicious source of protein, and works well in sweet and savory dishes.

Tip

Lemon balm is a lovely herb to grow in your garden. If you don't have it, try fresh mint leaves instead.

1	small ripe kiwifruit	1
6 tbsp	ricotta cheese	90 mL
2 tbsp	heavy or whipping (35%) cream	30 mL
1 tsp	lemon juice	5 mL
1	piece (about $\frac{1}{2}$ inch/1 cm long) gingerroot (see tip, below)	1
	Liquid sweetener (see page 158)	
1	sprig fresh lemon balm (see tip, at left)	1

1. Peel kiwi; cut lengthwise into wedges. Arrange on a plate in the shape of a flower.

2. In a bowl, stir together ricotta cheese, cream and lemon juice until smooth. Finely grate ginger; stir into ricotta mixture. Add sweetener to taste.

3. Spoon ricotta mixture into center of kiwi wedges. Wash and pat lemon balm leaves dry; pull leaves off stems. Garnish ricotta mixture with lemon balm leaves.

Prep Tip

A fine rasp grater is perfect for grating ginger. If you love ginger and often cook with it, it might be worthwhile to buy a special ginger grater. It strains out the fibrous parts of the root, leaving you with a smooth purée.

Nutrients per serving	
Calories	278
Fat	22 g
Carbohydrates	6 g
Protein	11 g

Amaranth and Quark Muesli

Muesli is a powerhouse of a breakfast dish. The combination of fresh fruit, oats and creamy quark is so pleasing.

Tips

Puffed amaranth is a bit like popcorn: the grains are heated and puff up into tiny, fluffy globes. Eating it in this form allows the body to more easily absorb its valuable nutrients, including high-quality protein, easily digestible carbohydrates, magnesium and iron.

Always choose full-fat versions of dairy products, such as quark and milk, when you're on the cancer-fighting diet. (Unless the recipe specifically calls for a low-fat version.) Your body needs the fat they contain to make energy.

1 tbsp	sesame seeds (see tip, below)	15 mL
2 tbsp	puffed amaranth (see tips, at left)	30 mL
1 tbsp	coarsely chopped flax seeds	15 mL
⅔ cup	quark (see tips, at left)	150 mL
2 tbsp	heavy or whipping (35%) cream	30 mL
	Ground cinnamon	
	Liquid sweetener (see page 158)	
1	piece (about 4 oz/125 g) honeydew melon, peeled, seeded and cut into bite-size pieces	1

1. In a dry nonstick skillet over medium heat, toast sesame seeds, shaking pan often, for 5 minutes or until golden and fragrant. Transfer to a small bowl; let cool slightly. Stir in amaranth and flax seeds.

2. In another bowl, stir quark with cream until smooth. Season to taste with cinnamon and sweetener. Fold in two-thirds of the amaranth mixture.

3. Spoon quark mixture into a cereal bowl. Garnish with melon and remaining amaranth mixture.

Prep Tip

To make breakfast assembly even simpler in the morning, toast three or four times the quantity of sesame seeds that you need. Then combine them with three or four times the puffed amaranth and flax seeds you need, and store them in an airtight container. This way, you can have the base for fresh muesli ready to go, on even the busiest mornings.

Nutrients per serving

Calories	487
Fat	33 g
Carbohydrates	24 g
Protein	24 g

Chilled Buttermilk with Mandarin Oranges

This cross between muesli and a smoothie is so easy to make. Depending on the season, you can replace the mandarin oranges with other fruits, such as fresh figs, apricots, nectarines or peaches.

Tip

Quark is a German fresh cheese that is similar to a French fresh cheese called fromage frais. If you can't find either, you can drain plain yogurt to make yogurt cheese and use that instead.

- **Blender**

1 tbsp	coarsely chopped hulled raw pumpkin seeds	15 mL
1	mandarin orange	1
1 cup	buttermilk	250 mL
2 tbsp	quark (see tip, at left)	30 mL
2 tbsp	lime juice	30 mL
1 tbsp	large-flake (old-fashioned) rolled oats	15 mL
	Liquid sweetener (see page 158)	

1. In a dry nonstick skillet over medium heat, toast pumpkin seeds, shaking pan often, for 5 minutes or until golden and fragrant. Remove from heat; let cool.

2. Peel mandarin orange and divide into segments, carefully removing the pith. In a blender, purée together two-thirds of the mandarin segments, buttermilk, quark and lime juice until smooth. Stir in oats; add sweetener to taste.

3. Pour buttermilk mixture into a bowl; garnish with remaining mandarin segments and toasted pumpkin seeds.

Nutrients per serving

Calories	242
Fat	9 g
Carbohydrates	23 g
Protein	15 g

Blueberry Buttermilk Shake

Makes 1 serving

**Prep time:
10 minutes**

Serve this thick, creamy beverage with a big, fat straw. It's a terrific breakfast for mornings when you don't have a lot of time to eat.

Tip

For a cool, creamy smoothie, use frozen berries instead of the fresh blueberries. Let them thaw for about 10 minutes at room temperature before puréeing them.

- **Blender**

⅔ cup	buttermilk	150 mL
7 tbsp	fresh blueberries (see tip, at left)	100 mL
1 tbsp	finely ground spelt bran (see tip, below)	15 mL
2 tsp	lemon juice	10 mL
2 tbsp	heavy or whipping (35%) cream	30 mL
	Liquid sweetener (see page 158)	

1. In a blender, purée together buttermilk, blueberries, spelt bran and lemon juice until smooth.

2. Add cream, and sweetener to taste. Blend again until incorporated.

3. Pour shake into a tall glass. Serve immediately.

Prep Tip

Look for spelt bran in health and bulk food stores. If it's a little coarser than you like in your smoothie, you can grind it more finely using a clean coffee grinder.

Nutrients per serving	
Calories	160
Fat	8 g
Carbohydrates	12 g
Protein	8 g

Cherry and Coconut Smoothie

Makes 1 serving

**Prep time:
15 minutes**

Coconut milk is so convenient to keep in your pantry. It's wonderful in curries, smoothies and much more.

Tips

For a tasty garnish, toast 2 tsp (10 mL) unsweetened shredded coconut in a small dry nonstick skillet, then sprinkle it over the finished drink.

For a tangier drink, add up to 2 tsp (10 mL) lime juice — or more, if you like.

● **Blender**

⅔ cup	canned unsweetened coconut milk (see tip, below)	150 mL
½ cup	frozen pitted sour cherries	125 mL
1 tbsp	unsweetened shredded coconut	15 mL
⅓ cup	milk	75 mL
1 tsp	lime juice, or to taste (see tips, at left)	5 mL
	Liquid sweetener (see page 158)	

1. Let cherries thaw at room temperature for 10 minutes. In a blender, purée together coconut milk, cherries and shredded coconut until smooth.

2. Add milk and lime juice, and sweetener to taste. Blend again until incorporated.

3. Pour smoothie into a tall glass. Serve immediately.

Shopping Tip

Make sure your canned coconut milk doesn't contain any added sugar or sweeteners. It should also be the full-fat, not the light, version to give your body the fat it needs to make energy.

Nutrients per serving	
Calories	136
Fat	8 g
Carbohydrates	10 g
Protein	3 g

Avocado Lassi

Makes 1 serving

Prep time: 10 minutes

Lassis, or yogurt-based drinks, are a feature of Indian cuisine. They are usually consumed to cool the fire of spicy curries. Here, an avocado gives this breakfast-time drink a decadent creaminess and plenty of healthy fat.

Tip

Look for fructose powder in health food stores or online. You can use it in place of sugar in many recipes, but you'll need less because it's sweeter.

- **Blender**

4	sprigs fresh basil	4
½	small ripe avocado	½
1 tbsp	lime juice	15 mL
⅔ cup	plain yogurt (see tip, below)	150 mL
⅓ cup	lightly carbonated mineral water	75 mL
1 tbsp	coarsely ground almonds	15 mL
1 tsp	fructose powder (see tip, at left)	5 mL

1. Wash and pat basil dry; pull leaves off stems. Set aside 2 leaves for garnish. Coarsely chop remaining basil leaves.

2. Pit, peel and coarsely chop avocado; place in a small bowl. Immediately drizzle with lime juice; toss to combine and prevent browning.

3. In a blender, purée together avocado mixture, chopped basil, yogurt, mineral water, almonds and fructose powder until smooth.

4. Pour lassi into a tall glass; garnish with reserved basil leaves. Serve immediately.

Substitution Tip

For a change of pace, try substituting kefir or buttermilk for the yogurt. The drink will have a slightly thinner consistency but will be just as refreshing.

Nutrients per serving

Calories	403
Fat	34 g
Carbohydrates	16 g
Protein	8 g

Two-Tone Mango Tofu Smoothie

Makes 1 serving

Prep time: 15 minutes

A layered smoothie is a fun way to start the day. The zippy ginger is an ideal partner to the sweet, juicy mango.

Tip

Well-stocked grocery stores often carry silken tofu. If you can't find it there, look in health food stores.

• **Blender**

½ cup	sliced ripe mango	125 mL
1 tsp	grated orange zest (see tip, below)	5 mL
2 tbsp	orange juice	30 mL
1 tbsp	lemon juice	15 mL
4 oz	silken tofu (see tip, at left), drained	125 g
½ tsp	ground ginger	2 mL
3	ice cubes, crushed	3
	Liquid sweetener (see page 158)	

1. In a blender, purée together mango, orange zest, orange juice and lemon juice until smooth. Pour mango purée into a tall glass.

2. Add tofu, ginger and ice to blender; add sweetener to taste. Purée until smooth.

3. Carefully pour tofu mixture into glass without disturbing mango purée to create two-toned effect. Serve immediately.

Shopping Tip

Always buy organic citrus fruit when you're grating zest. It is safer and cleaner to eat than conventionally grown citrus, which is sprayed with pesticides.

Nutrients per serving	
Calories	151
Fat	6 g
Carbohydrates	12 g
Protein	11 g

Vegetable Power Shake

**Prep time:
10 minutes**

*Don't wait until
lunchtime to eat
your vegetables. This
smoothie jump-starts
your day with a healthy
serving of them.*

Tips

Specially formulated
lactate drinks are a
good substitution for
the kefir if you can find
them. See page 162 for
more information.

Just 1 tsp (5 mL)
of flaxseed oil per
day covers your
daily requirement
of alpha-linolenic
acid, an essential
omega-3 fatty acid.

- **Blender**

1	organic mini cucumber (about 3½ oz/100 g), peeled	1
	Salt and freshly ground black pepper	
2 tsp	lemon juice	10 mL
1	mini red or orange bell pepper (see tip, below)	1
⅔ cup	kefir (see tips, at left)	150 mL
1 tbsp	large-flake (old-fashioned) rolled oats	15 mL
1 tsp	flaxseed oil (see tips, at left)	5 mL
3	sprigs fresh dill	3

1. Halve cucumber lengthwise; using a spoon, scrape out seeds. Cut cucumber halves into thin slices. Place in a small bowl. Season with salt to taste. Drizzle with lemon juice; let stand for 5 minutes.

2. Meanwhile, seed and chop red pepper. In a blender, purée together red pepper, cucumber with marinating liquid and kefir until smooth.

3. Add oats and flaxseed oil. Reserving a small sprig for garnish, remove dill sprigs from stems; add to blender. Season with salt and pepper to taste. Blend again until incorporated.

4. Pour shake into a tall glass. Garnish with reserved dill. Serve immediately.

Shopping Tip

Can't find mini bell peppers? Buy regular-size peppers and use one-third to one-half, depending on the size and your tastes.

Nutrients per serving	
Calories	217
Fat	11 g
Carbohydrates	16 g
Protein	12 g

Appetizers, Spreads and Baked Goods

Celeriac Fries with Mascarpone Dip

Makes 1 serving

**Prep time:
35 minutes**

*These crispy creations
are delicately celery-
flavored. They make
a tasty snack or
appetizer — just watch
your carb intake during
the rest of the day.*

Tip

Celeriac is a knobby
root vegetable that has a
wonderful celery flavor.
It is very large and has
unattractive roots all
over the outside, but
once it's peeled and
trimmed, the root reveals
crisp, delicate white
flesh inside.

Nutrients per serving	
Calories	985
Fat	90 g
Carbohydrates	24 g
Protein	21 g

- Bowl, filled with ice water
- Candy/deep-fry thermometer
- Plate, lined with paper towels

1	piece (8 oz/250 g) celeriac (see tip, at left)	1
2½ oz	mascarpone cheese	75 g
2 tbsp	milk	30 mL
	Grated zest of 1 organic lime	
1 tsp	lime juice	5 mL
	Salt and freshly ground black pepper	
	Cayenne pepper	
1	green onion (white and light green parts), thinly sliced	1
¼ cup	finely ground pecans	60 mL
2 tbsp	whole-grain spelt flour	30 mL
1	egg	1
	Oil for deep-frying (see page 162)	
	Lime wedges	

1. Trim and peel celeriac. Cut into ½-inch (1 cm) thick slices; cut slices into ¾-inch (2 cm) long sticks. In a saucepan of boiling salted water, blanch for 2 minutes. Using a slotted spoon, transfer to prepared bowl of ice water; let cool. Drain well.

2. Meanwhile, in a bowl, stir together cheese, milk, lime zest and lime juice until smooth; season to taste with salt, black pepper and cayenne pepper. Stir in green onion.

3. Sprinkle pecans and flour on separate plates. In a shallow dish, beat egg; season with salt and black pepper. Pat celeriac dry with paper towels. Dip celeriac into flour, then egg, then pecans, turning to coat all over and shaking off excess at each step.

4. In a large deep saucepan, heat oil over medium-high heat until a candy/deep-fry thermometer registers 350°F (180°C). In batches, add celeriac to oil; deep-fry, turning once, for 3 minutes or until golden brown and tender inside. Using a slotted spoon, transfer to prepared plate; let drain.

5. Serve fries with mascarpone dip and lime wedges.

Mushroom Fritters with Gorgonzola Dip

Deep-fried mushrooms are a real treat, and they're even more pleasing when they're dunked in a creamy blue cheese dip.

Tips

Gorgonzola is a creamy, versatile blue cheese, but you can certainly experiment with other blue cheeses if you prefer them.

This recipe makes a lot of batter, but you need that much to ensure the mushrooms are well coated. The nutrient values below don't include the batter that is discarded.

- Candy/deep-fry thermometer
- Plate, lined with paper towels

3 tbsp	milk	45 mL
2 tbsp	whole-grain spelt flour	30 mL
1 tbsp	ground almonds	15 mL
1	egg	1
	Salt and freshly ground black pepper	
2 oz	Gorgonzola cheese (see tips, at left)	60 g
¼ cup	heavy or whipping (35%) cream	60 mL
2 tsp	walnut oil (see tip, page 181)	10 mL
	Grated zest of 1 organic lemon	
	Oil for deep-frying (see page 162)	
4 oz	mushrooms	125 g
	Chopped fresh parsley	

1. In a bowl, stir together milk, flour, almonds and egg until smooth; season with salt and pepper. Let stand for 15 minutes.

2. Meanwhile, in another bowl, mash cheese with a fork; stir in cream, walnut oil and lemon zest until smooth. Season with salt and pepper to taste.

3. In a large deep saucepan, heat oil over medium-high heat until a candy/deep-fry thermometer registers 350°F (180°C).

4. Meanwhile, trim mushroom stems. Dip mushrooms into batter, turning to coat. In batches, add to oil; deep-fry, turning once, for 2 to 3 minutes or until golden brown. Using a slotted spoon, transfer mushrooms to prepared plate; let drain.

5. Serve mushrooms with Gorgonzola dip; garnish with parsley.

Nutrients per serving

Calories	765
Fat	66 g
Carbohydrates	17 g
Protein	26 g

Shrimp Fritters with Lime Dip

Makes 1 serving

**Prep time:
25 minutes**

If you love shrimp, these fritters will make your taste buds very happy. You can serve them with a simple green salad for a light dinner.

Tip

Lemongrass has very tough outer leaves that protect the flavorful core. Make sure to peel them off and discard them before you prepare the lemongrass. And since the inner leaves are still a bit fibrous, mincing them will ensure your shrimp fritters have the best texture.

* **Mini food processor**

5 oz	thawed frozen shrimp, peeled and deveined	150 g
½	stalk fresh lemongrass (see tip, at left)	½
1 tbsp	lime juice, divided	15 mL
1	egg white	1
	Salt and cayenne pepper	
2 tbsp	canola oil	30 mL
¼ cup	crème fraîche	60 mL
1	stalk celery	1
1	green chile pepper, seeded and minced	1

1. Finely chop shrimp. Trim and remove woody outer leaves from lemongrass; mince lemongrass. In a mini food processor, purée together shrimp, lemongrass, 2 tsp (10 mL) of the lime juice and half of the egg white (discard remaining half) until very finely chopped and mixture holds together when pressed. Season with salt and cayenne pepper.

2. In a nonstick skillet, heat oil over medium heat. Using 1 tbsp (15 mL) for each fritter, spoon shrimp mixture into skillet; press to flatten slightly. Fry patties, turning once, for 4 minutes or until golden, and shrimp is pink, firm and opaque.

3. Meanwhile, in a bowl, stir crème fraîche with remaining lime juice; season to taste with salt. Halve celery; mince half. Cut remaining celery into sticks. Stir minced celery and chile pepper into crème fraîche mixture. Serve with shrimp fritters and celery sticks.

Nutrients per serving	
Calories	557
Fat	46 g
Carbohydrates	3 g
Protein	32 g

Coconut Calamari with Avocado Dip

Golden, crispy and supremely satisfying, calamari is even more pleasing with this spicy avocado dip alongside.

Tip

Sambal oelek is a spicy Asian chile sauce. If you can't find it, substitute another Asian chile sauce or your favorite hot sauce.

½	ripe avocado (about 4 oz/125 g), peeled, pitted and finely chopped	½
1 tbsp	lime juice	15 mL
1 tbsp	crème fraîche	15 mL
½ tsp	sambal oelek (see tip, at left)	2 mL
1	green onion (white and light green parts), finely chopped	1
	Salt and freshly ground black pepper	
5 oz	cleaned squid (see tip, below)	150 g
3 tbsp	unsweetened shredded coconut	45 mL
1 tbsp	coconut flour (see tips, page 233)	15 mL
1	egg, lightly beaten	1
2 tbsp	olive oil	30 mL

1. In a bowl and using a fork, mash together one-third of the avocado, the lime juice, crème fraîche and sambal oelek. Stir in green onion and remaining avocado. Season to taste with salt and pepper.

2. Pat squid dry with paper towels; cut into rings. Season with salt and pepper. In separate shallow dishes, spread out shredded coconut, coconut flour and egg. Dip squid into flour, then egg, then coconut, turning to coat all over and shaking off excess at each step.

3. In a nonstick skillet, heat oil over medium heat. Add squid; fry, turning once, for 5 to 10 minutes or until golden brown and crisp. Serve squid with avocado dip.

Prep Tip

If you can, buy squid that's already been cleaned. It's more expensive, but it will save you time. If you can't find cleaned squid, buy whole squid and clean them at home. First, pull off the head, along with the innards. Cut off the tentacles just below the head; discard head and innards. Squeeze the tentacles at the top; remove and discard the hard beak. Squeeze the tube-shaped body; pull out and discard the transparent cuttlebone (it looks like a long piece of clear plastic). Slice the tube into rings, and the squid is ready to cook.

Nutrients per serving	
Calories	913
Fat	82 g
Carbohydrates	5 g
Protein	38 g

Camembert with Ramp Vinaigrette

Makes 1 serving

Prep time: 25 minutes

Camembert cheese is a pleasure on its own as an appetizer, but this healthy vinaigrette gives it even more depth of flavor.

Tip

Ramps are wild leeks, a great delicacy and a time-honored spring treat. In Germany, this recipe is made with wild garlic leaves (called Bärlauch), which are similar. Both are in season for only a short while.

1	round Camembert cheese (4 oz/125 g)	1
1	small red onion	1
1 tbsp	cider vinegar	15 mL
1 tbsp	lemon juice	15 mL
1 tbsp	canola oil	15 mL
1 tsp	flaxseed oil	5 mL
1 tsp	hot mustard	5 mL
	Salt and freshly ground black pepper	
3	ramp leaves (see tip, at left)	3

1. Cut cheese into slices; arrange on a plate. Halve and thinly slice red onion; sprinkle over cheese.

2. In a bowl, whisk cider vinegar with lemon juice until combined; whisk in canola oil, flaxseed oil and mustard until blended. Season to taste with salt and pepper.

3. Cut ramp leaves into very thin strips; stir into vinaigrette. Drizzle vinaigrette over cheese. Let stand for 10 minutes.

Substitution Tip

When you can find tender ramps at the store or farmer's market, turn them into homemade pesto and freeze it for later in the year. Substitute 1 tsp (5 mL) of the pesto for the leaves in this vinaigrette and garnish the dish with 1 tbsp (15 mL) chopped fresh chives.

Nutrients per serving	
Calories	422
Fat	32 g
Carbohydrates	3 g
Protein	30 g

Pear with Gorgonzola Cream

This is a sophisticated starter or side dish. A ripe pear really is the perfect partner for creamy, tangy blue cheese.

Tip

If you enjoy a fruit-and-cheese course after a meal, this dish also makes a refreshing alternative to dessert.

1 tbsp	chopped hazelnuts	15 mL
1/2	firm ripe pear (about 2 1/2 oz/75 g), peeled and cored	1/2
1 tbsp	lemon juice	15 mL
	Salt and freshly ground black pepper	
1 1/2 oz	Gorgonzola cheese (see tip, below)	45 g
2 tbsp	cream cheese	30 mL
1	leaf radicchio	1

1. In a dry nonstick skillet over medium heat, toast hazelnuts, shaking pan often, for 3 to 5 minutes or until fragrant and golden brown. Transfer to a plate; let cool.

2. Cut pear lengthwise into thin slices. Arrange on a plate; drizzle with lemon juice to prevent browning. Season to taste with salt and pepper.

3. In a small bowl and using a fork, mash Gorgonzola cheese; mash in cream cheese until smooth. Season to taste with salt and pepper. Spoon dollops of cheese mixture over pears.

4. Cut radicchio leaf into shreds; sprinkle over pear mixture. Garnish with hazelnuts.

Shopping Tip

Gorgonzola is a delicious option, but the creamy cheese mixture would be wonderful with many other blue cheeses. Look for local varieties and support artisanal cheesemakers in your area.

Nutrients per serving	
Calories	295
Fat	21 g
Carbohydrates	12 g
Protein	14 g

Parsnip Chips

These homemade chips will mean you'll never miss potato chips again. They are crisp and golden, and make a terrific snack.

Tip

These chips are wonderful with all sorts of spicy additions. Curry powder comes in a variety of types and heat levels. You can also experiment with different exotic salts. If you like, try paprika on them, too. It comes in sweet, hot and smoked varieties, which are all tasty.

- Sharp chef's knife or mandoline
- Plate, lined with paper towels

3½ oz	parsnip (about 1 large)	100 g
3 tbsp	coconut oil	45 mL
	Curry powder or salt (see tip, at left)	

1. If desired, peel parsnip (see tip, below). Using a sharp chef's knife or mandoline, slice parsnip as thinly as possible. Pat slices dry with paper towels.

2. In a deep saucepan, heat coconut oil over medium-high heat. Test the temperature by dipping the handle of a wooden spoon into the hot oil; if plenty of bubbles rise from the handle, the oil is the correct temperature.

3. Add parsnip slices to oil; fry, turning often, for about 5 minutes or until golden brown. Using a slotted spoon, transfer parsnips to prepared plate. Let drain.

4. Season chips to taste with curry powder.

Prep Tip

If your parsnips are young and tender, they don't really need to be peeled before you eat them. Older parsnips have a woodier texture, so those do need peeling. In either case, scrub them well to get any dirt out of the little crevices in the peel.

Nutrients per serving

Calories	250
Fat	27 g
Carbohydrates	2 g
Protein	1 g

Avocado Mascarpone Dip

Makes 2 servings

Prep time: 15 minutes

A ripe avocado has just the right silky texture for this dip. To check for ripeness, press the avocado with your thumb; it should yield to gentle pressure.

Tip

Mascarpone cheese is excellent in both sweet and savory dishes. It makes a wonderful base for crêpe fillings, and is lovely with fresh fruit and a pinch of healthy sugar (see page 158) for dessert.

- **Mini food processor or blender**

½	small ripe avocado (about 4 oz/125 g)	½
1 tbsp	lime juice	15 mL
2 oz	mascarpone cheese (see tip, at left)	60 g
1	small green onion (white and light green parts)	1
	Salt and freshly ground black pepper	
	Cayenne pepper	
	Grated organic lime zest	

1. Pit avocado; spoon out flesh and cut into chunks. In a mini food processor, purée together avocado, lime juice and cheese until smooth. Transfer to a bowl.

2. Trim and thinly slice green onion. Fold into avocado purée. Season with salt, black pepper, cayenne pepper and lime zest to taste.

Nutrients per serving	
Calories	207
Fat	21 g
Carbohydrates	1 g
Protein	2 g

Quark and Chive Spread

Makes 1 serving

**Prep time:
10 minutes**

Fresh chives are so easy to grow in the garden (or even in a pot on your windowsill). This dip is a good showcase for their fresh, oniony flavor.

Tip

Shelled hemp seeds are a nutritious addition to the cancer-fighting diet (see box, page 162). Look for them in health and bulk food stores. They have become very popular in recent years, and some brands are now available in supermarkets, as well.

¼ cup	quark (see tips, page 202)	60 mL
¼ cup	kefir (see tips, page 178)	60 mL
1 tsp	special oil mixture (see page 161)	5 mL
½ tsp	heavy or whipping (35%) cream	2 mL
½ tsp	shelled hemp seeds (see tip, at left)	2 mL
	Salt	
1½ tsp	snipped or chopped fresh chives (see tip, opposite)	7 mL

1. In a bowl, stir together quark, kefir, special oil mixture and cream until smooth and creamy.
2. Stir in hemp seeds. Season to taste with salt. Sprinkle with chives.

Serving Idea

This makes a nice, light spread for an open-faced sandwich on high-protein bread. Try it on a slice of homemade High-Protein Flaxseed Bread (recipe, page 206).

Nutrients per serving	
Calories	170
Fat	13 g
Carbohydrates	4 g
Protein	9 g

Radish and Cottage Cheese Spread

Makes 1 serving

**Prep time:
10 minutes**

Radishes are one of the first vegetables to pop up in gardens or at farmer's markets in the spring. They can be gritty, so make sure you scrub them well before you grate them.

Tip

Kitchen or poultry shears are the perfect tool for snipping fresh chives. They make the job so fast and easy.

½ cup	cottage cheese (see tip, below)	125 mL
3 tbsp	sour cream	45 mL
1 tbsp	special oil mixture (see page 161)	15 mL
3	radishes	3
1 tbsp	snipped or chopped fresh chives (see tip, at left), or to taste	15 mL

1. In a bowl, stir together cottage cheese, sour cream and special oil mixture.

2. Using the coarse side of a box grater, grate radishes. Stir into cottage cheese mixture along with chives.

Shopping Tip

Cottage cheese and sour cream come in different varieties, with different percentages of milk fat. Choose full-fat cottage cheese and sour cream when you're on the cancer-fighting diet, because your body needs the fat to create energy.

Nutrients per serving	
Calories	357
Fat	29 g
Carbohydrates	6 g
Protein	17 g

Sheep Cheese and Herb Spread

A mix of fresh herbs and walnuts (and a little garlic, if you like it), give this savory spread lots of personality. The crunch of the nuts is a nice contrast to the creamy texture.

Tips

Manouri cheese is a mildly flavored semisoft Greek cheese made from sheep's milk (or sometimes goat's milk). It is made from whey, like ricotta, but has a firmer texture. If you can't find it, you can substitute another fresh, mild cheese in this spread.

Quark is a German fresh cheese similar to the French cheese fromage frais. Choose the full-fat variety when you're on the cancer-fighting diet unless otherwise specified in a recipe.

2 oz	Manouri cheese (see tips, at left)	60 g
2 tbsp	quark (see tips, at left)	30 mL
2 or 3	sprigs fresh herbs, such as chervil, basil and/or parsley	2 or 3
4	walnut halves	4
1	small clove garlic, minced (optional)	1
	Salt and freshly ground black pepper	

1. In a bowl, and using a fork, mash cheese; stir in quark until smooth.

2. Wash herbs and shake dry; pull leaves off stems. Finely chop herbs and walnuts; stir into cheese mixture until combined.

3. Stir garlic (if using) into cheese mixture. Season to taste with salt and pepper.

Serving Idea

For a tasty open-faced sandwich, spread this mixture over a slice of High-Protein Flaxseed Bread (recipe, page 206) and top with slices of juicy, fresh tomato and fresh basil leaves.

Nutrients per serving	
Calories	210
Fat	19 g
Carbohydrates	3 g
Protein	7 g

Creamy Tuna Spread

This is a wonderful alternative to the usual mayonnaise-based tuna salads. Enjoy it on slices of high-protein bread for lunch or with homemade crackers for a protein-packed snack.

Tips

A kitchen scale is a terrific investment when you're watching portion sizes and carb content. Make sure you buy one with a tare button. That way, you can place a measuring cup on the scale and zero it, and the scale will weigh only the contents of the cup.

Make sure you choose full-fat cream cheese for this recipe. It has the fat your body needs on the cancer-fighting diet.

2 oz	drained canned tuna (see tip, below)	60 g
1	shallot	1
7 tbsp	cream cheese (see tips, at left)	100 mL
1 tsp	white balsamic vinegar	5 mL
	Salt and freshly ground black pepper	
1 tbsp	snipped or chopped fresh chives (see tip, page 201)	15 mL

1. Finely chop tuna and shallot. In a bowl, stir together tuna, shallot and cream cheese until smooth.

2. Stir in white balsamic vinegar; season to taste with salt and pepper. Sprinkle with chives.

Substitution Tip

This spread also tastes delicious if you make it with cooked trout fillets instead of tuna.

Nutrients per serving	
Calories	113
Fat	4 g
Carbohydrates	3 g
Protein	14 g

Paprika Cheese Spread

*Parmesan cheese adds
a delightful savoriness
to this creamy spread.
Avoid tubs of pregrated
Parmesan cheese, as
they often include
additives you don't want.*

Tip

Hungary is the traditional
home of paprika, and
the spice comes in many
varieties. The most
renowned type is sweet
(mild) rose paprika,
which is ground from
the highest-quality dried
red pepper flesh. There
are many other kinds,
including those made
from whole peppers
(including the seeds)
and those that have been
smoked. Paprika is very
popular in cooking and
easy to find.

3½ oz	ricotta cheese	100 g
2 tbsp	grated Parmesan cheese	30 mL
½ tsp	sweet paprika (see tip, at left)	2 mL
	Salt and freshly ground black pepper	
1	each mini red and green bell pepper	1

1. In a bowl, stir ricotta cheese with Parmesan cheese until creamy. Stir in paprika until blended. Season to taste with salt and pepper.

2. Halve and seed red and green peppers; finely chop. Stir into cream cheese mixture.

Variation

Bavarian-Style Paprika Cheese Spread: Replace ricotta and Parmesan cheeses with 3½ oz (100 g) ripe Camembert cheese and 2 tbsp (30 mL) butter, softened.

Serving Idea

For delicious canapés, spread the cheese mixture over slices of high-protein bread (see page 157), sprinkle with thinly sliced green onion and dust with a little more paprika. Cut into fingers or fancy shapes.

Nutrients per serving	
Calories	126
Fat	9 g
Carbohydrates	2 g
Protein	7 g

Easy Low-Carb Bread

Makes 5 loaves

Prep time: 45 minutes

These small quick loaves are simple to make and shape, and they're tasty with all kinds of toppings. Experiment with a mix of seeds according to your preferences. Add more or less depending on how crunchy you like your bread.

Tip

The seeds you add to the dough increase the protein and fiber content of the bread. Pumpkin seeds and flax seeds are especially healthy and delicious.

- Preheat oven to 350°F (180°C)
- Baking sheet, lined with parchment paper

⅔ cup	finely ground oat bran (see tip, page 175)	150 mL
7 tbsp	almond flour	100 mL
7 tbsp	chopped almonds	100 mL
7 tbsp	ground psyllium husks	100 mL
1 tsp	baking powder	5 mL
¼ tsp	salt	1 mL
¾ cup + 2 tbsp	sour cream (see tip, below)	200 mL
2	eggs	2
1 tbsp	canola oil	15 mL
	Mixed seeds (such as sesame, flax, pumpkin or sunflower seeds)	

1. In a large bowl, whisk together oat bran, almond flour, almonds, psyllium husks, baking powder and salt. In another bowl, stir together sour cream, eggs and canola oil. Stir into flour mixture just until combined.

2. Turn dough out onto floured work surface. Knead until smooth; knead in seeds. Shape dough into 5 loaves.

3. Arrange loaves on prepared baking sheet. Using a sharp knife, make several diagonal cuts into the top of each loaf. Bake in preheated oven for 25 minutes or until golden brown.

4. Transfer loaves to a wire rack; let cool.

Shopping Tip

Choose full-fat sour cream for the recipes in this book. It is the best choice for baking, and it contains healthy fat and the lactic acid–fermented milk that your body needs.

Nutrients per loaf

Calories	270
Fat	21 g
Carbohydrates	8 g
Protein	13 g

High-Protein Flaxseed Bread

Makes 1 loaf, about 20 slices (each about 1½ oz/45 g)

Prep time: 3¼ hours

Spelt is a relative of wheat, and thanks to its high gluten content, it is very well suited for baking. If you like, you can substitute whole-grain einkorn flour for the spelt flour.

Tip

In Germany, many breads are made with a traditional spice mixture called Brotgewürz, which usually contains caraway seeds, aniseed, fennel seeds and ground coriander. You can buy premade mixtures online from stores that specialize in German ingredients. Or you can experiment and make your own blend to taste.

- **12- by 4-inch (30 by 11 cm) loaf pan, greased**

1⅔ cups	whole-grain spelt flour	400 mL
1¼ cups	spelt bran	300 mL
¾ cup + 2 tbsp	buckwheat flour	200 mL
¾ cup + 2 tsp	dark rye flour	185 mL
½ cup	flax seeds, ground if desired (see tip, opposite)	125 mL
1	piece (1½ oz/45 g) fresh cake yeast (see tip, page 209)	1
1½ cups	buttermilk, heated to lukewarm, divided	375 mL
½ tsp	raw cane sugar	2 mL
2 tbsp	canola oil	30 mL
1½ tsp	bread spice mixture (see tip, at left), optional	7 mL
1¼ tsp	sea salt	6 mL

1. In a large bowl, whisk together spelt flour, spelt bran, buckwheat flour, rye flour and flax seeds. Make a well in the center and crumble in yeast. Add ⅓ cup (75 mL) of the buttermilk and sugar to well. Stir yeast mixture, incorporating a little flour from the edge of the well. Cover bowl and let stand in a warm place for 10 minutes or until yeast mixture is frothy.

2. Stir in remaining buttermilk, oil, bread spice mixture (if using) and salt until dough forms. Knead until dough is smooth. Cover and let rise in a warm place for 45 minutes.

3. Turn dough out onto floured work surface; knead until dough is smooth and elastic. Pat out dough, then roll up into cylinder, pinching ends to seal. Place in prepared loaf pan; pat top gently to smooth. Brush top lightly with water. Cover and let rise in pan for 30 minutes or until puffed up.

Nutrients per slice	
Calories	117
Fat	4 g
Carbohydrates	15 g
Protein	6 g

4. Meanwhile, preheat oven to 400°F (200°C). Place an ovenproof dish filled with boiling water on the bottom of preheated oven. Bake bread in center of oven for 1 hour or until golden brown all over.

5. Let cool in pan on a wire rack for 5 minutes. Transfer bread to rack; let cool completely.

Substitution Tip

Instead of flax seeds, try shelled hemp seeds or a mix of oily seeds, such as coarsely chopped hulled raw pumpkin seeds, sesame seeds or camelina seeds. Camelina (also known as gold-of-pleasure, wild flax or false flax) is an old-fashioned crop that was appreciated by the Celts for its healing properties. It also contains a large amount of omega-3 fatty acids.

Spelt and Nut Bread

Makes 1 loaf, about 25 slices (each about 1½ oz/45 g)

Prep time: 3 hours

This free-form loaf is rustic and studded with crunchy nuts and millet. It's wonderful toasted or topped with delicious spreads (see pages 200 to 204).

Tip

Look for whole-grain flours, and less-common soy and millet flours, at health food stores or in the natural foods aisle of the grocery store.

- **Baking sheet, lined with parchment paper**

2½ cups	whole-grain spelt flour (see tip, at left)	625 mL
¾ cup + 2 tbsp	soy flour	200 mL
¾ cup + 2 tbsp	millet flour	200 mL
1	piece (1½ oz/45 g) fresh cake yeast (see tip, opposite)	1
1⅔ cups	buttermilk, heated to lukewarm, divided	400 mL
1 tsp	raw cane sugar	5 mL
1	egg	1
1 cup	ground almonds	250 mL
6 tbsp	chopped walnuts	90 mL
2 tsp	sea salt	10 mL
¼ cup	chopped hazelnuts	60 mL

1. In a large bowl, whisk together spelt, soy and millet flours. Make a well in the center and crumble in yeast. Add ⅓ cup (75 mL) of the buttermilk and sugar to well. Stir yeast mixture, incorporating a little flour from the edge of the well. Cover bowl and let stand in a warm place for 15 minutes or until yeast mixture is frothy.

2. Stir in remaining buttermilk, egg, almonds, walnuts and salt until dough forms. Knead until dough is smooth. Cover and let rise in a warm place for 45 minutes.

3. Turn dough out onto floured work surface; knead until dough is smooth and elastic. Shape into an elongated loaf; place on prepared baking sheet. Using a damp, sharp knife, make three ¼-inch (0.5 cm) slashes in the top of the loaf. Brush top with a little more buttermilk; sprinkle with hazelnuts, pressing lightly to adhere. Cover and let rise for 30 minutes or until puffed up.

Nutrients per slice	
Calories	128
Fat	6 g
Carbohydrates	12 g
Protein	6 g

4. Meanwhile, preheat oven to 400°F (200°C). Place an ovenproof dish filled with boiling water on the bottom of preheated oven. Bake bread in center of oven for 50 minutes or until golden brown all over.

5. Let cool on pan on a wire rack for 5 minutes. Transfer bread to rack; let cool completely.

Substitution Tip

Fresh cake yeast is a staple for baking in Europe, and some stores in North America now carry it. It comes in different-size cubes, so use a digital scale to weigh the amount you need for this recipe. If you can't find it, you can substitute 3 packages (each 7 g) active dry yeast for the amount in this recipe.

Savory Cheese Crackers

Following the cancer-fighting diet doesn't mean giving up tasty snacks like these crackers. Try them with one of the spreads on pages 200 to 204.

Spotlight

Einkorn is an ancestor of today's hybrid wheat varieties. It has single-grain spikes, which give it its German name — *ein* means "one" and *korn* means "grain." It is experiencing a renaissance, especially among organic producers. Einkorn is high in protein (19 g in 3½ oz/100 g), essential amino acids and minerals. It has a delicate, nutty flavor and is highly nutritious due to the large amount of carotenoids it contains. These also give the flour its characteristic yellow color.

- Preheat oven to 350°F (180°C)
- Baking sheet, lined with parchment paper

¾ cup + 2 tbsp	ground psyllium husks	200 mL
¾ cup + 2 tbsp	finely ground oat bran (see tip, page 175)	200 mL
¾ cup	whole-grain einkorn flour (see spotlight, at left)	175 mL
1½ tsp	baking powder	7 mL
1½ tsp	salt	7 mL
1 tsp	sweet paprika	5 mL
1	egg	1
3½ oz	Emmental cheese, finely shredded	100 g
¾ cup	grated Parmesan cheese	175 mL
½ cup	heavy or whipping (35%) cream	125 mL
½ cup	cold butter, cubed	125 mL
1	egg yolk	1
1 tsp	water	5 mL
	Nuts (such as chopped pistachios, almonds, walnuts or hazelnuts), seeds (such as poppy seeds, caraway seeds or sesame seeds) or coarse salt (optional)	

1. In a large bowl, whisk together psyllium husks, oat bran, flour, baking powder, salt and paprika. Stir in egg, Emmental and Parmesan cheeses, and cream.

2. Knead in butter just until smooth dough forms. If dough is too sticky, refrigerate it for a few minutes before continuing.

3. Between sheets of parchment or waxed paper, roll out dough to about ½-inch (1 cm) thickness. Remove top paper; cut into 1½-inch (4 cm) squares. Arrange on prepared baking sheet.

4. In a small bowl, whisk egg yolk with water; brush over dough. Sprinkle dough with nuts (if using).

5. Bake in preheated oven for 20 minutes or until golden brown. Transfer crackers to a wire rack; let cool completely.

Nutrients per cracker	
Calories	70
Fat	6 g
Carbohydrates	3 g
Protein	3 g

Dietary Fiber Cookies

**Makes about
30 cookies**

Prep time: 1 hour

*Sure, you can buy
high-fiber biscuits at
the drugstore, but these
homemade savory
ones are so much
more delicious and
fun to make. Plus, you
don't have to worry
about added sugar
or preservatives.*

Tips

You can use whole flax
seeds instead of already
ground ones, but starting
with ones that are already
coarsely ground gives
you a head start in the
coffee grinder.

To crush caraway seeds
easily, place them on a
cutting board and press
down firmly on them
with the bottom of a
heavy saucepan. As they
crack, they'll become
more fragrant.

- Preheat oven to 350°F (180°C)
- Coffee or spice grinder
- Baking sheet, lined with parchment paper

1¾ cups	coarsely ground flax seeds (see tips, at left)	425 mL
¾ cup	sesame seeds	175 mL
1¾ cups	almond flour	425 mL
1½ cups	ground psyllium husks	375 mL
3 tbsp	each coriander seeds and crushed caraway seeds (see tips, at left)	45 mL
1 tbsp	baking soda	15 mL
1¾ tsp	salt	8 mL
1 tsp	baking powder	5 mL
1⅔ cups	water	400 mL
1	egg	1
2 tbsp	vinegar	30 mL

1. Using a clean coffee or spice grinder, finely grind flax seeds with sesame seeds. Transfer to a large bowl. Stir in almond flour, psyllium husks, coriander seeds, caraway seeds, baking soda, salt and baking powder.

2. In another bowl, whisk together water, egg and vinegar until foamy. Stir into flour mixture to form sticky dough, adding a little more water if necessary.

3. With moistened hands, form dough into about 2½-inch (6 cm) balls; arrange on prepared baking sheet, pressing to flatten. Using a damp, sharp knife, make an X in the top of each.

4. Bake in preheated oven for 30 minutes. Brush tops lightly with water; return to oven and bake for 15 minutes or until lightly browned and firm.

Nutrients per cookie	
Calories	75
Fat	5 g
Carbohydrates	1 g
Protein	7 g

Cheese Sticks with Poppy Seeds and Peanuts

Makes 40 pieces		

**Prep time:
1¼ hours**

This surprising combination of ingredients yields a deliciously crumbly treat you'll love. The sticks are wonderful as snacks or appetizers.

Tip

If you store these sticks in a tightly sealed airtight container in a cool place, they will stay fresh for about 2 weeks.

- Pastry blender
- Pastry wheel or pizza cutter
- 2 baking sheets, lined with parchment paper

1¼ cups	whole-grain spelt flour	300 mL
5 oz	Emmental cheese, finely shredded	150 g
⅔ cup	cold butter, cubed	150 mL
2 tbsp	water	30 mL
	Salt	
	Cayenne pepper	
1	egg yolk	1
2 tbsp	heavy or whipping (35%) cream	30 mL
2 tbsp	poppy seeds	30 mL
⅓ cup	unsalted peanuts, chopped	75 mL

1. In a large bowl, whisk flour with cheese. Using a pastry blender, cut in butter until in crumbs. Using a fork, briskly stir in water, and salt and cayenne pepper to taste, to form sticky dough. Turn out onto floured work surface and knead a few times to make smooth dough. Divide in half; wrap each in plastic wrap or waxed paper and refrigerate for 30 minutes or until chilled.

2. Preheat oven to 400°F (200°C). On floured work surface, roll out one half of the dough to ¼-inch (0.5 cm) thickness. Using a pastry wheel or pizza cutter, cut dough into ¾- by 3-inch (2 by 7.5 cm) rectangles. Place on one of the prepared baking sheets. Repeat with remaining dough. Place on remaining baking sheet.

3. In a small bowl, stir egg yolk with cream; brush over rectangles. Sprinkle poppy seeds over rectangles on one baking sheet. Sprinkle peanuts over rectangles on second baking sheet.

4. Bake in the top and bottom thirds of preheated oven, turning and switching pans halfway through, for 8 to 10 minutes or until golden brown.

5. Let cool completely on pans on wire racks.

Nutrients per piece	
Calories	69
Fat	6 g
Carbohydrates	3 g
Protein	2 g

Gorgonzola Scones

*If you like blue cheese,
these scones will be
your new favorites.
Little flecks of sun-dried
tomatoes give each bite
a slight sweetness that's
lovely with the cheese
and herbs.*

Tip

When a baking
recipe calls for milk,
be sure to use full-
fat (homogenized)
milk. It will give the
best results.

- Preheat oven to 400°F (200°C)
- 2-inch (5 cm) round biscuit cutter
- Baking sheet, lined with parchment paper

5 oz	Gorgonzola cheese (see tip, page 197)	150 g
6 tbsp	milk (see tip, at left), divided	90 mL
1/3 cup	canola oil	75 mL
1	egg	1
1 tsp	salt	5 mL
3/4 cup	dry-packed sun-dried tomatoes, finely chopped	175 mL
2 tbsp	coarsely ground flax seeds	30 mL
1 tbsp	chopped fresh thyme	15 mL
1 tbsp	chopped fresh parsley	15 mL
1 1/3 cups	whole-grain spelt flour	325 mL
2 tsp	cream of tartar	10 mL
1	egg yolk	1

1. Cut rind off cheese and discard; chop cheese. In a large bowl, stir together cheese, 1/4 cup (60 mL) of the milk, the oil, egg and salt until almost smooth. Stir in sun-dried tomatoes, flax seeds, thyme and parsley.

2. In another bowl, whisk flour with cream of tartar. Stir into cheese mixture to make ragged dough.

3. Turn dough out onto floured work surface. Knead just until smooth. Roll out dough to 3/4- to 1-inch (2 to 2.5 cm) thickness. Using a 2-inch (5 cm) round biscuit cutter, cut out scones, rerolling scraps once. Arrange on prepared baking sheet. In a small bowl, stir egg yolk with remaining milk; brush over scones.

4. Bake in preheated oven for 15 minutes or until golden brown. Transfer to a wire rack; eat warm or let cool to room temperature.

Nutrients per scone	
Calories	96
Fat	6 g
Carbohydrates	6 g
Protein	4 g

Blueberry and Nut Muffins

Blueberry muffins are usually packed with sugar and white flour, but this healthier version contains far fewer carbs. Indulge in them for breakfast or an afternoon treat with a cup of tea or coffee.

Tip

If you would like to make a gluten-free version of these muffins, you can substitute quinoa flour for the spelt flour.

- **Preheat oven to 350°F (180°C)**
- **12-cup muffin pan, greased or lined with paper liners**

¾ cup + 2 tbsp	whole-grain spelt flour (see tip, at left)	200 mL
1¼ cups	ground hazelnuts	300 mL
1¾ oz	soy flakes (see tips, below)	50 g
2 tsp	cream of tartar	10 mL
1	egg	1
¾ cup + 2 tbsp	buttermilk	200 mL
7 tbsp	canola oil	100 mL
3 tbsp	raw cane sugar	45 mL
½ tsp	vanilla powder (see tips, below)	2 mL
1⅓ cups	fresh or thawed frozen blueberries	325 mL

1. In a bowl, whisk together flour, hazelnuts, soy flakes and cream of tartar. In a large bowl, whisk together egg, buttermilk, oil, sugar and vanilla powder until smooth. Stir in flour mixture just until combined; fold in blueberries.

2. Spoon batter into prepared muffin cups, filling each about two-thirds full. Bake in preheated oven for 20 to 25 minutes or until golden brown and firm.

3. Transfer muffins to rack; let cool.

Variation

Carrot and Nut Muffins: Substitute 3 carrots (about 7 oz/210 g), coarsely grated, for the blueberrries, and 1 tsp (5 mL) grated organic lemon zest for the vanilla powder.

Shopping Tips

Soy flakes are steamed and rolled soybeans, and look similar to rolled oats. Look for them at health and bulk food stores.

Vanilla powder is simply ground dried vanilla beans. Buy pure versions, which contain no starch or preservatives. The powder adds an intense vanilla flavor to baking.

Nutrients per muffin	
Calories	214
Fat	16 g
Carbohydrates	12 g
Protein	5 g

Sandwiches and Soups

Horseradish and Smoked Salmon Sandwich

This is a deli classic that's also good for you. The horseradish is so flavorful, and you can add a little more if you like a spicier sandwich.

Tip

Choose full-fat cream cheese for this recipe. It's not only tastier than the light stuff but also better for you when you're following the cancer-fighting diet.

2 tbsp	cream cheese (see tip, at left)	30 mL
1 tsp	prepared horseradish	5 mL
	Salt and freshly ground black pepper	
1	organic mini cucumber	1
1	slice (about 1½ oz/45 g) high-protein bread (see page 157)	1
2	slices smoked salmon (about 1½ oz/45 g), see tips, below	2
	Fresh dill sprigs	

1. In a bowl, stir cream cheese with horseradish until smooth. Season to taste with salt and pepper. Slice cucumber.

2. Spread cream cheese mixture over bread; top with cucumber, overlapping slices. Top with smoked salmon.

3. Season to taste with pepper; garnish with dill sprigs.

Substitution Tips

If you like, you can substitute your favorite spreadable double-cream cheese, such as Boursin, for the cream cheese.

On the weekend, why not treat yourself to something a little more special? Instead of smoked salmon, top your sandwich with shrimp, smoked trout or caviar.

Nutrients per serving	
Calories	458
Fat	32 g
Carbohydrates	19 g
Protein	25 g

Open-Faced Avocado and Shrimp Sandwich

Avocados are the ultimate sandwich filling. They are creamy and rich tasting, and they offer a lot of healthy fat that your body needs.

Tip

Mashed avocado makes a nice spread for sandwiches on its own, as well. Try it as a replacement for mayonnaise.

½	small ripe avocado (about 4 oz/ 125 g), pitted (see tip, below)	½
3 tbsp	sour cream	45 mL
2 tsp	special oil mixture (see page 161)	10 mL
1 tsp	lemon juice	5 mL
2 tbsp	cooked small shrimp	30 mL
	Salt and freshly ground black pepper	
1	small slice (about 1 oz/30 g) high-protein bread (see page 157)	1

1. Using a spoon, scoop avocado flesh into a bowl. Using a fork, mash in sour cream, special oil mixture and lemon juice until smooth; stir in shrimp.

2. Season avocado mixture to taste with salt and pepper. Spread over bread.

Prep Tip

A ripe avocado should yield slightly to gentle pressure from your thumb. If it isn't quite ripe, you can still eat it, but you'll have to mash it a little more forcefully. To speed up the ripening process, enclose an avocado in a brown paper bag. It should be perfect in a day or so.

Nutrients per serving	
Calories	530
Fat	46 g
Carbohydrates	7 g
Protein	21 g

Egg Sandwich with Tomato Quark

When tomatoes are in season, this is the sandwich you want to make. Make sure you choose a juicy, brightly colored tomato for the best flavor, texture and nutrient value.

Tip

Quark is a German fresh cheese that is similar to a French fresh cheese called fromage frais. If you can't find either, you can drain plain yogurt to make yogurt cheese and use that instead.

1	egg	1
1 tsp	butter	5 mL
1	small slice (about 1 oz/30 g) high-protein bread (see page 157)	1
1	small ripe tomato (about 2 oz/60 g)	1
⅓ cup	quark (see tip, at left)	75 mL
2 tsp	special oil mixture (see page 161)	10 mL

1. In a saucepan, cover egg with cold water. Bring to a boil; boil for 10 minutes. Remove from heat; rinse egg under cold water. Let cool. Peel off shell.

2. Slice egg. Spread butter over bread; arrange egg slices over top.

3. Finely dice tomato. In a bowl, stir together quark, special oil mixture and tomato. Serve alongside egg sandwich.

Nutrients per serving

Calories	370
Fat	30 g
Carbohydrates	8 g
Protein	19 g

Open-Faced Radish, Cheese and Sprout Sandwich

Gruyère cheese is not only good for you on the cancer-fighting diet, but it also adds a touch of luxury to a lunchtime sandwich.

Tip

Rinse and drain sprouts well before adding them to sandwiches. Pat them dry lightly with a paper towel to keep them from making your sandwich soggy.

2 tbsp	quark (see tip, opposite)	30 mL
2 tsp	milk	10 mL
1 tsp	hot mustard	5 mL
	Salt	
1	slice (about 1½ oz/45 g) high-protein bread (see page 157)	1
1	handful white or red radish sprouts (see tips, below and left)	1
2	radishes	2
1	slice Gruyère cheese (about 1 oz/30 g)	1

1. In a bowl, stir together quark, milk and hot mustard until smooth. Season to taste with salt.

2. Spread quark mixture over bread. Set aside a few sprouts for garnish. Sprinkle remaining sprouts over quark mixture, pressing lightly to adhere.

3. Thinly slice radishes. Top sandwich with cheese, then radish slices. Garnish with reserved sprouts.

Shopping Tip

Sprouts from white (icicle) radish seeds are particularly spicy, and the mustard oils that make them spicy are also what make them so healthy. Mustard oils clear your sinuses and stimulate digestion, and their active ingredients are even said to prevent cancer. If you want a little milder flavor, use red (globe) radish sprouts instead. Look for fresh sprouts at farmer's markets and health food stores, which will have a good variety to choose from.

Nutrients per serving	
Calories	343
Fat	21 g
Carbohydrates	18 g
Protein	22 g

Apricot Quark Sandwiches

Makes 2 servings

**Prep time:
15 minutes**

This spread is sweet and creamy — just the thing for a quick breakfast or an energy-boosting lunch. It contains more carbs than some other spreads, so make sure you take that into account when you choose the rest of your meals for the day.

Tip

If apricots are not in season, you can make a similarly delicious spread with oranges.

2 tbsp	unsweetened shredded coconut	30 mL
²⁄₃ cup	quark (see tip, page 218)	150 mL
2 tbsp	heavy or whipping (35%) cream	30 mL
1 tsp	vanilla raw cane sugar (see tip, below)	5 mL
½ tsp	grated organic lemon zest	2 mL
2	ripe apricots (about 5 oz/150 g)	2
6	fresh mint leaves	6
2	slices (about 1½ oz/45 g each) high-protein bread (see page 157)	2

1. In a dry nonstick skillet over medium heat, toast coconut, shaking pan often, for 2 to 3 minutes or until fragrant and golden brown. Transfer to a bowl; let cool.

2. In another bowl, stir together quark, cream, vanilla sugar and lemon zest. Halve and pit apricots; cut 4 wedges and reserve for garnish. Dice remaining apricots; stir into quark mixture.

3. Wash mint leaves and pat dry. Cut 4 of the leaves into thin strips; stir into quark mixture along with half of the coconut.

4. Spread quark mixture over bread; sprinkle with remaining coconut. Garnish with reserved apricots and remaining mint leaves.

Prep Tip

If you can't find ready-made vanilla raw cane sugar, just make your own. Pour raw cane sugar into a jar and bury a vanilla bean (or two) in the mixture. Let it stand for a few days until the aroma permeates the sugar.

Nutrients per serving	
Calories	356
Fat	22 g
Carbohydrates	22 g
Protein	16 g

Egg and Chive Salad on Spelt Toast

Egg salad is another favorite sandwich filling that has all sorts of healthy fat and nutrients.

Tip

Look for small loaves of spelt bread in health food stores or the natural foods section of your supermarket. Make sure to check the label and watch the carbohydrate content (see page 157). Or bake a loaf of Spelt and Nut Bread (recipe, page 208) at home.

1	egg	1
1 tbsp	mayonnaise	15 mL
1 tbsp	snipped or chopped fresh chives (see tip, page 201), divided	15 mL
1	green onion (white and light green parts)	1
	Salt and freshly ground black pepper	
2	small slices (about 1 oz/30 g each) spelt bread (see tip, at left)	2

1. In a saucepan, cover egg with cold water. Bring to a boil; boil for 10 minutes. Remove from heat; rinse egg under cold water. Let cool. Peel off shell.

2. Cut 2 slices off egg and reserve for garnish. Finely chop remaining egg. In a bowl, stir together chopped egg, mayonnaise and 2 tsp (10 mL) of the chives.

3. Finely chop green onion; stir into egg mixture. Season to taste with salt and pepper.

4. Toast bread. Spread egg mixture over toast; sprinkle with remaining chives. Garnish with reserved egg slices.

Substitution Tip

This egg spread is tasty with fresh, crunchy vegetable additions, too. If you like, substitute 3 radishes, finely diced, or 1 small carrot, grated, for the green onion. Or just add them as extras along with the onion.

Nutrients per serving	
Calories	311
Fat	17 g
Carbohydrates	27 g
Protein	11 g

Broccoli Soup with Egg Garnish

Crisp sprouts and a tender soufflé-like egg garnish dress up this broccoli soup beautifully.

Tips

If you like something crunchy atop your soup, you can garnish it with toasted slivered almonds.

Don't eat the soup while it's still very hot. Let all of your dishes (especially soups and gratins) cool a little before you dig in. The heat can injure tender mucous membranes in your mouth, throat and esophagus. This can increase the likelihood of tumor cells forming in these areas.

- Preheat oven to 200°F (100°C)
- Small gratin dish, brushed with 1 tsp (5 mL) canola oil
- Roasting pan
- Immersion blender

2	small stalks broccoli	2
1	green onion (white and light green parts)	1
1	small tomato	1
1 tsp	butter	5 mL
1 cup	ready-to-use vegetable broth	250 mL
2 tbsp	chopped fresh parsley	30 mL
1 tbsp	heavy or whipping (35%) cream	15 mL
	Grated nutmeg	
	Salt and white pepper	
1 tbsp	broccoli sprouts	15 mL

Egg Garnish

1	egg	1
1 tbsp	heavy or whipping (35%) cream	15 mL
Pinch	grated nutmeg	Pinch
Pinch	salt	Pinch

1. **Egg Garnish:** In a bowl, whisk together egg, cream, nutmeg and salt; pour into prepared gratin dish. Place gratin dish in a roasting pan; fill roasting pan with enough hot water to come halfway up side. Bake in preheated oven for 45 minutes or until egg mixture is set and firm enough to cut.

2. Meanwhile, cut broccoli into florets; chop broccoli stems. Thinly slice green onion; core and dice tomato.

3. In a saucepan, melt butter over medium-high heat. Add green onion; sauté for 2 minutes or until translucent. Add broccoli and broth. Reduce heat to low and simmer for 20 minutes or until broccoli is tender.

4. Stir in parsley and cream. Using an immersion blender, purée soup until smooth. Season to taste with nutmeg, salt and pepper.

5. Cut egg garnish into bite-size pieces; arrange in a deep soup plate or bowl. Ladle soup over top; sprinkle with tomato and broccoli sprouts.

Nutrients per serving	
Calories	270
Fat	23 g
Carbohydrates	6 g
Protein	11 g

Tangy Zucchini Soup with Mixed Sprouts

Makes 1 serving

**Prep time:
20 minutes**

Sour cream gives this simple soup a bit of tang that's really pleasant. Soy flour is a great thickener and adds beneficial nutrients to the soup, as well.

Tips

Look for soy flour at health food stores or in the natural foods aisle of your supermarket.

Choose whatever sprouts suit your fancy, such as alfalfa, radish or broccoli sprouts. Or experiment with zippy onion sprouts for a change of pace.

• **Immersion blender**

1	zucchini	1
½	small carrot	½
1 tsp	soy flour (see tips, at left)	5 mL
¾ cup + 2 tbsp	ready-to-use chicken broth	200 mL
	Salt and freshly ground black pepper	
3 tbsp	sour cream (see tip, page 205)	45 mL
2 tsp	tomato paste	10 mL
¾ oz	mixed sprouts (see tip, below)	20 g

1. Using the coarse side of a box grater, grate zucchini. Using the fine side of a box grater, grate carrot.

2. Heat a dry saucepan over medium heat; add soy flour and cook, stirring, for about 5 minutes or until lightly browned. Standing back, pour in chicken broth (it will sizzle and spatter a bit); bring to a boil, stirring constantly.

3. Stir in zucchini; cook for 3 to 5 minutes or until soft. Season to taste with salt and pepper.

4. Stir in sour cream and tomato paste. Using an immersion blender, purée soup just until smooth.

5. Ladle soup into a deep soup plate or bowl. Just before serving, garnish with carrot and sprouts.

Prep Tip

A digital scale is great for measuring out the small amount of sprouts here. Since different sprouts are all different weights, this is a more accurate way to gauge the total serving size.

Nutrients per serving	
Calories	170
Fat	11 g
Carbohydrates	9 g
Protein	8 g

Cream of Fennel Soup

Orange zest and juice give this licorice-scented soup a bright, sunny flavor. Ground coriander adds a slightly lemony aroma, and you can add as much or as little of it as you like.

Tip

Freshly squeezed orange juice has the best flavor. Freeze any leftover juice to make more batches of this soup another day.

- **Immersion blender**

1	small bulb fennel	1
½ cup	ready-to-use vegetable broth	125 mL
2 tbsp	dry white wine or lemon juice	30 mL
2 tbsp	orange juice (see tip, at left)	30 mL
1 tsp	butter	5 mL
½ tsp	special oil mixture (see page 161)	2 mL
	Ground coriander	
	Freshly ground black pepper	
2 tbsp	heavy or whipping (35%) cream	30 mL
½ tsp	grated organic orange zest (see tip, below)	2 mL

1. Trim off fennel stems; reserve some of the feathery green fronds for garnish. Core and slice fennel thinly.

2. In a saucepan, combine broth and wine; bring to a boil. Add fennel; reduce heat and simmer for 10 to 15 minutes or until fennel is tender. Using an immersion blender, purée until smooth.

3. Add orange juice, butter and special oil mixture; stir until butter is melted. Season to taste with ground coriander and pepper.

4. Ladle soup into a deep soup plate or bowl. In another bowl, whip cream until stiff peaks form; spoon over soup. Garnish with orange zest and reserved fennel fronds.

Shopping Tip

Always choose organic citrus if you will be using the zest. It isn't contaminated with pesticides or other harmful chemicals.

Nutrients per serving	
Calories	220
Fat	15 g
Carbohydrates	6 g
Protein	4 g

Chilled Buttermilk Herb Soup with Parsnip Croutons

Makes 1 serving

Prep time: 45 minutes

Enjoy this soup on a hot summer day, when you can find all the fresh herbs you need in a farmer's market or your garden.

Tips

This soup is easy to prepare ahead. This makes it ideal for entertaining; just multiply the ingredients by the number of people you're serving.

Hot paprika is made from spicy red peppers, unlike sweet paprika, which is made from mild ones. Hot paprika gives this soup a little extra kick, but you can use the milder version if you prefer it.

- **Blender**

8 to 10	sprigs mixed fresh herbs (such as parsley, basil, dill and/or chervil)	8 to 10
¾ cup + 2 tbsp	buttermilk (see tip, below)	200 mL
⅓ cup	milk	75 mL
½ tsp	grated organic lemon zest	2 mL
2 tsp	lemon juice	10 mL
Pinch	hot paprika (see tips, at left)	Pinch
	Salt and freshly ground black pepper	
1	parsnip (about 3½ oz/100 g), peeled	1
2 tsp	butter	10 mL

1. Wash herbs and pat dry; pull leaves off stems. Reserve a few leaves for garnish; coarsely chop remaining leaves.

2. In a blender, purée together chopped herbs, buttermilk and milk until smooth. Stir in lemon zest, lemon juice and paprika. Season to taste with salt and pepper. Cover and refrigerate for 30 minutes or until chilled.

3. Meanwhile, cut parsnip into cubes. In a skillet, melt butter over medium heat. Add parsnip; fry, turning occasionally, for 5 minutes or until golden brown. Season to taste with salt.

4. Ladle soup into a deep soup plate or bowl; garnish with parsnip and reserved herbs.

Shopping Tip

Full-fat (3.25%) buttermilk can be harder to find in North America, but it's worth looking for. Besides containing extra fat, which your body needs during cancer treatments, it's richer, thicker and more delicious in this soup. If you can't find it, buy the highest-fat version you can find.

Nutrients per serving	
Calories	237
Fat	11 g
Carbohydrates	23 g
Protein	11 g

Romanesco Soup with Soft-Boiled Egg

Prep time: 35 minutes

This pretty green soup has a lovely, creamy egg served on top for both a hit of protein and a wonderful flavor.

Tip

Romanesco is the slightly alien-looking (but tasty!) green cousin of cauliflower. If you can't find it, you can simply replace it with cauliflower.

- **Immersion blender**

4 oz	romanesco (about one-quarter small head), see tip, at left	125 g
1	shallot	1
1 tbsp	butter	15 mL
¾ cup + 2 tbsp	ready-to-use vegetable broth	200 mL
¼ cup	heavy or whipping (35%) cream	60 mL
3 tbsp	dry white wine	45 mL
1	egg	1
	Salt and freshly ground black pepper	
2 or 3	fresh basil leaves	2 or 3

1. Cut romanesco into small florets. Peel and finely chop shallot. In a saucepan, melt butter over medium-high heat. Add shallot; sauté for 3 minutes or until translucent. Add romanesco; sauté for 2 to 3 minutes. Add broth, cream and wine; bring to a boil. Reduce heat to low; cover and simmer for 10 minutes.

2. Meanwhile, in another saucepan, cover egg with cold water. Bring to a boil; cook for 2 minutes or until soft-boiled (white will be solid and yolk will be runny). Remove from heat; rinse egg under cold water. Let cool slightly; carefully peel off shell.

3. Using an immersion blender, purée soup until smooth. Season to taste with salt and pepper.

4. Ladle soup into a deep soup plate or bowl. Cut top one-third of egg off to expose yolk (save top to eat with soup). Place egg in center of soup; season to taste with salt and pepper. Garnish soup with basil.

Nutrients per serving	
Calories	349
Fat	31 g
Carbohydrates	5 g
Protein	11 g

Carrot and Coconut Soup

You can make this soup as spicy as you like by changing the type or amount of curry powder you add. The mix of spices, herbs and coconut milk is incredibly tasty.

Tip

Refrigerate leftover coconut milk to use in smoothies, curries, or even cups of coffee or tea.

- **Immersion blender**

2 tsp	clarified butter (see tip, below)	10 mL
1	carrot, thinly sliced	1
1	piece (about ¾ inch/2 cm) gingerroot, finely chopped	1
1 tsp	hot or mild curry powder, or to taste	5 mL
1 cup	ready-to-use vegetable broth	250 mL
6 tbsp	canned coconut milk (see tip, at left)	90 mL
2 tsp	unsweetened shredded coconut	10 mL
3	sprigs fresh cilantro or parsley	3
1 tbsp	lime juice	15 mL
	Salt and freshly ground black pepper	

1. In a saucepan, heat clarified butter over medium-high heat. Add carrot and ginger; sauté for 2 to 3 minutes or until softened. Sprinkle curry powder over top; sauté for about 1 minute or until fragrant. Add broth and coconut milk; bring to a boil. Reduce heat to medium and simmer for 15 minutes.

2. In a dry nonstick skillet over medium heat, toast coconut, shaking pan often, for 2 to 3 minutes or until golden brown. Transfer to a bowl; set aside. Wash cilantro and pat dry; pull leaves off stems. Set aside leaves for garnish.

3. Using an immersion blender, purée soup until smooth. Stir in lime juice; season to taste with salt and pepper.

4. Ladle soup into a deep soup plate or bowl. Garnish with coconut and cilantro.

Prep Tip

Clarified butter is easy to make. Simply melt a chunk of butter in a small saucepan and simmer it for about 10 minutes without letting it brown. Remove from the heat and let it stand until the white milk solids settle in the bottom of the pan. The clear golden oil on top is the clarified butter.

Nutrients per serving

Calories	195
Fat	17 g
Carbohydrates	7 g
Protein	2 g

Yellow Pepper Soup with Shiitake Mushrooms

Makes 1 serving

**Prep time:
35 minutes**

A sautéed mushroom topping gives this wonderful soup a woodsy flavor that's so pleasing. Mascarpone cheese adds just a hint of creaminess.

Tip

Shiitake mushrooms are delicate and don't really like to be dunked in water for cleaning. You can brush them well to remove any grit, or wipe them with a damp paper towel before cutting them.

- **Immersion blender**

1 tbsp	olive oil	15 mL
1	yellow bell pepper, seeded and chopped	1
1	shallot, finely chopped	1
1	clove garlic, minced	1
1 tsp	hot paprika (see tips, page 225)	5 mL
¾ cup + 2 tbsp	ready-to-use vegetable broth	200 mL
⅓ cup	dry white wine	75 mL
½ tsp	dried rosemary	2 mL
1 tbsp	mascarpone cheese	15 mL
1 tsp	white balsamic vinegar	5 mL
	Salt and freshly ground black pepper	
1½ oz	fresh shiitake mushrooms (see tip, at left)	45 g

1. In a saucepan, heat oil over medium-high heat. Add yellow pepper, shallot and garlic; sauté for 3 to 4 minutes or until softened. Sprinkle paprika over top; sauté for 1 minute. Add broth, wine and rosemary; bring to a boil. Reduce heat to low and simmer for 10 minutes.

2. Using an immersion blender, purée soup until smooth. Stir in cheese and white balsamic vinegar; season to taste with salt and pepper. Return to boil; remove from heat.

3. Trim off and discard stems from shiitake mushrooms; cut caps into strips. In a dry nonstick skillet over high heat, sear mushrooms, turning constantly, for 2 to 3 minutes or until browned.

4. Ladle soup into a deep soup plate or bowl; sprinkle mushrooms over top.

Nutrients per serving	
Calories	246
Fat	18 g
Carbohydrates	13 g
Protein	5 g

Squash, Leek and Sausage Soup

This is actually more of a stew than a soup, but it is a hearty, warming dish that will take away the chill on a cold day.

Tip

Leeks can be really gritty, so make sure you separate the layers and wash well between them. Dirt likes to hide inside, and it will ruin the texture of the finished soup.

7 oz	red kuri squash (see tips, below)	210 g
1	small onion	1
½	red chile pepper	½
1 tbsp	olive oil	15 mL
1¼ cups	ready-to-use beef broth	300 mL
1	large leek (white and light green parts), see tip, at left	1
2	fully cooked sausages (about 3 oz/90 g each), such as frankfurters (see tips, below)	2
	Salt and freshly ground black pepper	
3	sprigs fresh parsley	3

1. Scrub squash well; cut in half and scrape out seeds. Cut squash into ¾-inch (2 cm) cubes. Finely chop onion. Seed chile pepper and cut into thin rings.

2. In a saucepan, heat oil over medium-high heat. Add onion and chile pepper; sauté for 1 to 2 minutes. Add squash; sauté for 3 minutes. Add broth; reduce heat to medium and simmer for 5 minutes.

3. Meanwhile, wash and trim leek. Cut leek and sausages diagonally into ¾-inch (2 cm) thick slices. Add leek and sausage to soup; simmer for 5 minutes or until leeks are softened and sausage is heated through. Season to taste with salt and pepper.

4. Wash parsley and pat dry; pull leaves off stems. Chop leaves. Ladle soup into a deep soup plate or bowl; sprinkle with parsley.

Substitution Tips

Red kuri squash is a sweet, flavorful Japanese winter squash that is similar to small pie pumpkins. You can substitute pie pumpkins or butternut squash if they are more readily available. (Just peel other squashes with tougher rinds before adding them to the recipe.) When it's not winter squash season, you can make this lovely soup with zucchini instead.

This soup can be customized with whatever cooked sausages you like. Check the list of Green-Light Foods (page 145) for other options to try.

Nutrients per serving	
Calories	608
Fat	45 g
Carbohydrates	11 g
Protein	28 g

Seafood Soup with Aïoli

Makes 2 servings

Prep time: 45 minutes

This soup is so delicious, it's designed to serve two so you can share it. The quick aïoli is good with all sorts of dishes, so keep the recipe handy.

Tips

Look for cans or bricks of ready-to-use fish broth near the seafood counter at your supermarket.

Frozen mixed seafood comes in convenient bags in the freezer or fish section of the supermarket. It contains shrimp, squid, shellfish (such as clams and mussels) and sometimes octopus. If you can't find it or want to make your own personal mix, no problem. Just use the same weight of your preferred combination of seafood.

1	onion	1
3	green onions (white and light green parts)	3
2	small carrots (about 2½ oz/ 75 g total)	2
¾ cup	cherry tomatoes	175 mL
1 tbsp	olive oil	15 mL
1 cup	ready-to-use fish broth (see tips, at left)	250 mL
8 oz	thawed frozen mixed seafood (see tips, at left), drained	250 g
	Salt and cayenne pepper	
½	bunch fresh dill, coarsely chopped	½

Aïoli

2 tbsp	mayonnaise	30 mL
1	small clove garlic, minced	1
1 tsp	lemon juice, or to taste	5 mL
	Salt and freshly ground black pepper	

1. **Aïoli:** In a bowl, stir together mayonnaise, garlic and lemon juice. Season to taste with salt and pepper. Cover and set aside in the refrigerator.

2. Finely dice onion. Cut green onions diagonally into ¾-inch (2 cm) long pieces. Quarter carrots lengthwise, then cut diagonally into ¾-inch (2 cm) pieces. Halve cherry tomatoes.

3. In a large saucepan, heat oil over medium-high heat. Add diced onion and carrots; sauté for 2 to 3 minutes or until softened. Add broth; bring to a boil. Reduce heat to medium and simmer for 5 minutes. Add seafood and green onions; simmer, uncovered, for 10 minutes.

4. Add cherry tomatoes; cook for 5 minutes or until seafood is cooked through. Season to taste with salt and cayenne pepper.

5. Stir dill into soup. Ladle soup into deep soup plates or bowls; top with aïoli.

Nutrients per serving	
Calories	258
Fat	16 g
Carbohydrates	6 g
Protein	22 g

Vegetarian Main Dishes

Gruyère-Topped Vegetable Skillet

This simple dish is great for weeknights, when you need something quick and healthy at the same time.

Tip

Change up the vegetables in this recipe according to what you like and what's in season. Parsnips, turnips, celery and mushrooms are all tasty options.

8 oz	mixed vegetables (such as romanesco, broccoli and/or cauliflower)	250 g
1 tsp	olive oil	5 mL
½	onion, finely chopped	½
½	clove garlic, minced	½
	Salt and freshly ground black pepper	
	Grated nutmeg	
½ cup	ready-to-use vegetable broth	125 mL
1¾ oz	Gruyère cheese, sliced	50 g
1 tbsp	chopped fresh parsley	15 mL

1. Trim and peel vegetables if necessary, depending on the variety. Cut into bite-size chunks or florets. In a saucepan, cover vegetables with salted water; bring to a boil. Cook for 5 minutes or until tender-crisp. Drain; keep warm.

2. Meanwhile, in a large nonstick skillet, heat oil over medium-high heat. Add onion and garlic; sauté for 3 to 5 minutes or until onion is starting to soften. Season to taste with salt, pepper and nutmeg.

3. Add broth; reduce heat to medium-low and simmer for 8 minutes. Stir in vegetables; arrange cheese over top. Remove from heat; let stand for 3 to 5 minutes or until cheese is melted. Sprinkle with parsley.

Nutrients per serving	
Calories	352
Fat	27 g
Carbohydrates	10 g
Protein	16 g

Savory Pancakes with Herbed Quark

Makes 1 serving

**Prep time:
25 minutes**

Who doesn't like pancakes for dinner? These healthy ones are filled with a smooth, creamy filling studded with fresh herbs and Emmental cheese.

Tips

Always choose full-fat versions of dairy products, such as quark and milk, when you're on the cancer-fighting diet (unless the recipe specifically calls for a low-fat version). Your body needs the fat they contain to make energy.

Coconut flour is popular because many people follow the Paleo Diet. Health food stores and many supermarkets carry it now.

2	eggs, separated	2
6 tbsp	full-fat quark (see tips, at left)	90 mL
1/4 cup	finely ground oat bran (see tips, page 175)	60 mL
1/4 cup	milk	60 mL
2 tbsp	whole-grain einkorn flour	30 mL
5 tsp	ground psyllium husks	25 mL
4 tsp	coconut flour (see tips, at left)	20 mL
Pinch	salt	Pinch
1 tbsp	coconut oil, divided	15 mL
1/4	small red bell pepper	1/4

Herbed Quark

3 tbsp	low-fat quark	45 mL
4 tsp	kefir	20 mL
1 tsp	special oil mixture (see page 161)	5 mL
1 tbsp	chopped fresh herbs (such as dill, chives and/or parsley)	15 mL
1/2 oz	Emmental cheese, shredded	15 g
	Salt and freshly ground black pepper	

1. In a large bowl, stir together egg yolks, full-fat quark, oat bran, milk, einkorn flour, psyllium husks, coconut flour and salt until smooth. In another bowl, beat egg whites until stiff peaks form; fold into egg yolk mixture.

2. In a nonstick skillet, heat 1 1/2 tsp (7 mL) of the coconut oil over medium heat; spoon in half of the batter; cook, turning once, for 4 minutes or until golden on both sides. Repeat with remaining coconut oil and batter.

3. **Herbed Quark:** In a bowl, stir together low-fat quark, kefir and special oil mixture until smooth. Stir in herbs and cheese; season to taste with salt and pepper.

4. Cut red pepper into thin strips. Spoon herbed quark onto pancakes; garnish with red pepper.

Nutrients per serving	
Calories	560
Fat	33 g
Carbohydrates	30 g
Protein	35 g

Nutty Mushroom Spaetzle

Makes 1 serving

**Prep time:
30 minutes**

Spaetzle is a rustic homemade pasta that is usually laden with carbs, thanks to all-purpose flour. This is a healthier, fiber-rich version you'll love.

Tips

There are spaetzle graters designed specifically for making this type of noodle. Look for them in specialty cooking stores.

If you're in the mood for a main dish with meat, try Beef and Pork Ragoût with Whole-Grain Spaetzle (recipe, page 250).

- **Coarse grater or colander with large holes (see tip, at left)**

1 tbsp	coconut oil	15 mL
4 oz	mushrooms, quartered	125 g
	Salt and freshly ground black pepper	
	Grated nutmeg	
2 tbsp	chopped hazelnuts	30 mL
1 tbsp	soy flour (see tips, page 223)	15 mL
¼ cup	ready-to-use vegetable broth	60 mL
½	clove garlic, crushed	½
2½ tsp	heavy or whipping (35%) cream	12 mL
½ oz	Emmental cheese, shredded	15 g
½ tsp	chopped fresh parsley	2 mL

Whole-Grain Spaetzle

2 tbsp	quark (see tips, page 233)	30 mL
1	egg	1
¼ cup	finely ground oat bran (see tip, page 175)	60 mL
2 tbsp	whole-grain einkorn flour	30 mL
Pinch	each salt and grated nutmeg	Pinch

1. In a nonstick skillet, heat coconut oil over medium-high heat. Add mushrooms; sauté for 5 minutes or until softened and golden. Season to taste with salt, pepper and nutmeg. Set aside.

2. In another dry nonstick skillet over medium heat, toast hazelnuts and soy flour, shaking pan often, for 5 minutes or until golden and fragrant. Add broth; bring to a boil. Reduce heat to low and simmer for 5 minutes. Stir in garlic; season to taste with salt and pepper.

3. Stir in cream; return to simmer. Stir in cheese until smooth; stir in mushrooms and parsley.

4. **Whole-Grain Spaetzle:** Meanwhile, in a bowl, stir together quark, egg, oat bran, flour, salt and nutmeg until a smooth dough forms. Bring a large saucepan of water to a boil; using a coarse grater or a colander held over water, grate or press dough into short pieces. Boil spaetzle for about 5 minutes or until they float to surface of water. Drain well. Serve topped with mushroom sauce.

Nutrients per serving	
Calories	466
Fat	29 g
Carbohydrates	25 g
Protein	27 g

Fennel Gratin

Prep time: 30 minutes

Gratins are the most wonderful dishes — cheesy, comforting and, in this case, packed with tender fennel and crunchy nuts.

Tip

Fennel is rich in natural carotenoids. The body can take up these fat-soluble vitamins only if you eat the vegetables that contain them with a little oil, butter or cream.

- Preheat oven to 425°F (220°C)
- 6-cup (1.5 L) gratin dish, greased with 1 tsp (5 mL) butter

2	small bulbs fennel (see tip, at left)	2
1 tsp	lemon juice	5 mL
¼ cup	heavy or whipping (35%) cream	60 mL
Pinch	freshly ground black pepper	Pinch
1 oz	Emmental cheese, shredded	30 g
½ tsp	nutritional yeast (see tip, below)	2 mL
1 tsp	chopped hazelnuts	5 mL
1 tsp	shelled hemp seeds (see tip, page 238)	5 mL

1. Trim and core fennel; discard stems. Chop a few delicate fronds; reserve for garnish. Using the coarse side of a box grater, grate fennel.

2. In a saucepan, bring salted water and the lemon juice to a boil. Add fennel; blanch for 1 minute. Reserving 2 tbsp (30 mL) of the cooking liquid, drain fennel well.

3. In a bowl, whip cream with pepper until stiff peaks form; fold in cheese. Alternately layer fennel and half of the cream mixture in prepared gratin dish.

4. In a small bowl, stir nutritional yeast with reserved cooking water; stir into remaining cream mixture. Pour over fennel in gratin dish. Sprinkle with hazelnuts and hemp seeds.

5. Bake in preheated oven for 10 minutes or until golden brown. Just before serving, garnish with reserved fennel fronds.

Shopping Tip

Nutritional yeast is not a live leavener, like the active-dry yeast you use in baking. It is a deactivated strain that's added to recipes to give them a higher vitamin and mineral content. Nutritional yeast also has a cheesy aroma, so it's terrific for boosting the flavor of savory dishes. Look for this ingredient at health food and bulk food stores.

Nutrients per serving	
Calories	400
Fat	33 g
Carbohydrates	8 g
Protein	16 g

Stuffed Mushrooms with Sage Pasta

Makes 1 serving

Prep time: 30 minutes

Stuffed mushrooms are usually served as an appetizer, but here they become the focus of the dish with sage-and-butter-topped pasta alongside.

Tips

If you don't want a strictly vegetarian dish, you can substitute chicken broth for the vegetable broth.

High-protein pasta (see page 157) contains fewer carbohydrates and more protein than regular white or whole-grain pastas. Look for it in health food stores or the health food aisle of well-stocked supermarkets.

- Preheat oven to 475°F (240°C)
- 6-cup (1.5 L) gratin dish, brushed with 1 tsp (5 mL) canola oil

2 oz	large white mushrooms	60 g
4 tsp	butter, divided	20 mL
½	small onion, finely chopped	½
1 oz	Gouda cheese, shredded	30 g
1 tbsp	chopped fresh parsley	15 mL
	Salt and freshly ground black pepper	
¼ cup	ready-to-use vegetable broth (see tips, at left)	60 mL
1 oz	high-protein pasta (see tips, at left)	30 g
3	fresh sage leaves	3
1 tsp	canola oil	5 mL

1. Trim mushrooms; using a sharp knife, remove stems to make hollow caps. Set aside mushroom caps. Finely chop mushroom stems.

2. In a nonstick skillet, melt 2 tsp (10 mL) of the butter over medium-high heat. Add onion and chopped mushroom stems; sauté for 3 to 5 minutes or until softened and golden.

3. Transfer onion mixture to a bowl; stir in cheese and parsley. Season to taste with salt and pepper. Spoon mixture into mushroom caps.

4. Arrange stuffed mushrooms in prepared gratin dish; pour in broth. Bake in preheated oven for 15 minutes or until mushroom caps are softened and cheese is melted.

5. Meanwhile, in a large pot of boiling salted water, cook pasta according to the package instructions until al dente. Drain well.

6. Meanwhile, wash sage leaves and pat dry. In a skillet, melt remaining butter over medium heat; fry sage leaves for 2 to 3 minutes or until crisp.

7. In a warmed serving bowl, combine canola oil and sage leaves. Toss with pasta to coat. Serve with stuffed mushrooms.

Nutrients per serving

Calories	300
Fat	21 g
Carbohydrates	8 g
Protein	26 g

Sesame Omelet with Shiitake Mushrooms

Fresh shiitake mushrooms are so good for you, and they add a wonderful, earthy flavor to this simple omelet.

Tips

If you don't have an ovenproof nonstick skillet, you can make one. Simply wrap the handle of a regular nonstick skillet in heavy-duty foil to protect it from the heat.

Tamari is a wheat-free version of soy sauce. It's a terrific addition to the cancer-fighting kitchen. Many brands are gluten free as well, but check the label to be sure.

- Preheat oven to 200°F (100°C)
- Ovenproof 9-inch (23 cm) nonstick skillet (see tips, at left)

2 oz	fresh shiitake mushrooms	60 g
3	sprigs fresh cilantro	3
2	eggs	2
1 tbsp	heavy or whipping (35%) cream	15 mL
1 tbsp	tamari or soy sauce (see tips, at left), divided	15 mL
1½ tbsp	canola oil, divided	22 mL
2 tsp	sesame seeds	10 mL
1	green onion (white and light green parts), sliced	1
1	piece (about ¾ inch/2 cm) gingerroot, minced	1
	Freshly ground black pepper	

1. Trim off and discard stems from shiitake mushrooms; halve caps. Wash cilantro and pat dry; pull leaves off stems.

2. In a bowl, whisk together eggs, cream and 1 tsp (5 mL) of the tamari. In an ovenproof 9-inch (23 cm) nonstick skillet, heat 1½ tsp (7 mL) of the oil over medium heat. Add sesame seeds; fry for 2 to 3 minutes or until golden brown.

3. Pour egg mixture into skillet; reduce heat to low and cook for 3 minutes or until eggs are set. Turn omelet; cook for 2 minutes or until golden on bottom. Keep warm in preheated oven.

4. In another nonstick skillet, heat remaining oil over medium-high heat. Add shiitake mushrooms; cook, turning often, for 1 to 2 minutes or until golden. Add green onion and ginger; fry for 1 minute. Drizzle remaining tamari over top; season to taste with pepper.

5. Serve mushroom mixture over omelet; garnish with cilantro.

Nutrients per serving	
Calories	435
Fat	35 g
Carbohydrates	10 g
Protein	19 g

Jerusalem Artichoke Gratin

Makes 1 serving

**Prep time:
1¼ hours**

Jerusalem artichokes are also called sunchokes, but they're not related to regular artichokes. They are, however, very delicious, especially in this gorgeous gratin.

Tips

Jerusalem artichokes don't require peeling, though you can peel them if you like. Just make sure to scrub them well to get all the dirt out of the little cracks in the skin.

Shelled hemp seeds are a nutritious addition to the cancer-fighting diet (see box, page 162). Look for them in health and bulk food stores. They have become very popular in recent years, and some brands are now available in supermarkets, as well.

- **Preheat oven to 350°F (180°C)**
- **6-cup (1.5 L) gratin dish**

1 tsp	butter	5 mL
¼ tsp	grated nutmeg	1 mL
7 oz	Jerusalem artichokes (see tips, at left)	210 g
¼ cup	ready-to-use vegetable broth	60 mL
¼ cup	heavy or whipping (35%) cream	60 mL
1	egg	1
½ tsp	herb salt (see tip, below)	2 mL
1½ tbsp	shelled hemp seeds (see tips, at left)	22 mL
1 oz	Gouda cheese, shredded	30 g

1. Rub butter all over inside of a 6-cup (1.5 L) gratin dish; sprinkle with nutmeg. Pat Jerusalem artichokes dry with paper towels; cut into ¼-inch (0.5 cm) thick slices. Arrange slices, overlapping, in gratin dish.

2. In a small bowl, whisk together broth, cream, egg and herb salt. Pour over Jerusalem artichokes; sprinkle with hemp seeds. Top with cheese.

3. Bake in preheated oven for 1 hour or until golden and Jerusalem artichokes are tender.

Shopping Tip

Herb salt is a blend of sea salt, spices, herbs and seaweed that's used to season foods. It contains less salt than plain table salt, and it adds a rich, herbal taste to cooking. You'll find it under the brand name Herbamare; look for it online and in some specialty food shops.

Nutrients per serving	
Calories	415
Fat	32 g
Carbohydrates	11 g
Protein	20 g

Tomatoes and Mushrooms en Papillote

This fancy-sounding method of cooking foods in a parchment paper packet couldn't be simpler. The packet holds in all the lovely juices from the tomatoes and mushrooms as they cook.

Tip

Fresh oyster mushrooms are very delicately flavored and delicious in this recipe. Look for mushrooms that are creamy white, without dark brown spots or any signs of wilting.

- Preheat oven to 400°F (200°C)
- 2 pieces parchment paper, each about 20 by 16 inches (50 by 40 cm), brushed with olive oil

3½ oz	small white mushrooms	100 g
2 oz	oyster mushrooms (see tip, at left)	60 g
5	cherry tomatoes	5
1	shallot, sliced	1
1	clove garlic, sliced	1
2	rounds soft goat cheese (about 1½ oz/45 g each)	2
1 tsp	chopped fresh rosemary	5 mL
2	sprigs fresh thyme	2
2 tbsp	olive oil	30 mL
	Salt and freshly ground black pepper	

1. Trim white mushroom stems; leave mushrooms whole or halve, depending on size. Cut oyster mushrooms into pieces. Halve cherry tomatoes.

2. Lay 1 piece of parchment paper on work surface; top with second piece of parchment paper. Scatter white and oyster mushrooms, cherry tomatoes, shallot and garlic in center of paper. Top with goat cheese; sprinkle with rosemary. Place thyme on top; drizzle with oil. Season to taste with pepper.

3. Fold and pleat edges of parchment paper to seal and form packet; place on a baking sheet. Bake in preheated oven for 15 to 20 minutes or until fragrant and vegetables are tender.

4. Open paper packets at the table, being careful of the steam inside; season with salt to taste.

Nutrients per serving	
Calories	533
Fat	48 g
Carbohydrates	5 g
Protein	17 g

Eggplant Piccata with Tomato Sauce

Makes 1 serving

Prep time: 35 minutes

For a complete meal, add a simple crisp salad and enjoy this combination with a glass of white wine. Just keep an eye on your daily carbohydrate limit.

Tip

Asian eggplants are long and slim, which allows you to make long, thin, pretty slices. Their thinner skins and gentle flavor are ideal for this piccata.

• **Immersion blender**

1	Asian eggplant (about 6 oz/175 g), see tip, at left	1
	Salt and freshly ground black pepper	
3 tbsp	olive oil, divided	45 mL
1	small onion, finely chopped	1
1	small clove garlic, minced	1
2 or 3	tomatoes (about 7 oz/210 g)	2 or 3
2 tbsp	water	30 mL
½ tsp	dried oregano	2 mL
1	egg	1
2 tbsp	grated Parmesan cheese	30 mL
2 tbsp	milk	30 mL
1 tbsp	whole-grain spelt flour	15 mL
2 tbsp	sour cream	30 mL

1. Trim off ends of eggplant; cut lengthwise into ½-inch (1 cm) thick slices. Season to taste with salt on both sides; let stand for 15 minutes.

2. Meanwhile, in a saucepan, heat 1 tbsp (15 mL) of the oil over medium-high heat. Add onion and garlic; sauté for 3 to 5 minutes or until softened.

3. Core and dice tomatoes; add tomatoes, water and oregano to pan. Reduce heat to low and simmer, stirring occasionally, for 10 minutes or until thickened and fragrant. Using an immersion blender, purée tomato sauce; season to taste with salt and pepper.

4. In a shallow dish, whisk together egg, cheese and milk. In a separate shallow dish, spread out flour. Pat eggplant dry with paper towels; season to taste with pepper on both sides. Dip eggplant into flour, then egg mixture, turning to coat all over and shaking off excess at each step.

5. In a nonstick skillet, heat remaining oil over medium heat. Add eggplant; fry, turning once, for 5 to 6 minutes or until golden brown and crisp. Serve with tomato sauce and sour cream.

Nutrients per serving	
Calories	533
Fat	42 g
Carbohydrates	20 g
Protein	17 g

Tomato and Cheese Omelet with Endive Salad

Makes 1 serving

Prep time: 20 minutes

A simple salad and a brightly flavored omelet are the perfect light dinner. They are excellent on a busy night when you have plenty to do besides cooking.

Tip

Curly endive is also known as chicory or frisée. It's a leafy green that adds a touch of refreshing bitterness to salads.

1	green onion (white and light green parts)	1
1	large tomato	1
2	eggs	2
3 tbsp	heavy or whipping (35%) cream	45 mL
	Salt and freshly ground black pepper	
1 tbsp	olive oil	15 mL
2 tbsp	shredded Gruyère cheese	30 mL

Endive Salad

2 tbsp	plain yogurt	30 mL
2 tsp	white wine vinegar	10 mL
	Salt and freshly ground black pepper	
2 or 3	leaves curly endive (see tip, at left)	2 or 3

1. **Endive Salad:** In a small bowl, stir yogurt with vinegar; season to taste with salt and pepper. Shred endive leaves; add to yogurt mixture and toss to coat. Set aside.

2. Cut green onion into 1-inch (2.5 cm) pieces. Core and cut tomato into $\frac{1}{2}$- to $\frac{3}{4}$-inch (1 to 2 cm) cubes. In a bowl, whisk eggs with cream; season with salt and pepper.

3. In a small nonstick skillet, heat oil over medium-high heat. Add tomato and green onion; sauté for 2 to 3 minutes. Season to taste with salt and pepper. Transfer to another bowl; keep warm.

4. Reduce heat to medium. Add egg mixture to skillet; cook, turning once, for 5 minutes or until eggs are set.

5. Transfer omelet to a plate; spoon tomato mixture over top. Sprinkle with cheese. Serve with endive salad.

Nutrients per serving	
Calories	477
Fat	40 g
Carbohydrates	7 g
Protein	23 g

Vegetable and Haloumi Stir-Fry

**Prep time:
30 minutes**

*Cheese in a stir-fry?
Yes, please! This is a
scrumptious change of
pace from Asian-style
stir-fries.*

Tip

Haloumi is a salty Cypriot
cheese that has become
very popular in recent
years. It doesn't melt
easily, so it's perfect for
grilling and pan-frying.
The cheese becomes
tender as it heats up but
never gets gooey.

- Grill pan

1	small zucchini (about 4 oz/125 g)	1
1	small yellow bell pepper	1
1½ tbsp	olive oil, divided	22 mL
1	shallot, finely chopped	1
1	clove garlic, minced	1
½ tsp	ground cumin	2 mL
	Salt and freshly ground black pepper	
½ cup	drained canned diced tomatoes	125 mL
2 tbsp	water	30 mL
1 tbsp	hot ajvar (see tip, opposite)	15 mL
4 oz	haloumi cheese (see tip, at left)	125 g

1. Trim and thinly slice zucchini. Halve and seed yellow
   pepper; cut into thin strips.

2. In a skillet, heat 1 tbsp (15 mL) of the oil over medium
   heat. Add shallot and garlic; fry for 3 to 4 minutes or until
   translucent. Add zucchini and yellow pepper; fry for 2 to
   3 minutes or until softened. Sprinkle cumin over top; season
   with salt and pepper to taste.

3. In a small bowl, stir together tomatoes, water and ajvar; stir
   into zucchini mixture. Reduce heat to low and simmer for
   5 minutes.

Nutrients per serving	
Calories	616
Fat	49 g
Carbohydrates	13 g
Protein	32 g

4. Meanwhile, cut cheese into $\frac{1}{2}$-inch (1 cm) thick slices. Brush a grill pan with remaining oil; heat over high heat. Sear cheese, turning once, for 2 to 3 minutes or until grill-marked.

5. Spoon vegetable mixture onto a plate; top with cheese.

Shopping Tip

Ajvar is a red pepper relish that's very popular in Eastern Europe and the Balkan region. It's made with roasted red bell peppers, garlic and various other ingredients. Families make this recipe in many different ways, and preserve jars of it at the end of the harvest for the coming winter. There are hot and mild varieties of ajvar, so choose whichever you prefer. You can find this treat in Eastern European markets and some well-stocked supermarkets.

Stir-Fried Asparagus and Tofu

White asparagus has a delicate, grassy flavor and is quite tender. If you can't find any at the grocery store, you can easily substitute regular green asparagus.

Tip

If you like, you can add up to 1 tbsp (15 mL) more tamari to the sauce for a saltier flavor.

3½ oz	firm tofu, drained (see spotlight, opposite)	100 g
2 tbsp	tamari or soy sauce, divided (see tip, at left)	30 mL
5 oz	white asparagus, trimmed and peeled	150 g
3	green onions (white and light green parts)	3
1	red chile pepper	1
1 tbsp	vegetable oil	15 mL
⅓ cup	ready-to-use vegetable broth	75 mL
	Salt and freshly ground black pepper	
1	handful bean sprouts, rinsed and drained	1
3 or 4	sprigs fresh cilantro	3 or 4

1. Cut tofu into ¾-inch (2 cm) cubes. In a bowl, pour 1 tbsp (15 mL) of the tamari over tofu, turning to coat.

2. Cut asparagus diagonally into thin slices. Trim and diagonally slice green onions into about 1½-inch (4 cm) pieces; halve white parts of green onions lengthwise. Halve chile pepper lengthwise, seed and cut into thin slices.

3. In a wok or large skillet, heat oil over medium-high heat. Pat tofu dry with paper towels. Add to wok; stir-fry for 2 to 3 minutes or until browned. Transfer to a plate; keep warm.

4. Add asparagus, green onions and chile pepper; stir-fry for 1 to 2 minutes. Add broth; cook for 5 minutes.

5. Add remaining tamari; season to taste with salt and pepper. Gently stir in tofu and bean sprouts; cook for 1 to 2 minutes or until heated through. Wash and pat cilantro dry; pull leaves off stems. Sprinkle leaves over stir-fry.

Nutrients per serving	
Calories	248
Fat	15 g
Carbohydrates	11 g
Protein	16 g

Spotlight

Tofu is now a staple in many kitchens. This yellowish white soybean-based protein source is made by adding a coagulant to soy milk, similar to the way rennet is added to animal milk to create cheese. It's pressed into blocks and comes in a variety of textures, from silken to firm, and styles, such as natural, smoked and seasoned with herbs. You'll find it in health food stores, Asian grocery stores and supermarkets.

Once you've opened the package, you can keep tofu covered in fresh water in the refrigerator for about 1 week. Remember to change the water daily. If you buy vacuum-packed tofu, you can freeze the unopened package for several weeks.

The protein content and nutritional value of tofu are comparable to those of meat and fish. It contains twice as much protein as fresh cow's milk cheeses, such as quark.

Thai Tofu Curry with Bok Choy

Prep time: 25 minutes

Red curry paste is fiery, but it's perfect for spicing up tender, mild tofu. If you don't have bok choy on hand, other greens or vegetables are tasty in the sauce.

Tip

Always make sure you buy real, full-fat coconut milk for curries like this. Also, read the label to be sure it is unsweetened.

5 oz	baby bok choy	150 g
1	small yellow bell pepper	1
1 tbsp	canola oil	15 mL
5 oz	firm tofu, drained and cubed	150 g
1	shallot, thinly sliced	1
1	clove garlic, thinly sliced	1
1 tsp	Thai red curry paste	5 mL
7 tbsp	ready-to-use vegetable broth	100 mL
1/3 cup	canned coconut milk (see tip, at left)	75 mL
1 tbsp	tamari or fish sauce (see tip, below)	15 mL
1 to 2 tsp	lime juice	5 to 10 mL
1/2 tsp	locust bean gum (see tip, page 290)	2 mL
Pinch	salt	Pinch
1 tbsp	chopped cashews	15 mL

1. Halve or quarter bok choy lengthwise, depending on size. Seed yellow pepper and cut into chunks.

2. In a wok or large heavy skillet, heat oil over medium-high heat. Add tofu and shallot; stir-fry for 2 to 3 minutes or until shallot starts to soften. Add yellow pepper; stir-fry for 3 minutes. Stir in garlic and curry paste; stir-fry for 1 minute. Stir in broth and coconut milk. Nestle bok choy into sauce; reduce heat to medium, cover and simmer for 3 to 4 minutes.

3. Stir in tamari, lime juice, locust bean gum and salt; cook for 1 or 2 minutes or until slightly thickened.

4. Ladle curry into a bowl; just before serving, sprinkle with cashews.

Substitution Tip

Using tamari in this curry makes it completely vegetarian, but fish sauce is more authentically Thai in flavor. Either is delicious, though.

Nutrients per serving	
Calories	356
Fat	22 g
Carbohydrates	19 g
Protein	20 g

Kohlrabi with Sesame Tofu

Makes 1 serving

**Prep time:
30 minutes**

Kohlrabi has a lovely flavor similar to cabbage and broccoli, but mild and a little peppery. It's full of nutrients and is a good source of fiber.

Tips

Firm tofu is a good choice for this recipe, because it will hold its shape as it's frying. More-delicate medium and soft tofu are better in dishes where they don't have to be moved too much.

Crème fraîche is the less-tangy cousin of sour cream. It gives sauces a rich, creamy taste and thickens them gently. If you have any left over, spoon it over fresh berries for a simple dessert.

5 oz	firm tofu, drained (see tips, at left)	150 g
1 tbsp	tamari or soy sauce (see tips, page 237)	15 mL
1	head kohlrabi	1
1 tbsp	butter	15 mL
⅓ cup	ready-to-use vegetable broth	75 mL
1 tbsp	crème fraîche (see tips, at left)	15 mL
1 tbsp	sesame seeds	15 mL
1 tbsp	canola oil	15 mL
	Salt and freshly ground black pepper	
1 tsp	lime juice	5 mL
½ tsp	grated organic lime zest	2 mL

1. Cut tofu crosswise into ½- to ¾-inch (1 to 2 cm) thick slices. Place in a shallow dish; drizzle with tamari. Trim and peel kohlrabi, reserving tender green leaves. Cut kohlrabi into large chunks, then slice thinly.

2. In a saucepan, melt butter over medium-high heat. Add kohlrabi slices; sauté for 3 minutes. Add broth; reduce heat to medium, cover and cook for 5 minutes.

3. Stir in crème fraîche; cook, uncovered, for 3 to 5 minutes or until sauce is thickened.

4. Meanwhile, pat tofu dry with paper towels. Sprinkle sesame seeds on a plate; press tofu into sesame seeds, turning to coat all over. In a small skillet, heat oil over medium heat. Add tofu; fry, turning once, for 4 to 6 minutes or until golden brown.

5. Season kohlrabi mixture to taste with salt and pepper; drizzle with lime juice. Cut reserved kohlrabi leaves into very thin strips; sprinkle shredded leaves and lime zest over kohlrabi mixture. Serve with sesame tofu.

Nutrients per serving	
Calories	443
Fat	37 g
Carbohydrates	10 g
Protein	18 g

Eggplant Carpaccio with Pecorino Cream

Makes 1 serving

Prep time: 20 minutes

Hot mustard gives the creamy sauce a nice bite that complements the tender eggplant and fresh tomatoes.

Tip

If you don't care for spicy foods, you can substitute another type of mustard for the hot mustard. Just check the label carefully to see how much sugar it contains, and steer clear of sweet and honey mustards.

- • **Plate, lined with paper towels**

1/2	eggplant (about 3 1/2 oz/100 g)	1/2
	Salt and freshly ground black pepper	
2 tbsp	olive oil	30 mL
2	plum tomatoes	2
1 tbsp	balsamic vinegar	15 mL
2 tbsp	grated Pecorino-Romano or Parmesan cheese	30 mL
2 tbsp	crème fraîche (see tips, page 247)	30 mL
1 tbsp	milk	15 mL
1 tsp	hot mustard (see tip, at left)	5 mL
1	small handful arugula, trimmed	1

1. Trim off stem end of eggplant and discard; cut eggplant into 1/4-inch (0.5 cm) thick slices. Season to taste with salt and pepper. In a large nonstick skillet, heat oil over medium heat; fry eggplant slices for 5 minutes or until golden. Transfer to prepared plate; let drain.

2. Core and cut tomatoes crosswise into thin slices. Alternately arrange eggplant and tomato slices, overlapping, on a plate; sprinkle with balsamic vinegar. Season to taste with salt and pepper.

3. In a bowl, stir together cheese, crème fraîche, milk and mustard until smooth; season to taste with salt and pepper. Spread over eggplant and tomatoes. Sprinkle arugula over top.

Nutrients per serving	
Calories	394
Fat	36 g
Carbohydrates	9 g
Protein	8 g

Beef, Veal and Lamb Main Dishes

Beef and Pork Ragoût with Whole-Grain Spaetzle

Makes 1 serving

**Prep time:
45 minutes**

*This spaetzle is so good,
it can be paired with all
sorts of saucy toppings.
Here it's crowned with
a rich meat ragoût
made with ground beef
and pork.*

Tip

Regular ground beef
and pork are definitely
not lean, which explains
in part why the calorie
count on this dish is so
high. But both contain
a large amount of the
protein and fat that you
need when you're on
the cancer-fighting diet.
This dish will boost your
strength for treatment
days ahead.

3 tbsp	olive oil	45 mL
1	small onion, chopped	1
1	clove garlic, minced	1
1 tbsp	butter	15 mL
1 tsp	sweet paprika	5 mL
½ tsp	dried oregano	2 mL
3½ oz	ground beef (see tip, at left)	100 g
3½ oz	ground pork	100 g
1 cup	ready-to-use chicken broth	250 mL
½ tsp	hot mustard (see tip, below)	2 mL
	Salt and freshly ground black pepper	
	Whole-Grain Spaetzle (recipe, page 234)	

1. In a large nonstick skillet, heat oil over medium-high heat. Add onion and garlic; sauté for about 5 minutes or until onion is translucent.

2. Add butter, paprika, oregano, ground beef and ground pork; sauté, breaking up with a spoon, until crumbly. Add chicken broth; reduce heat and simmer for 10 minutes or until beef and pork are no longer pink. Stir in mustard; season to taste with salt and pepper.

3. Serve ragoût over Whole-Grain Spaetzle.

Substitution Tip

Hot mustard will give this meat mixture a bit of a
kick. You can substitute mild mustard if you prefer;
just don't use sweet or honey mustard, as they contain
more carbohydrates.

Nutrients per serving

Calories	1,400
Fat	115 g
Carbohydrates	32 g
Protein	75 g

Asian Ground Beef Skillet

Makes 1 serving

Prep time: 20 minutes

Thick teriyaki sauce and sesame oil give this easy dinner a wonderful flavor. Using ground beef instead of chunks of steak makes the cooking quicker.

Tip

Thick teriyaki sauce is the right choice for this dish. Save bottles of thinner teriyaki marinade for steaks or chicken on the barbecue.

2	leeks (white and light green parts), about 8 oz (250 g) total	2
2 oz	fresh soybean sprouts or mung bean sprouts (see tips, below)	60 g
2 tbsp	canola oil	30 mL
8 oz	ground beef	250 g
3 tbsp	soy sauce	45 mL
2 tbsp	sesame oil	30 mL
1 tbsp	thick teriyaki sauce (see tip, at left)	15 mL

1. Slice leeks thinly. Rinse soybean sprouts well under cold running water; let drain.

2. In a nonstick skillet, heat canola oil over medium heat. Add ground beef; fry, breaking up with a spoon, until crumbly. Add leeks and soybean sprouts; cover and cook, stirring occasionally, for 3 to 5 minutes or until vegetables are tender-crisp and beef is no longer pink.

3. Stir in soy sauce, sesame oil and teriyaki sauce.

Substitution Tips

If you want to change this dish up, you can substitute mild white fish (such as pollock), shrimp or mixed seafood for the ground beef. Cook them as you would the beef, until they are firm and opaque.

Look for plump soybean sprouts at Korean markets or Asian grocery stores. If you can't find them, regular mung bean sprouts are easy to find in most supermarkets.

Nutrients per serving	
Calories	577
Fat	48 g
Carbohydrates	5 g
Protein	31 g

Steak with Creamy Roasted Parsnips

Makes 1 serving

Prep time: 40 minutes

Sometimes you just need a good steak. This simple skillet-seared one is so satisfying with the caramelized parsnips.

Tips

Sirloin grilling steaks are reasonably priced, so they're excellent for simple dinners like this. If you like, you can substitute any of your other favorite grilling steaks. Just use the same weight of meat for the recipe.

If your parsnips are young and tender, they don't really need to be peeled before you eat them. Older parsnips have a woodier texture, so those do need peeling. In either case, scrub them well to get any dirt out of the little crevices in the peel.

Nutrients per serving	
Calories	938
Fat	63 g
Carbohydrates	9 g
Protein	83 g

- **Preheat oven to 400°F (200°C)**

3	large parsnips (10 oz/300 g), peeled if desired (see tips, at left)	3
1 tbsp	olive oil	15 mL
1 tbsp	canola oil	15 mL
7 oz	beef sirloin grilling steak (see tips, at left)	210 g
¼ cup	heavy or whipping (35%) cream	60 mL
	Salt and freshly ground black pepper	
2 tbsp	shelled hemp seeds (see tip, page 238)	30 mL
2 oz	Gruyère cheese, shredded	60 g

1. Halve parsnips lengthwise; arrange on a baking sheet. Brush with olive oil; roast in preheated oven for 30 to 40 minutes or until tender.

2. Meanwhile, in a skillet, heat canola oil over high heat. Add steak; cook, turning once, until desired doneness. Transfer meat to a cutting board and cover with foil; keep warm.

3. Add cream to skillet; season to taste with salt and pepper. Heat over low heat for 2 minutes or until warmed through.

4. Meanwhile, in another dry skillet over medium heat, toast hemp seeds, shaking pan often, for 2 minutes or until fragrant. Stir into cream mixture.

5. Arrange parsnips on a plate with steak; drizzle parsnips with cream sauce and sprinkle with cheese.

Roast Beef with Tomatoes and Chopped Egg

Prep time: 15 minutes

This is a delicious dinner to make when you have leftover cooked roast beef. It's full of healthy protein.

Tips

You can also use deli roast beef to save time when making this dish. Ask at the deli counter if there are natural versions that are preserved without nitrates.

Kitchen or poultry shears are the perfect tool for snipping fresh chives. They make the job so fast and easy.

1	egg	1
¾ cup	cherry tomatoes	175 mL
3½ oz	cooked roast beef, thinly sliced (see tips, at left)	100 g
1 tsp	lemon juice	5 mL
2 tsp	canola oil	10 mL
	Salt and freshly ground black pepper	
1 tbsp	snipped or chopped fresh chives (see tips, at left)	15 mL
1 tbsp	crème fraîche	15 mL

1. In a saucepan, cover egg with cold water. Bring to a boil; boil for 10 minutes. Remove from heat; rinse egg under cold water. Let cool. Peel off shell; chop egg.

2. Halve cherry tomatoes; arrange on a plate with roast beef slices. In a bowl, whisk lemon juice with canola oil; season to taste with salt and pepper. Drizzle over beef.

3. Sprinkle chopped egg over beef; garnish with chives. Serve with crème fraîche.

Nutrients per serving	
Calories	435
Fat	33 g
Carbohydrates	4 g
Protein	31 g

Beef and Vegetable Stir-Fry

Makes 1 serving

**Prep time:
25 minutes**

Stir-fries are great for using up what's in the refrigerator. Check your crisper drawer to see what vegetables you have on hand, and substitute them for the romanesco and peppers in this recipe.

Tip

If you find you're missing having a starch alongside this stir-fry, you can add a healthy one. Serve the dish with 1½ oz (45 g) high-protein pasta, cooked according to the package directions.

4 oz	beef grilling steak, such as tenderloin or sirloin	125 g
2 tbsp	tamari or soy sauce (see tips, page 237)	30 mL
½	each small red and yellow bell pepper	½
3½ oz	romanesco (see tip, page 226) or broccoli	100 g
1 tbsp	peanut oil	15 mL
1 tsp	sesame oil	5 mL
⅓ cup	ready-to-use vegetable broth (see tip, below)	75 mL
	Salt and freshly ground black pepper	
1 tbsp	chopped peanuts	15 mL

1. Pat steak dry with paper towels. Cut into thin slices across the grain. In a bowl, toss steak with tamari to coat. Set aside.

2. Seed red and yellow peppers and cut into thin strips. Cut romanesco into small florets.

3. In a wok or large nonstick skillet, heat peanut oil and sesame oil over high heat. Reserving marinade, drain steak. Add steak to wok; stir-fry for 1 to 2 minutes or until browned. Transfer steak to a plate; set aside.

4. Add red and yellow peppers, and romanesco to wok; stir-fry for 3 minutes or until softened. Add broth and reserved marinade; cover and simmer for 3 minutes. Return steak to wok; cook for 2 minutes or until heated through.

5. Season to taste with salt and pepper; garnish with peanuts.

Storage Tip

You need only a small amount of broth for this recipe. Freeze the leftover broth in convenient recipe-size portions to use in other recipes later on.

Nutrients per serving	
Calories	413
Fat	25 g
Carbohydrates	10 g
Protein	35 g

Pepper Minute Steaks

Prep time: 25 minutes

Fast-fry steaks are ideal for nights when you're short on cooking time. Peppers give you a healthy dose of vitamin C and plenty of flavor.

Tip

If you can't find fast-fry steaks, ask the butcher to slice a regular steak into thin cutlet-style slices.

1	each small red and yellow bell pepper	1
3	sprigs fresh thyme	3
4	beef sirloin tip fast-fry steaks (about 1 oz/30 g each), see tip, at left	4
	Salt and freshly ground black pepper	
1½ tbsp	olive oil, divided	22 mL
1	small clove garlic, minced	1
3 tbsp	ready-to-use beef broth	45 mL
1 tbsp	balsamic vinegar	15 mL
1	handful arugula, trimmed (see tip, below)	1

1. Seed red and yellow peppers and cut into thin strips. Wash thyme and pat dry; pull leaves off stems. Finely chop thyme leaves. Pat steaks dry with paper towels; season with pepper on both sides.

2. In a skillet, heat 1 tbsp (15 mL) of the oil over medium heat. Add red and yellow peppers, and garlic; fry for 5 minutes or until peppers are softened. Add broth and vinegar; season to taste with salt and pepper. Cook for about 1 minute or until slightly thickened. Transfer pepper mixture to a plate; keep warm.

3. Add remaining oil to skillet and heat over medium-high heat. Add steaks and thyme; fry, turning once, for 1 to 2 minutes per side or until desired doneness. Add arugula to pepper mixture; toss to coat.

4. Arrange steak over pepper mixture; season to taste with salt, if desired.

Prep Tip

For even easier prep, you can use baby arugula in place of the mature leaves. Baby arugula has tender stems that don't need to be trimmed off before eating.

Nutrients per serving	
Calories	390
Fat	22 g
Carbohydrates	14 g
Protein	31 g

Spelt Crêpes with Avocado and Ground Beef

This Mexican-style twist on soft tacos gives you lower-carb, whole-grain goodness that tortillas don't provide.

Tip

For an extra delicious garnish, pull the leaves off half a bunch of fresh cilantro and sprinkle over the crêpes.

- Preheat oven to 200°F (100°C)

1 tbsp	olive oil	15 mL
8 oz	ground beef	250 g
1	onion, finely chopped	1
1 cup	drained canned diced tomatoes	250 mL
1 tsp	chili powder	5 mL
	Salt and freshly ground black pepper	
1	ripe avocado, halved, pitted and peeled	1
2	vine-ripened tomatoes	2
2 or 3	dashes hot pepper sauce	2 or 3

Whole-Grain Crêpes

⅓ cup	whole-grain spelt flour (see spotlight, opposite)	75 mL
1	egg	1
1	egg yolk	1
3 tbsp	milk	45 mL
3 tbsp	sparkling mineral water	45 mL
1 tbsp	butter, melted	15 mL
Pinch	salt	Pinch
	Clarified butter (see tip, page 227) for frying	

1. **Whole-Grain Crêpes:** In a bowl, stir together flour, egg, egg yolk, milk, mineral water, melted butter and salt just until smooth batter forms. Let stand for 30 minutes.

2. Meanwhile, in a nonstick skillet, heat oil over medium heat. Add ground beef; fry, breaking up with a spoon, for 5 minutes or until crumbly and no longer pink. Add onion; fry, stirring for 3 to 5 minutes or until translucent. Stir in diced tomatoes and chili powder; season to taste with salt and pepper. Reduce heat to low and simmer, uncovered, for 10 minutes.

Nutrients per serving	
Calories	840
Fat	66 g
Carbohydrates	20 g
Protein	41 g

Spotlight

Spelt is nutritionally similar to its close relative wheat, but it offers a few advantages. Spelt is easier to digest and contains more essential amino acids than wheat. It contains more essential minerals and has a more aromatic, nuttier flavor. It is also high in gluten, so it is great for baking. Spelt flour helps baked goods rise even when blended with gluten-free flours, such as those made from amaranth, quinoa and buckwheat.

3. In another nonstick skillet, heat a little bit of clarified butter over medium heat. Using one-quarter of the batter at a time and adding more clarified butter as necessary, cook 4 thin crêpes, turning once, for 2 to 3 minutes or until set. Transfer finished crêpes to a plate in preheated oven and keep warm.

4. Cut one half of the avocado into wedges; dice remaining avocado. Slice vine-ripened tomatoes. Gently fold diced avocado into beef mixture; season to taste with salt, pepper and hot pepper sauce.

5. Place crêpes on plates; fill with beef mixture. Garnish with avocado wedges and tomato slices.

Variation

Spelt Crêpes with Spinach and Cheese: Omit beef filling. Instead, heat 1 tbsp (15 mL) olive oil over medium-high heat. Add 8 oz (250 g) frozen leaf spinach, thawed; 1 onion, finely chopped; and 1 clove garlic, minced. Sauté for 5 to 8 minutes or until onion is softened. Stir in 3 tbsp (45 mL) crème fraîche and 1 1/2 oz (45 g) Gruyère cheese, shredded. Season to taste with salt, pepper and grated nutmeg. Fill crêpes with spinach mixture.

Sliced Fennel with Papaya and Bresaola

Makes 1 serving

Prep time: 40 minutes

This is a little like an antipasto platter. Enjoy it with a glass of red wine for a sophisticated but easy dinner.

Tip

Smoked salmon or trout will also work well in this dish in place of the bresaola.

1	small bulb fennel (about 5 oz/150 g)	1
1	small red onion	1
1	small red chile pepper	1
3 tbsp	orange juice	45 mL
2 tbsp	olive oil	30 mL
2 tbsp	lemon juice, divided	30 mL
	Salt and freshly ground black pepper	
½	ripe papaya (about 7 oz/210 g)	½
1 oz	sliced bresaola (see tip, below)	30 g

1. Core and quarter fennel, reserving a few of the feathery fronds for garnish. Thinly slice fennel and onion. Halve chile pepper lengthwise; seed and mince.

2. In a bowl, stir together orange juice, oil and 1 tbsp (15 mL) of the lemon juice; season to taste with salt and pepper. Add fennel, onion and chile pepper; toss to coat. Cover and let stand for 20 minutes to marinate.

3. Seed and peel papaya; cut lengthwise into slices. Arrange on a plate; drizzle with remaining lemon juice. Arrange fennel mixture and bresaola alongside papaya. Garnish with reserved fennel fronds.

Shopping Tip

Bresaola is an Italian salt-cured, aged, dried beef that is popular around the world. Look for it at specialty delicatessens or Italian grocery stores. If you like, you can substitute Bündnerfleisch, the delicious German version of air-dried beef.

Nutrients per serving	
Calories	356
Fat	23 g
Carbohydrates	9 g
Protein	15 g

Poached Veal with Tuna and Capers

In Italian, this unique dish is called vitello tonnato. The anchovies, tuna and capers give it a lovely saltiness, while the lemon brightens the flavor of the creamy sauce.

Tip

This dressing contains a raw egg yolk. If you are concerned about the food safety of raw eggs, substitute pasteurized liquid whole eggs for the yolk.

¼ cup	white wine	60 mL
1	leek (white and light green parts), coarsely chopped (see tip, below)	1
1	carrot, coarsely chopped	1
1	stalk celery, coarsely chopped	1
8 oz	lean veal roast	250 g
1	egg yolk (see tip, at left)	1
¼ cup	special oil mixture (see page 161)	60 mL
	Juice of 1 organic lemon	
½	can (6 oz/170 g) water-packed tuna, drained	½
1	anchovy fillet, minced	1
	Salt and freshly ground black pepper	
1 tbsp	drained capers	15 mL

1. In a saucepan, combine about 4 cups (1 L) lightly salted water, wine, leek, carrot and celery. Add veal; slowly bring to a boil. Reduce heat and simmer, uncovered, for about 1½ hours. Let cool in broth.

2. In a bowl, whisk egg yolk. Add special oil mixture in a thin stream, whisking constantly, until thickened. Gradually whisk in lemon juice.

3. Place tuna in a bowl; using a fork, break into chunks. Stir in anchovy and a little of the egg mixture. Press tuna mixture through a sieve; stir into remaining egg mixture. Season to taste with salt, if desired.

4. Drain veal; slice very thinly and arrange on a plate. Pour tuna mixture over top. Season to taste with pepper; garnish with capers.

Prep Tip

To make cleaning leeks easier, chop them before you wash them. Then, swish them in plenty of cold water, rubbing off the grit between the layers. Let the dirt settle to the bottom, then pick the leeks up without disturbing the water.

Nutrients per serving	
Calories	1,300
Fat	110 g
Carbohydrates	5 g
Protein	71 g

Veal Cutlets with Mâche Salad

Makes 1 serving

Prep time: 15 minutes

Tender veal is wonderful with this fruity, herby spring salad. If you can't find mâche, substitute another tender lettuce in the salad.

Tip

Mâche is also known as lamb's lettuce, corn salad or fetticus. It's a tender spring green with a mild, nutty taste.

½	green onion (white and light green parts)	½
3½ oz	mâche (see tip, at left)	100 g
½ tsp	raspberry vinegar	2 mL
½ tsp	walnut oil	2 mL
½ tsp	grapeseed oil	2 mL
Pinch	salt	Pinch
	Chopped fresh herbs (such as tarragon, lemon balm or fennel fronds)	
1½ tsp	chopped walnuts	7 mL
1½ tbsp	olive oil	22 mL
1	veal cutlet (see tip, below)	1

1. Slice green onion thinly. In a bowl, combine mâche and green onion.

2. In another bowl, whisk together raspberry vinegar, walnut oil, grapeseed oil and salt. Season to taste with fresh herbs. Pour over mâche mixture; toss to coat. Sprinkle with walnuts.

3. In a skillet, heat olive oil over medium-high heat. Add veal; fry, turning once, for 6 minutes or until desired doneness. Serve with salad.

Shopping Tip

Veal cutlets are often labeled with the Italian name scaloppine at the supermarket. They're the same cut.

Nutrients per serving	
Calories	612
Fat	19 g
Carbohydrates	5 g
Protein	106 g

Veal Saltimbocca with Leek Sauce

Saltimbocca means "jumps in your mouth," an appropriate description for this delicious, brightly flavored dish.

Tip

Prosciutto is the usual choice for this dish, but use extra-special Parma ham (a high-end version of this cured ham) if you can find it. It's worth the splurge.

- Meat mallet

2	thin veal cutlets (about 2 oz/60 g each)	2
	Salt and freshly ground black pepper	
2	slices prosciutto (see tip, at left)	2
2	fresh sage leaves	2
2	leeks (white and light green parts), about 8 oz (250 g) total	2
1 tbsp	butter	15 mL
1	clove garlic, minced	1
7 tbsp	ready-to-use chicken broth	100 mL
1/3 cup	heavy or whipping (35%) cream	75 mL
	Grated nutmeg	
2 tsp	canola oil	10 mL

1. Pat veal dry with paper towels; on a cutting board and using a meat mallet, pound to flatten slightly. Season with salt and pepper on both sides. Place 1 slice of the prosciutto and 1 sage leaf in the center of each cutlet. Roll up meat around filling; secure with a toothpick.

2. Cut leeks diagonally into 1/2-inch (1 cm) thick slices. In a skillet, melt butter over medium heat. Add leeks and garlic; fry for 1 minute. Add broth; reduce heat, cover and simmer for 5 minutes. Stir in cream; cook for 2 to 3 minutes or until thickened. Season to taste with salt, pepper and nutmeg.

3. Meanwhile, in another skillet, heat oil over medium heat. Add veal rolls; fry for 2 minutes. Turn rolls; fry for 2 minutes or until veal is no longer pink. Serve topped with leek sauce.

Nutrients per serving	
Calories	579
Fat	42 g
Carbohydrates	10 g
Protein	40 g

Veal Cutlets with Parsley and Nut Coating

You don't have to give up breaded cutlets if you coat them this way. The whole-grain and nut coating is crunchy and very tasty.

Tip

If you don't like turnips, these crispy cutlets are also delicious with kohlrabi. Peel and slice it the same as you would the turnips.

- **Plate, lined with paper towels**

2	white turnips (about 7 oz/ 210 g total), see tip, at left	2
1	carrot	1
1 tbsp	butter	15 mL
3 tbsp	ready-to-use vegetable broth	45 mL
3 tbsp	heavy or whipping (35%) cream	45 mL
	Salt and freshly ground black pepper	
½ tsp	locust bean gum (see tips, page 290)	2 mL
1	veal cutlet (about 5 oz/150 g)	1
2 tbsp	ground hazelnuts	30 mL
1 tbsp	chopped fresh parsley	30 mL
1 tbsp	whole-grain spelt flour	15 mL
1	egg white, lightly beaten	1
1 tbsp	canola oil	15 mL
1	lemon wedge	1

1. Peel and slice turnips and carrot. In a saucepan, melt butter over medium-high heat. Add turnips and carrot; sauté for 2 to 3 minutes. Add broth and cream; reduce heat to medium, cover and simmer for 6 to 7 minutes. Season to taste with salt and pepper; stir in locust bean gum. Cook for 1 minute or until slightly thickened.

2. Meanwhile, pat veal dry with paper towels; cut into 3 pieces. In a shallow dish, stir hazelnuts with parsley. In separate shallow dishes, spread out flour and egg white. Season veal with salt and pepper on both sides. Dip veal into flour, then egg white, then nut mixture, turning to coat all over and shaking off excess at each step.

3. In a skillet, heat oil over medium heat. Add veal; fry, turning once, for 2 to 3 minutes or until crisp and golden and veal is no longer pink. Transfer to prepared plate; let drain.

4. Serve cutlets with turnip mixture and lemon wedge.

Nutrients per serving	
Calories	653
Fat	43 g
Carbohydrates	20 g
Protein	42 g

Lamb Chops and Eggplant

Fresh rosemary and herbes de Provence dress up tiny lamb chops and give them a rich herbal edge. The tender eggplant and tomatoes makes this an easy complete meal.

Tip

Instead of lamb chops, you can substitute 7 oz (210 g) lamb tenderloin or lamb medallions in this recipe.

1	piece (5 oz/150 g) eggplant	1
2	tomatoes	2
1	strip organic lemon zest	1
1½ tsp	olive oil	7 mL
½	sprig fresh rosemary	½
2	lamb loin chops (see tip, at left)	2
	Salt and freshly ground black pepper	
½	clove garlic, minced	½
1 tbsp	water	15 mL
½ tsp	herbes de Provence	2 mL

1. In a saucepan of boiling salted water, cook eggplant for 20 minutes. Drain; let cool. Cut into thick slices.

2. Core and slice tomatoes. Cut lemon zest into thin shreds. Set aside.

3. In a skillet, heat oil with rosemary over medium heat. Add lamb chops; fry for 3 minutes per side or until desired doneness. Discard rosemary; season to taste with salt and pepper. Transfer lamb chops to a plate; keep warm.

4. Add eggplant, tomatoes, lemon zest, garlic, water and herbes de Provence to skillet; bring to a boil. Turn eggplant and tomato slices; cook for 2 minutes or until tomatoes are tender. Season to taste with salt and pepper.

5. Spoon eggplant mixture onto a plate; serve with lamb chops.

Nutrients per serving	
Calories	625
Fat	39 g
Carbohydrates	14 g
Protein	55 g

Lamb Tenderloin with Green Beans

Tender lamb and green beans are a classic combination. Here, they're topped with a dollop of yogurt for a creamy finish.

Tip

Fresh rosemary has a gentler flavor than dried rosemary. It's worth splurging on a package of it in the produce section. Even better is when you grow it in your own garden; it's always ready and waiting to be added to recipes.

• **Large bowl, filled with ice water**

4 oz	green beans	125 g
2	pieces lamb tenderloin (about 2 oz/60 g each)	2
	Salt and freshly ground black pepper	
1½ tbsp	olive oil, divided	22 mL
1	small red onion, thinly sliced	1
¼ cup	ready-to-use beef broth	60 mL
2 tsp	tomato paste	10 mL
1 tsp	chopped fresh rosemary (see tip, at left)	5 mL
1 tbsp	plain yogurt	15 mL

1. Trim and halve green beans crosswise. In a saucepan of boiling salted water, cook green beans for 8 to 10 minutes or until tender-crisp. Using a slotted spoon, transfer to prepared bowl of ice water; let cool. Drain well.

2. Pat lamb dry with paper towels; season with salt and pepper. In a skillet, heat 1 tbsp (15 mL) of the oil over high heat. Add lamb; fry for 2 to 3 minutes per side or until desired doneness. Wrap lamb in foil; keep warm.

3. Add remaining oil to skillet. Add onion; fry for 5 minutes or until translucent. Stir in broth and tomato paste; bring to a boil. Add green beans and rosemary; season to taste with salt and pepper.

4. Remove lamb from foil; pour any accumulated lamb juices over green bean mixture. Slice lamb diagonally; serve with bean mixture. Garnish with yogurt.

Nutrients per serving	
Calories	477
Fat	34 g
Carbohydrates	12 g
Protein	29 g

Pork and Poultry Main Dishes

Ham, Savoy Cabbage and Oyster Mushroom Fry

Makes 1 serving		

Prep time: 45 minutes		

Cabbage gets so sweet and tender when it's cooked. Matched with savory ham and mushrooms, it makes a healthy comfort food dish that's perfect for cool evenings.

Tip

Green cabbage is not as tender as savoy cabbage, but you can substitute it in this recipe with no problem.

- **Plate, lined with paper towels**

2 oz	oyster mushrooms	60 g
1 tsp	flaxseed oil	5 mL
2 oz	country-style ham (see tip, below), diced	60 g
½	onion, finely chopped	½
6 oz	savoy cabbage, cored and shredded (see tip, at left)	175 g
¼ cup	ready-to-use beef broth	60 mL
	Salt and freshly ground black pepper	
	Caraway seeds	
4 tsp	sour cream	20 mL
1 tbsp	chopped fresh parsley	15 mL

1. Remove and discard stems from oyster mushrooms; cut mushrooms into bite-size pieces. Set aside.

2. In a large nonstick skillet, heat oil over medium heat. Add ham and onion; fry, stirring, for 5 minutes or until onion is translucent. Add mushrooms; fry, stirring, for 5 minutes or until softened. Using a slotted spoon, transfer mushroom mixture to prepared plate; let drain.

3. Add cabbage to skillet; fry, stirring, for 5 minutes or until starting to soften. Add beef broth; season with salt, pepper and caraway seeds. Cook, stirring occasionally, for 20 minutes or until cabbage is wilted and soft. Return mushroom mixture to skillet. Stir to combine.

4. Spoon onto a plate; garnish with sour cream and parsley.

Shopping Tip

Country-style ham is smoked and dry-cured, so it has a texture similar to prosciutto. It's very popular in the southern United States; the Smithfield brand of country-style ham is well known. For this recipe, buy a chunk of the ham, rather than slices, because you want little cubes of it throughout the stir-fry.

Nutrients per serving	
Calories	220
Fat	12 g
Carbohydrates	7 g
Protein	21 g

Bacon and Leek Quiche

Makes 4 servings

Prep time: 1 hour

Gouda cheese, leeks and bacon make a divine filling for a simple quiche. Made with bran and almond flour, the crust is much healthier than ones made with refined wheat flour.

Tips

Finely ground oat bran is perfect for making this crust. It should have the texture of flour, rather than flakes.

If you can't find goat's milk Gouda, substitute regular Gouda cheese instead.

- Preheat oven to 350°F (180°C)
- 9-inch (23 cm) springform pan

1 cup	finely ground oat bran (see tips, at left)	250 mL
1 cup	almond flour	250 mL
1⅔ cups	sour cream, divided	400 mL
3 tbsp	canola oil, divided	45 mL
Pinch	each salt and freshly ground black pepper	Pinch
8 oz	leeks (white and light green parts), about 3	250 g
4 oz	bacon, diced	125 g
4	eggs	4
5 oz	goat's milk Gouda cheese, shredded (see tips, at left)	150 g
	Grated nutmeg	

1. In a large bowl, whisk oat bran with almond flour. In another bowl, whisk together half of the sour cream, 2 tbsp (30 mL) of the canola oil, salt and pepper; stir into flour mixture, kneading with hands if too stiff, to form a smooth dough.

2. On a floured work surface, roll out dough to about 10-inch (25 cm) circle. Fit into a 9-inch (23 cm) springform pan, pressing dough up side of pan slightly to form a lip. Set aside.

3. Slice leeks thinly. In a skillet, heat remaining oil over medium heat. Add bacon; fry for 2 to 3 minutes or until fat starts to melt. Add leeks; fry, stirring often, for 5 minutes or until leeks are softened. Remove from heat.

4. In a bowl, whisk together eggs, cheese and remaining sour cream. Season with salt, pepper and nutmeg.

5. Scatter leeks and bacon over dough; pour egg mixture over top. Bake in preheated oven for 20 minutes or until filling is set and crust is golden. Let cool slightly before serving.

Nutrients per serving	
Calories	314
Fat	46 g
Carbohydrates	18 g
Protein	32 g

Ham and Cauliflower Frittata

Makes 1 serving		
Prep time: 30 minutes		

This is one of those simple dinners you can make without even thinking. You won't need a whole head of cauliflower to make this quiche, so steam leftover florets to enjoy as a vegetable the next night.

Tips

Serrano ham is a wonderful Spanish cured ham that's extremely popular around the world. If you can't find any, you can substitute prosciutto or country-style ham.

Garden cress is an herb with tiny leaves that's often sold alongside sprouts. If you can't find it, try another type of sprout you like, such as broccoli or radish sprouts.

- **Bowl, filled with ice water**

½	small head cauliflower (5 oz/ 150 g), cut into florets	½
3	eggs	3
	Salt and freshly ground black pepper	
	Grated nutmeg	
2 tbsp	olive oil	30 mL
1	small onion, thinly sliced	1
1½ oz	serrano ham (see tips, at left), finely diced	45 g
2 tbsp	sour cream	30 mL
1	handful garden cress (see tips, at left)	1

1. In a large saucepan of boiling salted water, blanch cauliflower for 5 minutes. Using a slotted spoon, transfer to prepared bowl of ice water; let cool. Drain well.

2. In a bowl, whisk eggs; season with salt, pepper and nutmeg. In a small nonstick skillet, heat oil over medium-high heat. Add onion; sauté for 3 to 5 minutes or until translucent. Add serrano ham and cauliflower; sauté for 1 to 2 minutes.

3. Pour egg mixture over cauliflower mixture. Reduce heat to low, cover and cook for 6 to 8 minutes or until frittata is set. Turn; cook for 1 to 2 minutes or until bottom is golden and set.

4. Spoon sour cream into a small bowl; season to taste with salt and pepper. Garnish sour cream with garden cress; serve with frittata.

Variation

Cheesy Ham and Cauliflower Frittata: Use an ovenproof skillet to make frittata. Sprinkle finished frittata with 2 tbsp (30 mL) shredded Gruyère cheese; broil for 6 to 7 minutes or until cheese is melted and bubbly.

Nutrients per serving	
Calories	603
Fat	49 g
Carbohydrates	8 g
Protein	34 g

Figs with Serrano Ham and Goat Cheese

This is a lovely little cheese-and-charcuterie plate designed for one. Serve it with a slice of Spelt and Nut Bread (recipe, page 208) if you like.

Tip

Strawberries are another wonderful complement to the cured ham and goat cheese in this recipe. If you like, replace one of the figs with two or three fresh strawberries. Hull and halve the strawberries before arranging them on the plate.

2	ripe fresh figs (see tip, at left)	2
1	round (about 1 oz/30 g) soft goat cheese, such as Picandou	1
2 tsp	balsamic vinegar	10 mL
	Salt and freshly ground black pepper	
3	slices serrano ham (about 1½ oz/45 g)	3
2	sprigs fresh basil	2

1. Cut figs lengthwise into sixths. Decoratively arrange figs and cheese on a plate.

2. Drizzle balsamic vinegar over figs and cheese; season to taste with salt and pepper.

3. Arrange serrano ham slices decoratively around figs and cheese. Wash basil sprigs and pat dry; pull leaves off stems. Garnish dish with basil leaves.

Nutrients per serving	
Calories	192
Fat	10 g
Carbohydrates	10 g
Protein	14 g

Bacon and Vegetable Quiche

**Makes
12 servings**

**Prep time:
2½ hours**

*This quiche calls for
a simple homemade
pastry that you can use
as a base for any sort
of quiche or savory pie
you like. This one is
big enough to serve at
a party.*

Tip

Ground nuts are even
more perishable than
their whole counterparts.
To keep them fresh,
store them in a tightly
sealed airtight container
in the freezer for up to
6 months.

- Pastry blender
- 10-inch (25 cm) springform pan, greased

8 oz	carrots (about 4)	250 g
7 oz	celery (about 4 stalks)	210 g
2	leeks (white and light green parts), about 8 oz (250 g) total	2
5	slices bacon (3½ oz/100 g)	5
1 tbsp	canola oil	15 mL
	Salt and freshly ground black pepper	
	Grated nutmeg	
3	eggs	3
¾ cup + 2 tbsp	heavy or whipping (35%) cream	200 mL
3½ oz	Gruyère cheese, shredded	100 g

Pastry

1¼ cups	whole-grain spelt flour	300 mL
1¼ cups	ground hazelnuts (see tip, at left)	300 mL
½ tsp	salt	2 mL
1	egg	1
2 tbsp	cold water	30 mL
⅔ cup	cold butter, cubed	150 mL

1. **Pastry:** In a large bowl, whisk together flour, hazelnuts and salt. In another bowl, whisk egg with cold water. Using a pastry blender, cut butter into flour mixture until in crumbs. Using a fork, stir in egg mixture to make ragged dough. Knead a few times until dough comes together and is smooth. Wrap in plastic wrap and refrigerate for 1 hour.

2. Meanwhile, cut carrots, celery and leeks into ½-inch (1 cm) pieces. Finely chop bacon.

Nutrients per serving	
Calories	380
Fat	33 g
Carbohydrates	12 g
Protein	9 g

3. In a large nonstick skillet, heat oil over medium-high heat. Sauté bacon for about 5 minutes or until crisp. Add carrots, celery and leeks; sauté for 7 minutes or until softened. Season to taste with salt, pepper and nutmeg.

4. Preheat oven to 400°F (200°C). On a floured work surface, roll out dough into a 12-inch (30 cm) circle. Fit into prepared springform pan, pressing up side of pan slightly to make a 1-inch (2.5 cm) lip. Using a fork, prick pastry in a few places. Bake in preheated oven for 12 to 15 minutes or until light golden. Let cool slightly in pan on a wire rack.

5. Sprinkle bacon and vegetables over crust. In a bowl, whisk together eggs, cream and cheese; season with salt and pepper. Pour over vegetable mixture. Bake in preheated oven for 25 to 30 minutes or until filling is set.

Serving Idea

Wedges of quiche are delicious hot or cold. Serve any leftover slices for lunch or dinner the next day with a fresh tossed salad.

Simmered Pork Tenderloin with Vegetables

Pork tenderloin is meaty and lean, with lots of protein. Partnered with lovely harvest vegetables, it's a dinner that's fancy enough for company (if you want to share).

Tips

Choose full-fat cream cheese for this recipe. It gives the topping richness and much better flavor than reduced-fat cream cheese would.

Increase the horseradish to 2 tsp (10 mL) if you want a spicier topping.

1	stalk celery	1
1	large leek (white and light green parts), about 3 oz (90 g)	1
1	small carrot	1
2	Jerusalem artichokes (see tip, page 238), peeled	2
2 cups	ready-to-use beef broth	500 mL
5 oz	pork tenderloin	150 g
	Salt and freshly ground black pepper	
¼ cup	cream cheese (see tips, at left)	60 mL
2 tbsp	heavy or whipping (35%) cream	30 mL
1 tsp	prepared horseradish, or to taste (see tips, at left)	5 mL

1. Cut celery, leek and carrot into ¼-inch (0.5 cm) thick slices. Cut Jerusalem artichokes into chunks. In a large saucepan, bring broth to a boil. Add celery, carrot and Jerusalem artichokes; reduce heat to low and simmer for 10 minutes.

2. Add pork to broth mixture; cover and simmer for 10 minutes or until pork is no longer pink, adding leek during final 2 minutes of cooking time. Season to taste with salt and pepper.

3. In a small bowl, stir together cream cheese, cream and horseradish until smooth. Transfer pork to a cutting board; let rest for 2 to 3 minutes. Cut into slices.

4. Using a slotted spoon, transfer vegetables to a plate; serve with pork, seasoning to taste with salt and pepper. Spoon a little of the broth mixture over top; serve with cream cheese mixture alongside to dollop on top.

Nutrients per serving	
Calories	715
Fat	25 g
Carbohydrates	27 g
Protein	76 g

Chicken Curry

Curries often taken a long time to simmer, but this one is quick enough for a light weeknight meal. It even has a bit of apple to give the dish some natural sweetness.

Tip

Bone-in skin-on chicken breasts are less expensive than boneless skinless ones. You can easily pull off the skin and cut around the bones to save a bit of money.

1	onion	1
1	carrot	1
¼	apple, peeled and cored (see tip, below)	¼
1	boneless skinless chicken breast (see tip, at left)	1
1 tsp	canola oil	5 mL
½ tsp	curry powder	2 mL
½ tsp	turmeric	2 mL
	Salt and freshly ground black pepper	
4 tsp	ready-to-use chicken broth	20 mL

1. Cut onion into thin rings and carrot into long thin strips. Finely dice apple. Pat chicken dry with paper towels; cut into bite-size pieces.

2. In a nonstick skillet, heat oil over medium-high heat. Add chicken, onion, carrot and apple; sauté for about 5 minutes or until onion is softened.

3. Sprinkle with curry powder and turmeric; season with pepper. Add broth; reduce heat, cover and simmer for 20 minutes or until chicken is no longer pink inside. Season to taste with salt and pepper.

Shopping Tip

Choose a firm, crisp, tart apple for this curry. Try Granny Smith, Empire or your favorite heirloom variety. Enjoy the leftover apple for dessert or as a snack.

Nutrients per serving	
Calories	210
Fat	6 g
Carbohydrates	9 g
Protein	32 g

Provençal-Style Chicken Skillet

Makes 1 serving

Prep time: 40 minutes

Stewed tomatoes, olives, green pepper and garlic give this dish a decidedly southern French feel. It's extra nice with a slice of high-protein bread to mop up the tasty sauce.

Tip

You can easily substitute boneless skinless turkey breast for the chicken breast in this recipe.

¼	small green bell pepper	¼
1	boneless skinless chicken breast (see tip, at left)	1
1½ tsp	olive oil	7 mL
1	small onion, finely chopped	1
1	small clove garlic, minced	1
1 cup	dry red wine	250 mL
7 tbsp	ready-to-use beef broth	100 mL
3 tbsp	canned stewed tomatoes (see tip, opposite)	45 mL
	Salt and freshly ground black pepper	
	Dried thyme	
4	black olives (see tip, opposite), pitted and coarsely chopped	4
1 tbsp	chopped fresh parsley	15 mL

1. Seed green pepper and cut into thin strips. Pat chicken dry with paper towels; cut into bite-size pieces.

2. In a nonstick skillet, heat oil over medium-high heat. Add chicken; sauté for about 5 minutes or until starting to turn golden. Transfer chicken to a plate; keep warm.

3. Add onion and garlic to skillet; sauté for about 2 minutes or until starting to soften. Add green pepper; sauté for 2 to 4 minutes or until starting to soften. Add wine, broth and tomatoes; bring to a boil.

Nutrients per serving	
Calories	250
Fat	13 g
Carbohydrates	5 g
Protein	25 g

Tip

Olives are a food you can eat freely on the cancer-fighting diet (see Green-Light Foods list, page 144). There are so many different types of olives and ways of preparing them. They can add variety and interest to many dishes and are a terrific, satisfying snack.

4. Return chicken to skillet; reduce heat and simmer, uncovered, for 15 minutes or until most of the liquid is evaporated and chicken is no longer pink inside. Season to taste with salt, pepper and thyme. Stir in olives.

5. Spoon chicken mixture onto a plate; garnish with parsley just before serving.

Storage Tip

You'll have leftover canned stewed tomatoes, but don't let them go to waste. Freeze them in recipe-friendly portions in airtight containers.

Asian Chicken en Papillote

Makes 1 serving

**Prep time:
35 minutes**

*A simple French
steaming technique
yields moist, juicy
chicken and tender
veggies without a lot of
fuss. This is certainly a
dish that's fancy enough
for entertaining.*

Tip

Dark toasted sesame
oil is common in Asian
grocery stores, and most
large supermarkets
carry it, too. It has a
wonderful, rich flavor
and is so good for you.

- Preheat oven to 350°F (180°C)
- Two 16-inch (40 cm) squares parchment paper, brushed with canola oil
- Kitchen string

2½ oz	fresh shiitake mushrooms (see spotlight, at right)	75 g
3½ oz	napa cabbage, trimmed and shredded	100 g
1	boneless skinless chicken breast	1
	Salt and freshly ground black pepper	
1 tbsp	canola oil	15 mL
3 tbsp	ready-to-use vegetable broth	45 mL
1 tbsp	tamari or soy sauce (see tips, page 237)	15 mL
2 tsp	sesame oil (see tip, at left)	10 mL
3 or 4	sprigs fresh cilantro	3 or 4

1. Trim off and discard stems from shiitake mushrooms; halve caps. In a bowl, toss mushroom caps with cabbage. Pat chicken dry with paper towels; season with salt and pepper on both sides.

2. In a skillet, heat canola oil over high heat. Add chicken; cook, turning once, for 2 minutes per side or until lightly browned. Transfer chicken to a plate.

3. Lay 1 piece of parchment paper on work surface; top with second piece of parchment paper. Scatter mushrooms and cabbage in center of paper. Top with chicken; drizzle with broth, tamari and sesame oil. Fold and pleat edges of parchment paper to seal and form packet; tie loosely with kitchen string. Place on a baking sheet. Bake in preheated oven for 10 to 15 minutes or until chicken is no longer pink inside.

Nutrients per serving	
Calories	402
Fat	23 g
Carbohydrates	8 g
Protein	36 g

Tip

Napa cabbage is an Asian-style cabbage with tender leaves and chewy but edible ribs. If you can't find any, try Chinese cabbage or even savoy cabbage.

4. Meanwhile, wash cilantro and shake dry; pull leaves off stems. Arrange packet on a plate; open, being careful of the steam inside. Garnish with cilantro leaves.

Spotlight

Shiitake mushrooms are not just tasty; they also offer a number of positive health benefits. Eating them regularly strengthens the heart and a weakened immune system. They are also said to be antiviral, antiallergenic, antibacterial and anti-inflammatory. Some scientists have discovered that shiitakes can work against tumors, lower cholesterol and blood pressure, and alleviate migraines and circulation problems. In addition, shiitake mushrooms are one of the few plant-based sources of ergosterol, a precursor to vitamin D. Plus, they contain valuable protein, fiber, minerals (especially iron, calcium, potassium and zinc) and B vitamins. This should all be reason enough to put them on the table more often.

Coriander and Pepper–Crusted Chicken

Makes 1 serving

Prep time: 25 minutes

Coriander and peppercorns give chicken a slightly spicy, slightly citrusy crust with a crunchy texture.

Tip

Fruit vinegars are a wonderful way to add a little sweet-tart note to sauces and salads. Look for a variety of them at farmer's markets, where they're made with local fruit. Try raspberry, blueberry or other berry varieties in this dish.

- Coffee grinder, or mortar and pestle
- Grill pan

1	boneless skinless chicken breast	1
	Salt and freshly ground black pepper	
1 tsp	black peppercorns	5 mL
1 tsp	coriander seeds	5 mL
1 tbsp	olive oil	15 mL
⅓ cup	drained canned diced tomatoes	75 mL
2 tsp	tamari or soy sauce (see tips, page 237)	10 mL
1 tsp	fruit vinegar (see tip, at left)	5 mL
1	clove garlic, crushed	1
1 or 2	pinches curry powder	1 or 2
1	small head Belgian endive, cored and separated into leaves	1

1. Pat chicken dry with paper towels; season with salt. In a clean coffee grinder, coarsely grind peppercorns with coriander seeds. Transfer to a shallow dish; press chicken into peppercorn mixture to coat all over.

2. In a grill pan, heat oil over medium heat. Add chicken; fry, turning once, for 7 to 10 minutes or until golden brown and chicken is no longer pink inside. Transfer chicken to a cutting board; cover with foil and let stand for 2 minutes.

3. Meanwhile, in a small saucepan, stir together tomatoes, tamari, vinegar and garlic. Add curry powder; bring to a boil. Reduce heat to low and simmer for 2 to 3 minutes or until heated through and slightly thickened. Season to taste with salt and pepper.

4. Arrange endive on a plate. Cut chicken diagonally into slices; serve with endive and tomato mixture.

Nutrients per serving	
Calories	295
Fat	13 g
Carbohydrates	6 g
Protein	34 g

Chicken with Marinated Asparagus

*Enjoy this simple
chicken and vegetable
combination with a
glass of dry white wine.
It's a delicious way to
end the day.*

Tip

Any chopped nuts or
seeds would be delicious
on this dish. Try chopped
almonds, pecans or
pumpkin seeds instead
of the sunflower seeds.

3½ oz	asparagus, trimmed (see tip, page 280)	100 g
2 tsp	butter	10 mL
1	shallot, finely chopped	1
	Salt and white pepper	
2 tbsp	olive oil, divided	30 mL
1 tbsp	white wine vinegar	15 mL
2 tsp	white balsamic vinegar	10 mL
1 tsp	pumpkin seed oil	5 mL
2	boneless skinless chicken breasts	2
2 oz	mixed salad greens, torn into bite-size pieces	60 g
2 tsp	hulled sunflower seeds (see tip, at left)	10 mL

1. Peel bottom third of each asparagus spear; slice asparagus thinly. In a skillet, melt butter over medium-high heat. Add shallot and asparagus; sauté for 3 to 4 minutes or until asparagus is tender. Remove from heat; season to taste with salt and pepper.

2. In a bowl, whisk together 1 tbsp (15 mL) of the olive oil, white wine vinegar, white balsamic vinegar and pumpkin seed oil. Add asparagus mixture; toss to coat. Let stand to marinate.

3. Pat chicken dry with paper towels; season with salt and pepper. Add remaining oil to skillet; heat over medium-high heat. Add chicken; fry, turning once, for 7 to 10 minutes or until golden brown and no longer pink inside.

4. Cut chicken diagonally into slices. Arrange salad greens on a plate; top with asparagus and chicken. Garnish with sunflower seeds.

Nutrients per serving	
Calories	587
Fat	48 g
Carbohydrates	6 g
Protein	31 g

Turkey Ham and Ricotta Rolls with Asparagus

Makes 1 serving

Prep time: 25 minutes

This is another dinner that's excellent for packing and taking with you on a busy night. Put it in a bag with an ice pack to keep everything nice and cool.

Tip

The bottoms of asparagus stems can be very woody and unpleasant to eat. Trim or snap off those ends, about 1 inch (2.5 cm) up from bottom. Discard them, or freeze them and save for making vegetable stock.

7 oz	asparagus, trimmed (see tip, at left)	210 g
1 tbsp	white balsamic vinegar	15 mL
1 tbsp	lemon juice	15 mL
1 tbsp	olive oil	15 mL
	Salt and freshly ground black pepper	
1	tomato, cored, seeded and finely chopped	1
4	black olives, pitted and chopped	4
1	small green onion (white and light green parts), finely chopped	1
6 tbsp	ricotta cheese	90 mL
1 tbsp	grated Parmesan cheese	15 mL
4	slices turkey ham (about 2 oz/60 g)	4
3	fresh basil leaves	3

1. Peel bottom third of each asparagus spear; cut spears diagonally into 1½-inch (4 cm) pieces. In a saucepan of boiling salted water, cook asparagus for 6 minutes or until tender-crisp. Drain well.

2. In a bowl, whisk together vinegar, lemon juice and oil; season to taste with salt and pepper. Add asparagus; toss to coat. Let stand to marinate.

3. In another bowl, stir together tomato, olives and green onion; stir in ricotta cheese and Parmesan cheese until smooth. Season to taste with salt and pepper.

4. Lay turkey ham slices on a work surface; spread ricotta mixture over top. Roll up meat around filling.

5. Serve rolls with marinated asparagus; garnish with basil leaves.

Nutrients per serving	
Calories	434
Fat	32 g
Carbohydrates	9 g
Protein	27 g

Turkey Kabobs with Tomato Salsa

Makes 1 serving

Prep time: 25 minutes

Juicy kabobs are a hit, especially with this zesty tomato and zucchini salsa. Make this dish in the summer when fresh produce is at its peak.

Tip

The salsa is even tastier if you add 1 tbsp (15 mL) chopped fresh cilantro.

- Metal or soaked wooden skewers (see tip, below)

1	large vine-ripened tomato, cored, seeded and finely chopped	1
1	green onion (white and light green parts), thinly sliced	1
4	black olives, pitted and finely chopped	4
1 tbsp	lime juice	15 mL
	Salt and freshly ground black pepper	
3½ oz	boneless skinless turkey breast	100 g
1	small zucchini (about 3½ oz/100 g)	1
¼	red bell pepper	¼
1 tbsp	olive oil	15 mL

1. In a bowl, stir together tomato, green onion, olives and lime juice; season to taste with salt and pepper.

2. Pat turkey dry with paper towels; cut into ¾-inch (2 cm) cubes. Cut zucchini into ¾-inch (2 cm) thick slices. Seed red pepper and cut into ¾-inch (2 cm) pieces. Alternately thread turkey, zucchini and red pepper onto prepared skewers; season with salt and pepper.

3. In a large nonstick skillet, heat oil over medium heat. Fry kabobs, turning often, for 10 minutes or until golden brown and turkey is no longer pink inside. Serve with tomato salsa.

Prep Tip

Wooden or bamboo skewers are convenient to use, but their ends can char when exposed to high heat. To solve this problem, soak the skewers in water for about 30 minutes prior to using them.

Nutrients per serving	
Calories	263
Fat	14 g
Carbohydrates	6 g
Protein	27 g

Duck and Mushroom Skillet

*Want to treat yourself
to a gourmet meal that's
also good for you? Look
no further than this
meltingly tender duck
with exotic mushrooms.*

Tip

Fino sherry is a very dry,
pale sherry that's quite
different from sweeter,
well-aged sherries. If you
can't find it, dry white
wine makes a good
substitute in this recipe.

6 oz	boneless skin-on duck breast	175 g
3½ oz	mixed fresh mushrooms (such as chanterelle, portobello and cremini mushrooms)	100 g
1	shallot	1
2 tsp	clarified butter (see tip, page 227)	10 mL
	Salt and freshly ground black pepper	
2 tsp	whole-grain spelt flour	10 mL
2 tbsp	fino dry sherry (see tip, at left)	30 mL
⅓ cup	ready-to-use chicken broth	75 mL
⅓ cup	heavy or whipping (35%) cream	75 mL
3	sprigs fresh thyme	3

1. Skin duck breast, reserving skin for garnish, if desired (see serving idea, below). Pat duck dry with paper towels; thinly slice. Coarsely chop mushrooms. Thinly slice shallot.

2. In a skillet, heat clarified butter over high heat. Add duck; fry for 2 to 3 minutes or until browned and just a hint of pink remains inside. Transfer duck to plate; season with salt and pepper.

3. Add shallot to skillet; reduce heat to medium-high and sauté for 5 to 7 minutes or until translucent. Add mushrooms; sauté for 2 to 3 minutes. Sprinkle with flour; sauté for 1 to 2 minutes. Add sherry; cook, stirring, for 2 to 3 minutes. Add broth and cream; reduce heat to medium and cook, stirring, for 2 minutes.

4. Return duck and any accumulated juices to skillet; cook until warmed through. Season to taste with salt and pepper.

5. Wash thyme and shake dry; pull leaves off stems. Garnish duck mixture with thyme leaves.

Serving Idea

For a crunchy, decadently delicious garnish, dice 1½ oz (45 g) duck skin and fry it in a dry skillet until crispy. Sprinkle over finished dish.

Nutrients per serving	
Calories	616
Fat	44 g
Carbohydrates	13 g
Protein	77 g

Fish and Seafood Main Dishes

Spinach and Smoked Salmon Quiche

Makes 4 servings

Prep time: 1 hour

Spinach and smoked salmon are an ideal pairing, especially in quiche. Even people who aren't watching their carbohydrate intake will love this dish's rich taste.

Tips

If you're a fan of heartier flavors, replace the mozzarella cheese with raclette cheese and the spinach with dinosaur kale.

Oat bran may be coarsely or finely ground. The finely ground version may be labeled as a hot cereal or as oat bran powder; either will work in this recipe.

- **Preheat oven to 350°F (180°C)**
- **9-inch (23 cm) springform pan**

1 cup	finely ground oat bran (see tips, at left)	250 mL
1 cup	almond flour	250 mL
¼ tsp	each salt and freshly ground black pepper	1 mL
1⅔ cups	sour cream, divided	400 mL
3 tbsp	canola oil	45 mL
1 tbsp	olive oil	15 mL
7 oz	frozen leaf spinach, thawed and drained	210 g
5	slices smoked salmon (about 3½ oz/100 g), cut into strips	5
3½ oz	mozzarella cheese, shredded	100 g
4	eggs	4
	Grated nutmeg	
	Hot pepper flakes	

1. In a bowl, whisk together oat bran, almond flour, salt and pepper. In another bowl, whisk half of the sour cream with the canola oil. Stir into flour mixture just until soft dough forms. Knead a few times until dough is smooth. On a floured work surface, roll out dough to about 10-inch (25 cm) circle. Fit into a 9-inch (23 cm) springform pan, pressing dough up side of pan slightly to form a lip. Set aside.

2. In a saucepan, heat olive oil over medium heat. Add spinach; cook, stirring, for about 5 minutes or until heated through. Stir in smoked salmon; remove from heat and let cool slightly.

3. In a bowl, stir together remaining sour cream, cheese and eggs; stir in spinach mixture. Season with salt, pepper, nutmeg and hot pepper flakes.

4. Spread spinach mixture in crust; bake in preheated oven for about 20 minutes or until filling is set and crust is until golden.

Nutrients per serving	
Calories	644
Fat	48 g
Carbohydrates	17 g
Protein	35 g

Savoy Cabbage and Smoked Salmon

Smoked salmon is a convenient food you should indulge in. Here, it's paired with quickly sautéed cabbage for a complete meal in no time.

Tip

Herb salt is a blend of sea salt, spices, herbs and seaweed that's used to season foods. It contains less salt than plain table salt, and it adds a rich, herbal taste to cooking. You'll find it under the brand name Herbamare; look for it online and in some specialty food shops.

6 oz	savoy cabbage	175 g
1 tbsp	canola oil	15 mL
1	onion, finely chopped	1
2 tbsp	water	30 mL
4 tsp	heavy or whipping (35%) cream	20 mL
1 tbsp	horseradish cream (see tip, below)	15 mL
	Herb salt (see tip, at left)	
10	slices smoked salmon (about 7 oz/210 g)	10

1. Core and shred cabbage. In a nonstick skillet, heat oil over medium-high heat. Add onion; sauté for about 5 minutes or until translucent. Add cabbage; sauté for 2 minutes. Add water; cook, stirring, for about 10 minutes or until cabbage is tender-crisp.

2. In a bowl, stir heavy cream with horseradish cream until smooth; stir into cabbage mixture. Season to taste with herb salt.

3. Spoon cabbage mixture onto a plate; top with smoked salmon. Serve immediately.

Shopping Tip

Horseradish cream is a condiment often served with cold meats or fish in Europe; you might also find it under the name creamed horseradish. It usually contains whipping cream, sour cream or mayonnaise. It is different than prepared horseradish, which contains only grated horseradish and vinegar.

Nutrients per serving	
Calories	480
Fat	30 g
Carbohydrates	7 g
Protein	45 g

Porcini "Risotto" with Smoked Salmon

*This tasty take on
the famous rice dish
contains no rice at all.
Grated celeriac replaces
the rice and adds tons of
vitamins and minerals to
the recipe.*

Tips

Dried porcini
mushrooms come in
irregularly sized slices,
so a digital scale is handy
for measuring them for
this recipe.

Celeriac is a knobby
root vegetable that has a
wonderful celery flavor.
It is very large and has
unattractive roots all
over the outside, but
once it's peeled and
trimmed, the root reveals
crisp, delicate white
flesh inside.

1 cup	water	250 mL
⅛ oz	dried porcini mushrooms (see tip, at left)	3 g
1 tbsp	canola oil	15 mL
1 tsp	butter	5 mL
3 tbsp	finely chopped onion	45 mL
2 tbsp	minced garlic	30 mL
1 tbsp	dry white wine	15 mL
1 tbsp	ready-to-use chicken broth	15 mL
3½ oz	celeriac (see tips, at left)	100 g
2½ tbsp	grated Parmesan cheese	37 mL
4	slices smoked salmon (about 2½ oz/75 g)	4
	Freshly ground black pepper	

1. In a bowl, combine water with porcini mushrooms; let soak for 2 hours.

2. Reserving soaking liquid, drain mushrooms. In a saucepan, heat oil and butter over medium-high heat. Add onion and garlic; sauté for 5 minutes or until translucent. Stir in white wine; add soaked porcini mushrooms and broth. Bring to a boil; boil for 1 to 2 minutes or until slightly reduced.

3. Meanwhile, peel celeriac; using a box grater, grate celeriac finely until in pieces about the size of rice grains. Stir grated celeriac into broth mixture, adding enough of the reserved mushroom soaking liquid to just cover bottom of pan.

4. Reduce heat, cover and simmer, stirring occasionally, for about 10 minutes or until celeriac is tender. Stir in cheese; remove from heat and let stand for 5 minutes.

5. Cut smoked salmon into strips. Spoon "risotto" onto a plate; top with smoked salmon. Season to taste with pepper.

Nutrients per serving	
Calories	307
Fat	21 g
Carbohydrates	7 g
Protein	21 g

Salmon Pancake Rolls

**Prep time:
1¾ hours**

*These rolls make a
terrific portable lunch
for busy days. Pack
them in your lunch
box with an ice pack
to keep them cool until
serving time.*

Tip

Gravlax is Scandinavian
cured salmon. It has a
similar texture to that
of cold-smoked salmon
(also called lox), but it
is not smoked. If you
like, you can substitute
smoked salmon for it in
this recipe.

- **Preheat oven to 200°F (100°C)**

7 tbsp	buttermilk	100 mL
¼ cup	whole-grain spelt flour	60 mL
1	egg	1
1 tbsp	butter, melted	15 mL
	Salt and freshly ground black pepper	
2 tsp	olive oil, divided	10 mL
1 tbsp	cream cheese, softened	15 mL
1 tbsp	crème fraîche	15 mL
2 tsp	prepared horseradish	10 mL
1	handful arugula, trimmed	1
4	thin slices gravlax (about 2½ oz/75 g), see tip, at left	4

1. In a bowl, stir together buttermilk, flour, egg, butter, and salt and pepper, to make a smooth batter. Let stand for 15 minutes.

2. In a small nonstick skillet, heat 1 tsp (5 mL) of the oil over medium heat; spoon in half of the batter and spread to make thin pancake. Cook for 4 to 5 minutes; turn and cook for 4 to 5 minutes or until golden brown. Transfer to a baking sheet; keep warm in preheated oven. Repeat with remaining oil and batter.

3. Meanwhile, in a bowl, stir together cream cheese, crème fraîche and horseradish; season to taste with salt and pepper.

4. Spread cheese mixture over pancakes. Sprinkle arugula over top; top each pancake with 2 slices of the gravlax. Roll up pancake around filling and wrap tightly in plastic wrap; refrigerate for 1 hour. To serve, cut pancake rolls diagonally into 3 slices each.

Nutrients per serving	
Calories	691
Fat	45 g
Carbohydrates	35 g
Protein	36 g

Smoked Trout with Radish-Ricotta Dip

Enjoy this meal on a steamy summer evening. It's ideal for nights when it's too hot to cook.

Tips

Choose full-fat ricotta for this recipe. It's creamy and delicious, and it adds plenty of healthy fat to your diet.

Look for smoked trout fillets at the fish counter of the supermarket. Hot-smoked salmon fillets are a nice alternative.

1 tbsp	chopped almonds	15 mL
2 oz	ricotta cheese (see tips, at left)	60 g
1 tbsp	heavy or whipping (35%) cream	15 mL
1 tsp	lemon juice	5 mL
4	radishes	4
	Salt and freshly ground black pepper	
1	head Belgian endive	1
1 tbsp	balsamic vinegar	15 mL
1 tbsp	olive oil	15 mL
1	smoked trout fillet (about 5 oz/ 150 g), see tips, at left	1
1 tbsp	snipped or chopped fresh chives (see tips, page 253)	15 mL

1. In a dry nonstick skillet over medium heat, toast almonds, shaking pan often, for about 5 minutes or until golden brown. Transfer to a bowl; let cool.

2. Meanwhile, in another bowl, stir together cheese, cream and lemon juice until smooth. Finely chop radishes. Stir radishes and almonds into cheese mixture; season to taste with salt and pepper.

3. Halve endive lengthwise and core; cut halves crosswise into 1-inch (2.5 cm) pieces. In a large bowl, whisk vinegar with oil; season to taste with salt and pepper. Add endive; toss to coat.

4. Arrange trout fillet on a plate; serve with radish dip and endive salad. Garnish with chives.

Serving Idea

For an extra hit of fresh flavor, sprinkle a handful of radish sprouts over the ricotta dip.

Nutrients per serving	
Calories	463
Fat	31 g
Carbohydrates	7 g
Protein	38 g

Pesto Catfish with Sautéed Vegetables

Makes 1 serving

Prep time: 30 minutes

Catfish is meaty, substantial and filling. Here, it's accented by an easy-to-make pesto topping and sautéed veggies.

Tip

You can substitute any similarly textured fish for the catfish. Check the Green-Light Foods list on page 146 for healthy options.

- Preheat oven to 400°F (200°C)
- 6-cup (1.5 L) gratin dish, lightly brushed with oil
- Mini food processor

1 tsp	olive oil	5 mL
½ tsp	lemon juice	2 mL
	Salt and freshly ground black pepper	
1	catfish fillet (3½ oz/100 g)	1
½	each carrot and small zucchini	½
½ tsp	butter	2 mL
½	small onion, finely chopped	½
1 tbsp	ready-to-use vegetable broth	15 mL
3 tbsp	sour cream	45 mL
Pinch	herb salt (see tip, page 285)	Pinch
½ tsp	special oil mixture (see page 161)	2 mL

Pesto

1	handful fresh basil sprigs	1
1 tsp	pine nuts or chopped almonds	5 mL
2½ tsp	grated Parmesan cheese	12 mL
1 tsp	olive oil	5 mL

1. In a bowl, stir olive oil with lemon juice; season to taste with salt and pepper. Pat fish dry with paper towels; arrange fish in prepared gratin dish. Brush with oil mixture.

2. **Pesto:** Wash basil sprigs and pat dry; pull leaves off stems. In a mini food processor, pulse basil leaves with pine nuts until finely chopped; pulse in cheese. With machine running, add oil in steady stream until combined. Spread over fish. Bake in preheated oven for 15 minutes or until fish flakes easily when tested with a fork.

3. Meanwhile, cut carrot and zucchini lengthwise into thin strips. In a nonstick skillet, melt butter over medium-high heat. Add carrot and onion; sauté for 2 minutes. Add broth; simmer for 3 minutes. Add zucchini; simmer for 3 minutes or until zucchini is tender-crisp. Stir in sour cream and herb salt.

4. Arrange fish and zucchini mixture on a plate. Drizzle with special oil mixture.

Nutrients per serving	
Calories	374
Fat	30 g
Carbohydrates	4 g
Protein	22 g

Catfish with Lemon Spinach

This dish is wonderful with any firm-fleshed white fish you like. The pine nuts add a crunchy, nutty note that's really appealing.

Tip

Pine nuts can be quite expensive. If you like, you can substitute chopped almonds for them in this dish. But since you need only 1 tbsp (15 mL), they're worth the splurge for their wonderful flavor.

1½ tsp	butter	7 mL
1	shallot, finely chopped	1
1 tbsp	pine nuts (see tip, at left)	15 mL
1	catfish fillet (7 oz/210 g)	1
	Salt and freshly ground black pepper	
1 tbsp	olive oil	15 mL
⅓ cup	ready-to-use chicken broth	75 mL
⅓ cup	heavy or whipping (35%) cream	75 mL
½ tsp	locust bean gum (see tip, below)	2 mL
5 oz	baby spinach	150 g
	Grated zest of 1 organic lemon	

1. In a nonstick skillet, melt butter over medium heat. Add shallot and pine nuts; cook, stirring, for 2 to 3 minutes or until shallot is starting to soften.

2. Meanwhile, pat fish dry with paper towels; cut into strips. Season with salt and pepper. In another nonstick skillet, heat oil over medium heat. Add fish; cook for 1 to 2 minutes.

3. Add broth and cream to fish; stir in locust bean gum. Cook, stirring occasionally, for 3 to 4 minutes or until sauce is slightly thickened and fish is opaque and flakes easily when tested with a fork. Season to taste with salt and pepper.

4. Meanwhile, stir spinach into pine nut mixture. Increase heat to medium-high; sauté for 1 to 2 minutes or until spinach is wilted. Stir in lemon zest; season to taste with salt and pepper. Serve with fish.

Shopping Tip

Locust bean gum is also called carob bean gum. It is a natural plant thickener that you can use when you're on the cancer-fighting diet (see page 147). Look for it in health food stores.

Nutrients per serving	
Calories	506
Fat	41 g
Carbohydrates	6 g
Protein	29 g

Sesame-Coated Fish with Spinach and Tomatoes

Sesame seeds create a crunchy, satisfying crust on this tender fish. The warm spinach and tomatoes is the ideal complement.

Tip

This is another recipe that's excellent with all sorts of fish. Change the recipe up and try salmon fillets, trout fillets or any firm white fish you like. Check the Green-Light Foods list (page 146) for ideas.

1	green onion (white and light green parts)	1
4	cherry tomatoes	4
1 tbsp	canola oil	15 mL
1 tsp	sesame oil	5 mL
2½ oz	baby spinach	75 g
1½ tbsp	tamari or soy sauce (see tips, page 237), divided	22 mL
	Freshly ground black pepper	
1	catfish fillet (about 5 oz/150 g), see tip, at left	1
1	egg yolk	1
1 tbsp	sesame seeds	15 mL
1 tbsp	heavy or whipping (35%) cream	15 mL
2 tsp	butter	10 mL

1. Thinly slice green onion diagonally. Quarter cherry tomatoes. Set aside.

2. In a nonstick skillet, heat canola oil and sesame oil over medium heat. Add green onion and spinach; cover and cook for 2 to 3 minutes or until spinach is wilted. Remove from heat; drizzle with 1 tbsp (15 mL) of the tamari. Season to taste with pepper. Stir in cherry tomatoes; let cool slightly.

3. Meanwhile, pat fish dry with paper towels; drizzle with remaining tamari. In a bowl, stir together egg yolk, sesame seeds and cream; add fish, turning to coat.

4. In a small nonstick skillet, melt butter over medium-high heat. Add fish; fry, turning once, for 4 to 6 minutes or until golden brown, and fish is opaque and flakes easily when tested with a fork. Serve with spinach mixture.

Nutrients per serving	
Calories	497
Fat	41 g
Carbohydrates	6 g
Protein	26 g

Pan-Fried Salmon with Broccoli

Simple and elegant is the name of the game with this meal. Look for sustainably caught wild salmon for the best flavor and nutrition.

Tip

Marinades that contain raw fish or meat should be cooked if you're planning to consume them. This one contains fish, so simmering it for a few minutes is enough. If you're using a marinade that has contained raw poultry or meat, boil it for 5 minutes before digging in. It should reach 165°F (74°C) to kill any bacteria.

1 tsp	olive oil	5 mL
	Juice of ½ lemon	
1	skin-on salmon fillet (7 oz/210 g)	1
2 tsp	butter	10 mL
	Salt	
8 oz	broccoli, trimmed and cut into florets	250 g
	Chopped fresh chives and parsley	
1	lemon wedge	1

1. In a bowl, stir olive oil with lemon juice; add fish. Let stand for 20 minutes to marinate.

2. In a nonstick skillet, melt butter over low heat. Reserving marinade, add fish, skin side down; cook, turning once, for 8 to 12 minutes or until golden brown. Pour reserved marinade over fish (see tip, at left); cook for 2 to 3 minutes or until fish is opaque and flakes easily when tested with a fork. Season to taste with salt.

3. Meanwhile, in a saucepan of boiling salted water, cook broccoli for 5 to 10 minutes or until tender-crisp. Drain.

4. Transfer fish and broccoli to a plate; drizzle with pan juices in skillet. Garnish with chives, parsley and lemon wedge.

Nutrients per serving	
Calories	420
Fat	24 g
Carbohydrates	6 g
Protein	44 g

Spinach and Salmon Skillet

A little bit of your special oil mixture is the crowning glory on this simple supper. The oil adds high-quality fats and a rich flavor to the tender fish.

Tip

If you don't feel like trimming off larger spinach stems, use the same weight of baby spinach. You can consume the slender stems because they are so tender.

1	tomato	1
1	small skin-on salmon fillet (3½ oz/100 g)	1
1 tsp	lemon juice	5 mL
	Salt and white pepper	
1 tbsp	canola oil, divided	15 mL
½	small onion, finely chopped	½
7 oz	fresh spinach, trimmed and shredded (see tip, at left)	210 g
2 tsp	special oil mixture (see page 161)	10 mL
1 tsp	turmeric	5 mL

1. Core and cut tomato into eighths. Pat fish dry with paper towels; drizzle lemon juice over top. Season with salt.

2. In a nonstick skillet, heat 1 tsp (5 mL) of the canola oil over medium-high heat. Add fish, skin side down; fry for 4 minutes. Turn; reduce heat to low and cook for 2 minutes or until fish is opaque and flakes easily when tested with a fork. Transfer to a plate; keep warm.

3. Add remaining canola oil to skillet; heat over medium-high heat. Add onion; sauté for 2 minutes or until starting to soften. Add spinach and tomato. Reduce heat to medium; cook, stirring, for 3 to 5 minutes or until spinach is wilted and tender. Stir in special oil mixture and turmeric; season to taste with salt and pepper. Serve with fish.

Nutrients per serving	
Calories	290
Fat	20 g
Carbohydrates	4 g
Protein	24 g

Salmon with Cabbage and Orange

Makes 1 serving

Prep time: 30 minutes

Orange makes this dish so bright and citrusy. It's perfect for a gloomy evening, when you need a boost.

Tip

Sliced fennel bulb makes a nice substitute for the cabbage if you like it.

- **Preheat oven to 200°F (100°C)**

1	skin-on salmon fillet (7 oz/210 g)		1
2 tsp	lemon juice		10 mL
	Salt and freshly ground black pepper		
1½ tbsp	olive oil, divided		22 mL
1	sprig fresh rosemary		1
7 oz	green cabbage, finely shredded		210 g
	Zest and juice of 1 organic orange		
1 tbsp	cold butter		15 mL
	Cayenne pepper		

1. Pat fish dry with paper towels; drizzle with lemon juice. Season with salt and black pepper. In a nonstick skillet, heat 1½ tsp (7 mL) of the oil over medium heat. Add rosemary and fish, skin side down; fry for 5 minutes. Turn; fry for 2 minutes or until fish is opaque and flakes easily when tested with a fork. Transfer to an ovenproof plate, discarding rosemary; keep fish warm in preheated oven.

2. Add remaining oil to skillet. Add cabbage; fry, stirring often, for 2 minutes or until wilted. Season to taste with salt and black pepper. Add cabbage to plate in oven.

3. Add orange juice to skillet; cook, stirring up brown bits from bottom of pan, for 1 to 2 minutes. Add orange zest; cook, stirring occasionally, for 5 minutes or until sauce is reduced by half.

4. Stir butter into sauce until melted and smooth. Season to taste with salt and cayenne pepper.

5. Remove cabbage and fish from oven; drizzle sauce over top.

Nutrients per serving	
Calories	693
Fat	52 g
Carbohydrates	13 g
Protein	42 g

Fish and Parsnip Fries

Makes 1 serving

Prep time: 30 minutes

This is a healthier take on fish and chips that you can't get in a restaurant. It has the typical crispy beer batter you expect, but with fewer carbohydrates.

Tips

A number of breweries now make reduced-carbohydrate beers. Look for a refreshing Pilsner-style one for this recipe. It will help make the batter light and crispy.

Wild Atlantic cod that's caught using the hook-and-line method is the most sustainable choice.

- Preheat oven to 475°F (240°C)
- Candy/deep-fry thermometer
- Plate, lined with paper towels
- Baking sheet, lined with parchment paper

3 tbsp	ground almonds	45 mL
1 tsp	finely ground oat bran (see tips, page 284)	5 mL
1 tsp	baking powder	5 mL
Pinch	each salt and freshly ground black pepper	Pinch
3 tbsp	low-carb Pilsner-style beer (see tips, at left)	45 mL
1	egg	1
1	parsnip, peeled if desired (see tips, page 252)	1
	Coconut oil for deep-frying	
1	cod fillet (about 4 oz/125 g), see tips, at left	1

1. In a large bowl, whisk together ground almonds, oat bran, baking powder, salt and pepper; stir in beer and egg until smooth. Let stand for 15 minutes.

2. Meanwhile, cut parsnip into thick sticks; pat dry with paper towels. In a large deep saucepan, heat coconut oil over medium-high heat until a candy/deep-fry thermometer registers 350°F (180°C). Add parsnip sticks to oil; deep-fry, turning once, for 3 minutes. Transfer to prepared plate; let drain.

3. Dip fish into batter, turning to coat. Add to oil; deep-fry, turning once, for 2 to 3 minutes or until golden brown. Transfer to prepared baking sheet; bake in preheated oven for about 10 minutes or until fish is opaque and flakes easily when tested with a fork.

4. Meanwhile, deep-fry parsnip sticks again for about 3 minutes or until golden brown and crisp. Serve with fish.

Prep Tip

A large, tall-sided saucepan works well for deep-frying small amounts, but you can use a stand-alone deep-fryer if you prefer.

Nutrients per serving	
Calories	270
Fat	13 g
Carbohydrates	6 g
Protein	29 g

Red Mullet with Vegetable Quinoa

This dish is a tasty way to enjoy gluten-free quinoa for dinner. It's an enjoyable addition to the cancer-fighting menu.

Tip

You can use fresh or thawed frozen red mullet in this dish. The vegetable quinoa also tastes delicious with pike, perch or gilthead sea bream.

1	skin-on red mullet fillet (5 oz/150 g)	1
2 tsp	lemon juice	10 mL
	Salt and freshly ground black pepper	
1	small onion	1
1	carrot	1
1	small red bell pepper	1
1/2	zucchini (3 1/2 oz/100 g)	1/2
2 tbsp	olive oil, divided	30 mL
2 tbsp	quinoa	30 mL
7 tbsp	ready-to-use vegetable broth	100 mL
	Hot paprika (see tips, page 225)	
1 tbsp	chopped fresh parsley	15 mL

1. Pat fish dry with paper towels; drizzle with lemon juice. Season with salt and pepper. Finely chop onion, carrot, red pepper and zucchini.

2. In a saucepan, heat 1 tbsp (15 mL) of the oil over medium-high heat. Add onion; sauté for 5 minutes or until translucent.

3. Meanwhile, rinse quinoa in hot water; drain well. Add quinoa, carrot, red pepper and zucchini to pan; cook, stirring, for 1 minute. Add broth; bring to a boil. Reduce heat to low, cover and simmer for 15 minutes or until vegetables and quinoa are tender.

4. Meanwhile, in another skillet, heat remaining oil over medium-high heat. Add fish, skin side down; fry for 2 minutes. Turn; fry for 2 minutes or until fish is opaque and flakes easily when tested with a fork. Season to taste with salt, pepper and paprika.

5. Serve quinoa mixture with fish; garnish with parsley.

Nutrients per serving	
Calories	506
Fat	41 g
Carbohydrates	6 g
Protein	29 g

Pollock Fillet on Fennel and Tomatoes

Makes 1 serving

**Prep time:
45 minutes**

Gouda cheese is a surprising (and surprisingly delicious!) addition to this saucy fish. The foil packet makes this recipe perfect for nights when you don't want to wash extra dishes.

Tip

If you can't find pollock, substitute any tender white fish you like. Check the Green-Light Foods list (page 146) for ideas.

- Preheat oven to 400°F (200°C)
- Bowl, filled with ice water
- Long rectangle of foil, brushed with oil

1	bulb fennel (about 7½ oz/225 g)	1
1	stalk celery	1
2	plum tomatoes	2
1	pollock fillet (5 oz/150 g), see tip, at left	1
2 tsp	lemon juice	10 mL
	Salt and freshly ground black pepper	
1	thick slice Gouda cheese (about 1½ oz/45 g)	1

1. Trim and core fennel, reserving some of the delicate fronds for garnish; slice fennel thinly. Cut celery diagonally into ¾-inch (2 cm) pieces. In a saucepan of boiling salted water, blanch fennel and celery for 2 minutes. Using a slotted spoon, transfer fennel and celery to prepared bowl of ice water; let cool. Drain well.

2. Core and slice tomatoes. Pat fish dry with paper towels; drizzle with lemon juice. Season with salt and pepper.

3. Arrange fennel, celery and half of the tomato slices on prepared foil; top with fish. Cover with remaining tomato slices; season with salt and pepper. Top with cheese; seal foil around contents to form packet.

4. Roast, directly on rack, in preheated oven for 20 to 25 minutes or until fish is opaque and flakes easily when tested with a fork.

5. Open foil packet, being careful of the steam inside; arrange fish mixture on a plate. Garnish with reserved fennel fronds.

Nutrients per serving	
Calories	383
Fat	19 g
Carbohydrates	10 g
Protein	43 g

Ocean Perch with Saffron Sauce

Makes 1 serving

Prep time: 30 minutes

Saffron is one of the world's most expensive spices, and for good reason. The best brands are hand harvested from millions of crocuses. Fortunately, you need only a tiny bit to season this wonderful fish.

Tip

Stirring little pats of cold butter into a sauce makes it silky and a little bit shiny. It adds a wonderful texture to an already tasty topping for the fish and vegetables.

• **Immersion blender**

1	carrot	1
1	large leek (white and light green parts), about 3½ oz (100 g)	1
1	ocean perch fillet (5 oz/150 g)	1
1 tbsp	olive oil	15 mL
1	clove garlic, minced	1
7 tbsp	ready-to-use fish broth or chicken broth	100 mL
7 tbsp	heavy or whipping (35%) cream, divided	100 mL
5 or 6	saffron threads	5 or 6
	Salt and freshly ground black pepper	
7 oz	celeriac (see tips, page 286), peeled and diced	210 g
1 tbsp	chopped fresh parsley	15 mL
1 tbsp	cold butter, cubed (see tip, at left)	15 mL

1. Cut carrot and leek into thin strips. Pat fish dry with paper towels; cut in half crosswise.

2. In a nonstick skillet, heat oil over medium-high heat. Add carrot, leek and garlic; sauté for 2 minutes. Add broth, ⅓ cup (75 mL) of the cream and saffron; season to taste with salt and pepper. Nestle fish into liquid; reduce heat to low, cover and simmer for 8 minutes or until fish is opaque and flakes easily when tested with a fork.

3. Meanwhile, in a saucepan of boiling salted water, cook celeriac for 8 minutes or until tender. Drain; using an immersion blender, purée celeriac with remaining cream. Season to taste with salt and pepper; stir in parsley.

4. Using a slotted spoon, transfer fish and vegetables to a plate; keep warm. Season cooking liquid to taste with salt and pepper; whisk in butter, a cube at a time, until melted and smooth. Pour sauce over fish and vegetables. Serve with celeriac purée.

Nutrients per serving	
Calories	632
Fat	47 g
Carbohydrates	14 g
Protein	37 g

Bream with Summer Vegetables

This is a delicious dish to make after a trip to the farmer's market in late summer. Enjoy it with a glass of red or rosé wine.

Tip

Gilthead sea bream is a delicious, sustainable fish choice. It is raised in Canada in closed systems, so it has less impact on the environment. This species is also considered the most delicious type of sea bream, with mild, tender flesh.

½	zucchini (about 5 oz/150 g)	½
3	green onions (white and light green parts)	3
½ cup	cherry tomatoes	125 mL
1	skin-on gilthead sea bream fillet (5 oz/150 g), see tip, at left	1
2 tsp	lemon juice	10 mL
	Salt and freshly ground black pepper	
2 tbsp	olive oil, divided	30 mL
3 tbsp	ready-to-use vegetable broth	45 mL
2 tsp	chopped fresh oregano (or ½ tsp/2 mL dried oregano)	10 mL
2 tsp	basil pesto (homemade or jarred)	10 mL

1. Using a vegetable peeler, cut zucchini lengthwise into thin slices. Cut green onions diagonally into ¾- to 1-inch (2 to 2.5 cm) lengths. Halve cherry tomatoes. Set aside.

2. Pat fish dry with paper towels; drizzle with lemon juice. Season with salt and pepper.

3. In a nonstick skillet, heat 1 tbsp (15 mL) of the oil over medium-high heat. Add fish, skin side down; fry for 4 minutes or until crisp and golden. Turn; fry for 2 minutes or until fish is opaque and flakes easily when tested with a fork.

4. Meanwhile, in another nonstick skillet, heat remaining oil over high heat. Add zucchini and green onions; sauté for 2 minutes. Add cherry tomatoes, broth and oregano; sauté for 2 minutes or until zucchini is tender. Season to taste with salt and pepper.

5. Transfer fish and zucchini mixture to a plate; serve with pesto.

Nutrients per serving	
Calories	405
Fat	30 g
Carbohydrates	8 g
Protein	25 g

Mediterranean Foil-Baked Trout

Trout is meaty and satisfying. Here, it's baked in a simple foil packet, which keeps the fish moist and tender, and makes cleanup easy.

Tip

If you can't find mini bell peppers, use the same weight of regular bell peppers, in assorted colors.

- **Preheat oven to 425°F (220°C)**
- **12-inch (30 cm) long piece of foil, brushed with olive oil**

1	whole trout (about 12 oz/375 g), cleaned (see tip, below)	1
	Salt and freshly ground black pepper	
3	sprigs fresh thyme	3
1	clove garlic, thinly sliced	1
2	slices organic lemon	2
3½ oz	yellow, orange and red mini bell peppers (see tip, at left)	100 g
5	pimento-stuffed olives, sliced	5
1 tbsp	drained capers	15 mL

1. Pat fish dry, inside and outside, with paper towels; season inside and outside with salt and pepper. Wash thyme and pat dry. Stuff fish cavity with thyme, garlic and lemon slices.

2. Seed peppers and cut into thin rings. Place trout on prepared foil; top with peppers, olives and capers. Seal foil around trout to make packet; place on a baking sheet.

3. Bake in preheated oven for 30 minutes or until fish is opaque and flakes easily when tested with a fork. Open packet at the table, being careful of the steam inside.

Shopping Tip

When you're buying a whole fish that's cleaned and ready to cook, there are signs of freshness you should watch for. The eyes should be clear, not milky; and the gills should be bright red, not brownish. The scales should also be shiny. The skin and the flesh should both bounce back when you press a finger against them. One last thing is certain: if fish smells fishy, it is definitely not fresh.

Nutrients per serving

Calories	345
Fat	18 g
Carbohydrates	4 g
Protein	41 g

Shrimp-Stuffed Zucchini

Makes 1 serving

Prep time: 40 minutes

Stuffed vegetables are always fun, and this recipe is a terrific way to use up zucchini if they're overrunning your garden.

Tip

Crème fraîche is a wonderful, creamy, less-tangy alternative to sour cream. Use leftovers as a simple topping on berries for dessert.

- Preheat oven to 400°F (200°C)
- 6-cup (1.5 L) gratin dish, greased with 1 tsp (5 mL) butter

1	zucchini (about 8 oz/250 g)	1
1 tbsp	canola oil	15 mL
1	small onion, finely chopped	1
3 tbsp	crème fraîche (see tip, at left)	45 mL
2 oz	deveined peeled small shrimp	60 g
1 tsp	chopped fresh dill	5 mL
	Salt and freshly ground black pepper	
2½ tbsp	grated Parmesan cheese	37 mL

1. Halve zucchini lengthwise. Using a spoon, scrape out flesh, leaving a thin wall around edge. Set aside zucchini shells. Finely chop zucchini flesh.

2. In a nonstick skillet, heat oil over medium-high heat. Add onion and zucchini flesh; sauté for 2 minutes or until starting to soften. If pan is dry, add a little water; sauté for 2 to 3 minutes or until onion is softened. Remove from heat. Stir in crème fraîche, shrimp and dill; season with salt and pepper.

3. Arrange zucchini shells in prepared gratin dish; spoon filling into shells. Sprinkle with cheese. Bake in preheated oven for about 25 minutes or until shrimp are pink, firm and opaque, and tops are golden brown.

Nutrients per serving	
Calories	348
Fat	28 g
Carbohydrates	8 g
Protein	16 g

Lemony Shrimp with Spinach

*Shrimp is so easy on
a busy night. It takes
very little time to cook,
and it's satisfying paired
with leafy greens, like
this spinach.*

Tip

The shrimp in
supermarkets are often
farmed. When buying
them, look for brands
with an organic label
whenever possible. They
are fed only organic feed
and naturally occurring
plankton; no artificial
additives, antibiotics
or growth hormones
are used.

3	cherry tomatoes	3
1	clove garlic	1
2 tsp	canola oil, divided	10 mL
1	package (10 oz/283 g) frozen leaf spinach, thawed and drained	1
	Salt and freshly ground black pepper	
1 tsp	chile oil (see tip, below)	5 mL
7 oz	thawed frozen jumbo shrimp (see tip, at left), peeled and deveined	210 g
½	organic lemon, sliced thinly	½

1. Halve cherry tomatoes. Cut garlic into paper-thin slices.

2. In a saucepan, heat 1 tsp (5 mL) of the canola oil over medium-high heat. Add garlic; sauté for 1 minute or until fragrant. Add cherry tomatoes; fry for 1 to 2 minutes or until starting to soften. Add spinach; reduce heat to medium, cover and cook, stirring occasionally, for 5 to 7 minutes or until heated through. Season to taste with salt and pepper.

3. In a nonstick skillet, heat remaining canola oil and chile oil over high heat. Add shrimp; cook, turning once, for 3 to 5 minutes or until shrimp are pink, firm and opaque. Season to taste with salt and pepper.

4. Transfer shrimp to a plate; serve with spinach mixture. Garnish shrimp with lemon slices.

Shopping Tip

Chile oil is simply a base oil that's had hot red chiles steeped in it. Look for ready-made bottles of it at Asian grocery stores.

Nutrients per serving	
Calories	475
Fat	22 g
Carbohydrates	11 g
Protein	54 g

Shrimp and Scrambled Eggs

Makes 1 serving

**Prep time:
10 minutes**

*This is an easy supper
you can make in a flash.
If you like, serve it with
one slice of High-Protein
Flaxseed Bread (recipe,
page 206).*

Tips

Look for cooked
deveined peeled shrimp
in the freezer section
of the supermarket. All
they require is thawing,
and they're ready to eat.
If you like them warm,
sauté them in a little
more butter for just a
minute or so until they're
heated through.

2	eggs	2
2 tbsp	heavy or whipping (35%) cream	30 mL
	Salt and freshly ground black pepper	
2 tsp	butter	10 mL
1	leaf lettuce, such as Boston or green leaf	1
2 oz	thawed frozen cooked small shrimp (see tips, at left)	60 g
1	handful garden cress (see tips, page 311)	1

1. In a bowl, whisk eggs with cream; season with salt and pepper. In a small nonstick skillet, melt butter over medium-low heat. Pour in egg mixture; cook, stirring and pushing eggs to form large soft curds, for 3 to 5 minutes or until set.

2. Arrange lettuce on a plate; top with scrambled eggs and shrimp. Garnish with garden cress.

Substitution Tip

You can substitute thawed frozen crayfish tails for the shrimp, cooking them according to the package instructions. Or, for a meaty alternative, substitute chopped ham or prosciutto.

Nutrients per serving	
Calories	348
Fat	27 g
Carbohydrates	2 g
Protein	24 g

Scallops on Mixed Greens

Makes 1 serving

Prep time: 20 minutes

Big, juicy sea scallops are quick to cook and packed with nutrients. Here, they top a refreshing green salad that's accented with crunchy almonds.

Tip

If you can't find or don't care for scallops, substitute jumbo shrimp.

3 oz	mixed salad greens (such as mâche, curly endive and/or arugula)	90 g
1	shallot, finely chopped	1
1 tbsp	white wine vinegar	15 mL
1 tbsp	orange juice	15 mL
1 tbsp	grapeseed oil	15 mL
	Salt and freshly ground black pepper	
3	sea scallops (about 3½ oz/100 g), see tip, below	3
2 tsp	butter	10 mL
1 tbsp	sliced almonds	15 mL
1 tbsp	crème fraîche	15 mL

1. Arrange salad greens on a large plate. In a bowl, whisk together shallot, vinegar, orange juice and oil; season to taste with salt and pepper. Drizzle over greens.

2. Pat scallops dry with paper towels; season with salt and pepper. In a small skillet, melt butter over medium-high heat. Add scallops; cook for 2 minutes per side or until golden brown and opaque in center. Transfer to a plate; keep warm.

3. Add almonds to skillet; sauté for 1 to 2 minutes or until golden brown. Arrange scallops on salad; sprinkle with almonds. Serve with crème fraîche.

Shopping Tip

Look for what fishmongers call dry scallops. They are natural and unprocessed, and don't contain any artificial ingredients. Wet scallops are often injected with preservatives, which make them absorb more water; these scallops look plump, but the water cooks off quickly, leaving you with less-than-delicious results.

Nutrients per serving

Calories	381
Fat	35 g
Carbohydrates	7 g
Protein	10 g

Salads and Side Dishes

Spicy Asian Salad with Chicken

This salad makes a delicious dinner, complete with protein, vegetables and fruit. All you need is dessert afterward!

Tip

When you're seeding and chopping a chile pepper, it's a good idea to wear gloves. The hotter the pepper, the thicker the gloves should be to protect you from the hot chile oil inside.

1	boneless skinless chicken breast (about 5 oz/150 g)	1
1	piece (¾ inch/2 cm) gingerroot, minced	1
4 tsp	tamari or soy sauce, divided	20 mL
1	piece (about 3½ oz/100 g) cucumber, peeled	1
1	star fruit (about 4 oz/125 g), see tip, page 325	1
1	red chile pepper (see tip, at left)	1
1½ tbsp	olive oil, divided	22 mL
1 tbsp	rice vinegar or fruit vinegar	15 mL
1 tbsp	chopped peanuts	15 mL
3	sprigs fresh cilantro	3
	Freshly ground black pepper	

1. Pat chicken dry with paper towels; cut into ¾-inch (2 cm) cubes. In a bowl, toss together chicken, ginger and 2 tsp (10 mL) of the tamari. Let stand to marinate.

2. Meanwhile, slice cucumber and star fruit; arrange decoratively on a plate. Halve chile pepper; seed and cut into thin shreds. Set aside for garnish.

3. In another bowl, whisk together 1 tbsp (15 mL) of the oil, vinegar and remaining tamari; drizzle over cucumber and star fruit.

4. In a small nonstick skillet, heat remaining oil over medium-high heat. Add chicken with marinade, and peanuts; cook, stirring, for 5 to 10 minutes or until sauce is reduced and chicken is no longer pink inside.

5. Spoon chicken mixture over salad. Wash and pat cilantro dry; pull leaves off stems. Garnish chicken mixture with cilantro leaves and chile pepper; season to taste with pepper.

Nutrients per serving	
Calories	434
Fat	23 g
Carbohydrates	15 g
Protein	38 g

Jerusalem Artichoke Salad with Tofu Dressing

Makes 1 serving

Prep time: 25 minutes

A little like potatoes but a lot less carb-heavy, Jerusalem artichokes make a terrific salad. The tofu dressing is creamy, with lots of good-for-you protein.

Tip

Use up leftover silken tofu in breakfast beverages, such as Two-Tone Mango Tofu Smoothie (recipe, page 189).

- **Immersion blender with tall cup**

8 oz	Jerusalem artichokes (see spotlight, below)	250 g
1½ tbsp	olive oil, divided	22 mL
	Salt and freshly ground black pepper	
5	radishes	5
1½ tbsp	white balsamic vinegar, divided	22 mL
2½ oz	silken tofu (see tip, at left), drained	75 g
2 tbsp	heavy or whipping (35%) cream	30 mL
2 tsp	hot mustard	10 mL
2 oz	mâche (see tip, page 260)	60 g
2	handfuls garden cress (see tips, page 311)	2

1. Peel Jerusalem artichokes; cut diagonally into thin slices. In a nonstick skillet, heat 1 tbsp (15 mL) of the oil over medium-high heat. Add Jerusalem artichokes; fry, turning once, for 7 to 8 minutes or until golden brown. Transfer to a plate; season to taste with salt and pepper.

2. Trim and quarter radishes. In a bowl, whisk 1 tbsp (15 mL) of the vinegar with remaining oil; season to taste with salt and pepper. Add warm Jerusalem artichokes and radishes, turning to coat.

3. In a tall cup and using an immersion blender, purée together tofu, cream, mustard and remaining vinegar; season to taste with salt and pepper.

4. Arrange mâche on a plate; top with Jerusalem artichoke mixture. Drizzle with tofu dressing; garnish with garden cress.

Spotlight

Jerusalem artichokes do not contain starch. Instead, they contain up to 16% inulin (see page 75), which helps slow down the rise in blood sugar after a meal. They have a nutty, slightly sweet taste reminiscent of artichokes. Store them in the crisper drawer of your refrigerator. Revive slightly withered tubers by soaking them in cold water.

Nutrients per serving	
Calories	370
Fat	27 g
Carbohydrates	16 g
Protein	15 g

Belgian Endive and Shrimp Salad

Belgian endive has a pleasantly bitter edge, which is a nice contrast to the slightly sweet shrimp and creamy dressing.

Tip

If you don't like Belgian endive, replace it with a similar amount of lettuce, such as green or red leaf.

1	small head Belgian endive (see tip, at left)	1
1 oz	cooked small shrimp (see tip, page 303)	30 g
2 tsp	kefir (see tip, below)	10 mL
1 tsp	chopped fresh dill	5 mL
1 tsp	special oil mixture (see page 161)	5 mL
	Salt and freshly ground black pepper	
1 tbsp	hulled raw pumpkin seeds	15 mL

1. Core endive; separate into leaves. Arrange in a circle on a plate; arrange shrimp in center of circle.

2. In a bowl, whisk together kefir, dill and special oil mixture. Season to taste with salt and pepper. Drizzle over endive.

3. In a dry nonstick skillet over medium heat, toast pumpkin seeds, shaking pan often, for 5 minutes or until fragrant and golden brown. Coarsely chop pumpkin seeds; sprinkle over endive and shrimp.

Shopping Tip

Kefir is a fermented milk drink that's full of healthy bacteria your digestive system needs. You can find it in many supermarkets today, but it's also possible to make your own at home using a starter culture.

Nutrients per serving	
Calories	135
Fat	10 g
Carbohydrates	3 g
Protein	8 g

Salade Niçoise with Anchovies

Makes 1 serving

**Prep time:
25 minutes**

*Anchovies are a salty,
guilty pleasure for
some people — but they
are good for you, too.
Here, they add depth of
flavor to a version
of the classic, hearty
salade Niçoise.*

Tip

If you don't care for
anchovies, substitute
your favorite smoked fish
or canned tuna.

- Bowl, filled with ice water

2½ oz	green beans, trimmed	75 g
1	parsnip	1
1	head mini romaine lettuce (see tip, page 321)	1
1	tomato	1
1	hard-boiled egg, peeled	1
4	anchovy fillets (see tip, at left)	4
4	green olives	4
1 tbsp	white wine vinegar	15 mL
1 tbsp	water	15 mL
1 tbsp	olive oil	15 mL
½	clove garlic, crushed	½
	Salt and freshly ground black pepper	

1. Halve green beans; peel and slice parsnip. In a saucepan of boiling salted water, cook beans for 5 minutes. Add parsnip; cook for 3 minutes or until vegetables are tender-crisp. Using a slotted spoon, transfer vegetables to prepared bowl of ice water; let cool. Drain well.

2. Tear lettuce into bite-size pieces. Core tomato; cut tomato and egg into wedges. Arrange lettuce, beans, parsnip, tomato, egg, anchovies and olives on a plate.

3. In a bowl, whisk together vinegar, water, oil and garlic; season to taste with salt and pepper. Drizzle over salad.

Nutrients per serving	
Calories	348
Fat	21 g
Carbohydrates	20 g
Protein	20 g

Green Parsnip Salad with Smoked Mackerel

Of course, parsnips aren't green, but the combination of fresh herbs, cucumber and green onion gives this salad a fresh flavor and an inviting hue.

Tip

This salad would also be scrumptious with smoked trout or a hot-smoked salmon fillet.

4 oz	parsnips (about 1½ large)	125 g
2	sprigs fresh parsley	2
1	sprig fresh basil	1
1	organic mini-cucumber	1
1	clove garlic, halved	1
1½ tbsp	olive oil	22 mL
1 tbsp	red wine vinegar	15 mL
1 tbsp	water	15 mL
	Salt and freshly ground black pepper	
1	green onion (white and light green parts), thinly sliced	1
1	smoked peppered mackerel fillet (about 4 oz/125 g), see tip, at left	1

1. Peel and thinly slice parsnips. In a saucepan of boiling salted water, blanch for 2 minutes. Drain well.

2. Wash parsley and basil sprigs and pat dry; pull leaves off stems. Finely chop leaves. Set aside.

3. Using a vegetable peeler, peel strips of skin off cucumber, leaving decorative stripes. Halve cucumber lengthwise; using a spoon, scrape out seeds. Slice cucumber crosswise.

4. Rub cut sides of garlic over inside of a salad bowl; add oil, vinegar and water. Whisk to combine; season to taste with salt and pepper. Add parsnips, cucumber and green onion; gently toss to coat.

5. Arrange salad on a plate; serve with mackerel. Garnish with chopped parsley and basil.

Nutrients per serving	
Calories	491
Fat	34 g
Carbohydrates	17 g
Protein	28 g

Ham Rolls on Arugula

This reimagined chef's salad is the best dinner to take with you on a busy night. Packed in an airtight container, it's portable and, best of all, full of healthy nutrients that takeout options don't provide.

Tips

These ham rolls also make a wonderful appetizer if you have guests for dinner. Simply multiply the amounts of ingredients to make enough for the group.

Garden cress is an herb with tiny leaves that's often sold alongside sprouts. If you can't find it, try another type of sprout you like, such as broccoli or radish sprouts.

3	slices deli ham (about 3 oz/90 g)	3
2½ oz	fresh mozzarella cheese, sliced	75 g
	Salt and freshly ground black pepper	
1 tbsp	olive oil	15 mL
½	small yellow bell pepper, cut in thin strips	½
1	handful garden cress (see tips, at left)	1
1	handful arugula, trimmed	1

1. Place ham slices on a work surface; fold each in half lengthwise. Arrange cheese in center of ham; season to taste with salt and pepper. Drizzle with oil.

2. Arrange yellow pepper and garden cress over cheese. Firmly roll up ham around filling, skewering with a toothpick if desired.

3. In an airtight container, arrange arugula; top with ham rolls. Seal container and refrigerate until ready to eat.

Variation

Ham Rolls with Arugula Salad: If you have time to sit down and eat, make the arugula into a simple dressed salad. In a bowl, whisk together 1 tbsp (15 mL) olive oil, 2 tsp (10 mL) balsamic or other vinegar, and a pinch each of salt and freshly ground black pepper; toss with arugula.

Nutrients per serving	
Calories	473
Fat	35 g
Carbohydrates	3 g
Protein	37 g

Tomato Salad with Sheep's Milk Feta

Makes 1 serving

**Prep time:
15 minutes**

*Make this salad at
the height of tomato
season in August
and September, when
field tomatoes are at
their juiciest.*

Tip

This salad is one where
you'll want to splurge
and use your best high-
quality extra-virgin olive
oil. Some oils have a
fruity taste; these are
ideal on a simple salad
like this.

2	tomatoes	2
½	small onion, thinly sliced	½
4	black olives, pitted and halved	4
1 tsp	herbes de Provence	5 mL
1 tsp	balsamic vinegar	5 mL
1 tsp	olive oil (see tip, at left)	5 mL
1 tsp	special oil mixture (see page 161)	5 mL
	Salt and freshly ground black pepper	
1 oz	sheep's milk feta cheese (see tip, below)	30 g
1 tbsp	chopped fresh basil	15 mL

1. Core and slice tomatoes. Decoratively arrange tomato and onion slices on a plate; garnish with olives.

2. In a bowl, whisk together herbes de Provence, vinegar, olive oil and special oil mixture; season to taste with salt and pepper. Drizzle over tomato salad.

3. Crumble cheese; sprinkle over salad. Garnish with basil.

Shopping Tip

Authentic feta cheese is made in Greece with sheep's milk, or a combination of sheep's and goat's milk. In North America, some feta-style cheeses are made with cow's milk. They are still delicious, with the briny flavor of the original, but they are technically not feta.

Nutrients per serving	
Calories	170
Fat	16 g
Carbohydrates	3 g
Protein	5 g

Mâche Salad with Green Peppercorn Dressing

Makes 1 serving

**Prep time:
15 minutes**

Cured ham and figs are a match made in heaven. Here, they're made even more scrumptious with the addition of briny green peppercorns and savory shaved Parmesan cheese.

Tip

Green peppercorns are pickled in brine. You'll find jars or cans of them in the pickle aisle of the supermarket, near the capers.

1	ripe fresh fig (see tip, below)	1
2 oz	mâche	60 g
2 tbsp	orange juice	30 mL
1 tbsp	olive oil	15 mL
1 tbsp	balsamic vinegar	15 mL
	Salt and freshly ground black pepper	
1 tsp	drained jarred green peppercorns (see tip, at left)	5 mL
6	slices country-style ham (see tip, page 266)	6
¾ oz	Parmesan cheese	20 g

1. Cut fig into wedges; decoratively arrange fig wedges and mâche on a plate.

2. In a bowl, whisk together orange juice, oil and vinegar; season to taste with salt and pepper. Stir in green peppercorns.

3. Tuck ham slices into salad. Using a vegetable peeler or the coarse side of a box grater, shave or shred cheese over salad. Drizzle dressing over top.

Substitution Tip

When figs aren't in season, other fruits will work well in this salad. The peppery flavor of the mâche is a nice match with berries or currants. Substitute two or three fresh strawberries, hulled, or 2 to 3 tbsp (30 to 45 mL) red currants for the fig.

Nutrients per serving	
Calories	310
Fat	19 g
Carbohydrates	7 g
Protein	25 g

Kohlrabi and Mozzarella Salad

Makes 1 serving

**Prep time:
20 minutes**

*This is an interesting
combination that you
don't often hear of. But
the tender-crisp kohlrabi
and the delicate cheese
are happy partners.*

Tip

In the summertime,
when juicy tomatoes
are in season, use them
instead of the kohlrabi.

- **Bowl, filled with ice water**

1	head kohlrabi (about 6 oz/175 g), see tip, at left	1
4 oz	fresh mozzarella cheese (see tip, below)	125 g
2 tsp	sesame seeds	10 mL
1 tbsp	olive oil	15 mL
1 tbsp	white balsamic vinegar	15 mL
2 tsp	lemon juice	10 mL
	Salt and freshly ground black pepper	

1. Reserving leaves for garnish, trim and peel kohlrabi. Cut kohlrabi into 1/4-inch (0.5 cm) thick slices. In a saucepan of boiling salted water, blanch kohlrabi slices for 2 minutes or until tender-crisp. Using a slotted spoon, transfer kohlrabi slices to prepared bowl of ice water; let cool. Drain well.

2. Meanwhile, pat cheese dry with paper towels; cut it into 1/4-inch (0.5 cm) thick slices.

3. In a small dry nonstick skillet over medium heat, toast sesame seeds, shaking pan often, for 3 to 5 minutes or until fragrant and golden brown. Transfer to a plate; let cool.

4. Alternately arrange kohlrabi and mozzarella slices, overlapping, on a plate. In a bowl, whisk together oil, vinegar and lemon juice; season to taste with salt and pepper. Drizzle over salad.

5. Cut kohlrabi leaves into thin strips; garnish salad with sesame seeds and kohlrabi leaves.

Shopping Tip

Make sure you buy a ball of fresh mozzarella, which is
packed in liquid at the deli counter. Drier, yellow pizza
mozzarella is not the right texture for this fresh salad.

Nutrients per serving	
Calories	504
Fat	40 g
Carbohydrates	8 g
Protein	27 g

Spinach with Almond-Coated Goat Cheese

These rounds of goat cheese are coated with crunchy nuts and served on a bed of wilted spinach. They make a lovely starter or a light-tasting lunch.

Tip

Frozen spinach contains a lot of moisture, so let it stand in a fine-mesh sieve to drain as it thaws. Before you cook the spinach, you can press or squeeze handfuls of it to ensure the excess liquid is removed.

2 tbsp	sliced almonds	30 mL
1 tbsp	butter	15 mL
1/2	small onion, finely chopped	1/2
1	package (10 oz/283 g) frozen leaf spinach, thawed and drained (see tip, at left)	1
	Salt and freshly ground black pepper	
	Grated nutmeg	
2	rounds (about 1/2-inch/1 cm thick) soft goat cheese	2

1. In a dry nonstick skillet over medium heat, toast almonds, shaking pan often, for 5 minutes or until fragrant and golden brown. Transfer to a plate; let cool.

2. In another nonstick skillet, melt butter over medium heat. Add onion; cook, stirring, for 5 minutes or until translucent. Add spinach; cover and cook, stirring often, for 5 to 7 minutes or until heated through. Season to taste with salt, pepper and nutmeg.

3. Spoon spinach mixture onto a plate. Gently press cheese into toasted almonds, turning to coat; arrange over spinach.

Nutrients per serving	
Calories	570
Fat	47 g
Carbohydrates	4 g
Protein	32 g

Mâche Salad with Goat Cheese

Makes 1 serving

Prep time: 10 minutes

Also called lamb's lettuce or corn salad, mâche is a tender spring green you'll love in salads. Here, it's a tasty partner to mushrooms and soft goat cheese.

Tip

Plain white mushrooms are lovely in this salad, but you can try more exotic cremini mushrooms if you like. They are simply small portobello mushrooms, with the same rich flavor.

1 oz	mushrooms (see tip, at left)	30 g
1 tsp	shelled hemp seeds	5 mL
1 tbsp	kefir (see tip, page 308)	15 mL
2 tsp	special oil mixture (see page 161)	10 mL
1 tsp	heavy or whipping (35%) cream	5 mL
½ tsp	lemon juice	2 mL
½	clove garlic, crushed	½
1 tbsp	chopped fresh herbs (such as parsley or chives)	15 mL
	Salt	
2 oz	mâche (see tip, below)	60 g
3½ oz	soft goat cheese, sliced	100 g

1. Thinly slice mushrooms. In a dry nonstick skillet over medium heat, toast hemp seeds, shaking pan often, for 3 to 4 minutes or until fragrant. Transfer to a plate; let cool.

2. In a bowl, whisk together kefir, special oil mixture, cream and lemon juice. Stir in garlic and herbs; season to taste with salt.

3. Arrange mâche and mushrooms on a plate. Drizzle with kefir mixture; sprinkle with hemp seeds. Top with cheese.

Prep Tip

Wash all greens thoroughly to make sure you remove any grit and bacteria. A salad spinner is an excellent investment, and it's wonderful for drying washed herbs as well as greens.

Nutrients per serving	
Calories	640
Fat	51 g
Carbohydrates	2 g
Protein	46 g

Greek-Style Salad

Makes 1 serving

Prep time: 10 minutes

In North America, Greek salads tend to contain lettuce, but this lettuce-less version is closer to the real thing you'll eat in Greece.

Tip

Use whatever type of black olives you like best in this salad, from briny kalamata olives to oily sun-dried olives.

3	small vine-ripened tomatoes	3
1	organic mini cucumber	1
	Salt and freshly ground black pepper	
2 oz	feta cheese (see tip, page 312)	60 g
4	black olives (see tip, at left)	4
2 tsp	lemon juice	10 mL
2 tsp	olive oil	10 mL
	Hot pepper flakes (optional)	

1. Core and slice tomatoes. Using a vegetable peeler, peel strips of skin off cucumber, leaving decorative stripes. Cut cucumber into slices. Alternately arrange tomato and cucumber slices, overlapping, on a plate; season to taste with salt and pepper.

2. Dice cheese; arrange cheese and olives on top of tomato and cucumber slices.

3. In a bowl, whisk lemon juice with oil; season to taste with salt and pepper. Drizzle over salad; season to taste with hot pepper flakes (if using).

Serving Idea

This Mediterranean salad also makes a delicious small meal if you combine it with a slice of High-Protein Flaxseed Bread (recipe, page 206) or Spelt and Nut Bread (recipe, page 208).

Nutrients per serving

Calories	292
Fat	22 g
Carbohydrates	8 g
Protein	14 g

Avocado Grapefruit Salad

Makes 1 serving

**Prep time:
15 minutes**

These two fruits are not normally partners, but they are wonderful in this creative salad. The smoked mozzarella on top gives it a decadent finish.

Tips

Scamorza is similar to smoked mozzarella cheese. It's a rich, pulled-curd cheese that's formed into a gourd shape (like caciocavallo) and smoked. Use it for this salad if you can find it.

Walnut oil is highly perishable. Keep it in the refrigerator to prevent it from going rancid.

1 tbsp	pine nuts	15 mL
½	pink grapefruit (about 6 oz/175 g)	½
2 tsp	walnut oil (see tips, at left)	10 mL
	Salt and freshly ground black pepper	
½	ripe avocado, peeled and pitted	½
¾ oz	smoked mozzarella cheese (see tip, below), shredded	20 g

1. In a dry nonstick skillet over medium heat, toast pine nuts, shaking pan often, for 5 minutes or until fragrant and golden brown. Transfer to a plate; let cool.

2. Meanwhile, peel grapefruit, completely removing white pith. Using a sharp paring knife and working over a bowl to catch juice and segments, cut between membranes to separate flesh into segments. Reserving 1 tbsp (15 mL) of the grapefruit juice, drain grapefruit segments (use remaining juice for another recipe).

3. In a bowl, whisk reserved grapefruit juice with oil; season to taste with salt and pepper.

4. Cut avocado lengthwise into thin slices; arrange grapefruit and avocado on a plate. Drizzle oil mixture over top. Sprinkle with cheese; garnish with pine nuts.

Substitution Tip

If you're not a fan of smoked cheese or want a different flavor, substitute 2 oz (60 g) soft goat cheese for the mozzarella and crumble it over the salad.

Nutrients per serving	
Calories	510
Fat	47 g
Carbohydrates	12 g
Protein	8 g

Herbed Goat Cheese and Radicchio Salad

Goat cheese is so easy to dress up. Here, it's rolled in fresh parsley and chives and served with a tangy-sweet salad of radicchio and arugula.

Tip

Add a slice of High-Protein Flaxseed Bread (recipe, page 206), and you'll have a very satisfying light lunch.

1 tbsp	hulled raw pumpkin seeds	15 mL
5	sprigs fresh chives	5
3	sprigs fresh parsley	3
	Salt and freshly ground black pepper	
2	rounds (about 1 oz/30 g each) soft goat cheese, such as Picandou	2
½	small head radicchio (about 2½ oz/75 g)	½
1	handful arugula, trimmed	1
1 tbsp	cider vinegar	15 mL
1 tbsp	orange juice	15 mL
1 tbsp	grapeseed oil	15 mL
2 tsp	pumpkin seed oil	10 mL

1. In a dry nonstick skillet over medium heat, toast pumpkin seeds, shaking pan often, for 5 minutes or until fragrant and golden brown. Transfer to a plate; let cool. Finely chop pumpkin seeds.

2. Wash chives and parsley and pat dry; pull leaves off parsley stems. Finely chop parsley leaves and chives. In a bowl, stir together parsley, chives and pumpkin seeds; season to taste with salt and pepper. Gently press cheese into herb mixture to coat all over, pressing so that herb mixture adheres. Reserve any remaining herb mixture for garnish.

3. Core radicchio; tear radicchio and arugula into bite-size pieces. Arrange on a plate; top with cheese.

4. In a bowl, whisk together vinegar, orange juice and grapeseed oil; season to taste with salt and pepper. Drizzle vinegar mixture and pumpkin seed oil over salad; garnish with reserved herb mixture.

Nutrients per serving	
Calories	424
Fat	38 g
Carbohydrates	4 g
Protein	17 g

Marinated Mushroom and Bell Pepper Salad

A mix of exotic mushrooms and colorful bell pepper create a salad that's ultra-tasty and ultra-nutritious.

Tip

Shiitake mushrooms have very hard stems that are unpleasantly chewy. Trim them off and save them for making vegetable stock.

4 oz	small king trumpet mushrooms (see spotlight, opposite)	125 g
2 oz	shiitake mushrooms (see tip, at left)	60 g
1 tbsp	olive oil	15 mL
1	red or orange bell pepper, sliced	1
1	shallot, finely chopped	1
1	clove garlic, minced	1
	Salt and freshly ground black pepper	
4 tsp	lemon juice, divided	20 mL
1 tsp	grapeseed oil	5 mL
1	head mini romaine lettuce (see tip, opposite)	1
2 tbsp	mayonnaise	30 mL
1 tsp	hot mustard	5 mL
½	bunch fresh chives	½

1. Cut king trumpet mushrooms in half crosswise. Trim off and discard stems from shiitake mushrooms; halve or quarter caps.

2. Heat a dry nonstick skillet over high heat. Add king trumpet and shiitake mushrooms; sauté for 4 to 5 minutes or until browned. Add olive oil, red pepper, shallot and garlic; sauté for 2 minutes or until softened. Season to taste with salt and pepper. Transfer mushroom mixture to a bowl. Drizzle with 1 tbsp (15 mL) of the lemon juice, and grapeseed oil; let stand for 5 minutes to marinate.

Nutrients per serving	
Calories	478
Fat	40 g
Carbohydrates	16 g
Protein	11 g

Tip

Look for mini romaine lettuce at gourmet stores. If you're a gardener, there are nice heirloom varieties of this lettuce you can grow in your garden.

3. Meanwhile, tear lettuce into bite-size pieces. Arrange on a plate. In a bowl, stir together mayonnaise, mustard and remaining lemon juice; season to taste with salt and pepper.

4. Wash chives and pat dry; thinly slice. Set aside 1 tsp (5 mL) for garnish; stir remaining chives into mushroom mixture. Spoon mushroom mixture over lettuce. Drizzle with mayonnaise mixture; sprinkle with reserved chives.

Spotlight

King trumpet mushrooms (*Pleurotus eryngii*) are rising stars among cultivated mushrooms. They are related to oyster mushrooms, so they are sometimes call king oyster mushrooms. However, they look and taste more like cèpes. King trumpet mushrooms have firm, white flesh that tastes spicy and nutty; they are low in calories, and rich in protein and fiber. You can use both the stems and the caps, so there is hardly any waste. Try king trumpet mushrooms in just about any dish that calls for mushrooms.

Brussels Sprouts with Walnut Crumbs

Makes 1 serving

Prep time: 20 minutes

These tiny cabbages are excellent when cooked till just tender-crisp and topped with rich walnut crumbs. Make a larger batch to share at holiday meals.

Tip

Aleppo pepper is a famous seasoning used in the Mediterranean region and the Middle East. It is made by grinding dried peppers and is moderately spicy. It also has smoky, cumin-like notes, which make it a very nice addition to recipes. If you can't find it, you can substitute hot pepper flakes in this dish, adding them to taste.

8 oz	Brussels sprouts	250 g
2 tbsp	crème fraîche	30 mL
4 tsp	lime juice, divided	20 mL
¼ tsp	Aleppo pepper flakes (see tip, at left)	1 mL
	Salt and freshly ground black pepper	
3	sprigs fresh parsley	3
1 tbsp	butter	15 mL
1 tbsp	chopped walnuts (see tip, below)	15 mL
	Grated organic lime zest	

1. Using a sharp paring knife, cut a thin slice off the bottom of each Brussels sprout core; discard slices. Peel off outer leaves and discard. Cut an X in bottom of each core. In a saucepan of boiling salted water, cook Brussels sprouts for 7 minutes or until tender-crisp. Drain well.

2. Meanwhile, in a bowl, stir together crème fraîche, 2 tsp (10 mL) of the lime juice and Aleppo pepper; season to taste with salt. Wash and pat parsley dry; pull leaves off stems. Chop leaves finely; stir into crème fraîche mixture. Set aside.

3. In a skillet, melt butter over medium heat. Add walnuts; cook, stirring, for 1 to 2 minutes or until golden brown. Stir in remaining lime juice; season to taste with salt, black pepper and lime zest.

4. In a bowl, toss Brussels sprouts with walnut mixture to combine. Serve with crème fraîche mixture.

Shopping Tip

Buy whole nuts or nut halves rather than packaged chopped nuts. Walnuts are especially prone to going rancid. Store them in the freezer and chop only what you need for a particular recipe.

Nutrients per serving	
Calories	333
Fat	27 g
Carbohydrates	9 g
Protein	11 g

Desserts

Mango Coconut Ice Pops

Makes 6 servings

**Prep time:
2¼ hours**

*These tropical delights
are so refreshing on
a hot afternoon when
you need a cool, sweet
treat. They are so much
healthier than the
sugary pops you'll find
in the freezer section at
the supermarket.*

Tip

Fresh seasonal fruits are
delicious alternatives
to the mango juice in
these pops. You can chop
and fold just about any
fresh fruit into the cream
mixture. Try berries,
peaches, apricots,
mangos, pineapple or
cherries. Keep an eye,
however, on the overall
sugar content of the fruit
you choose. An easy
guideline to follow is
to use nine parts cream
mixture to one part fruit.

* **6 ice-pop molds, or ice cream maker**

¾ cup + 2 tbsp	heavy or whipping (35%) cream	200 mL
7 tbsp	mango juice (see tip, at left)	100 mL
2 tbsp	unsweetened shredded coconut (see tip, below)	30 mL
	Sweetener (see page 158)	

1. In a bowl, beat cream until stiff peaks form. Fold in mango juice until combined; fold in coconut. Sweeten to taste with sweetener.

2. Spoon cream mixture into ice-pop molds and freeze for 2 hours or until firm. Alternatively, freeze cream mixture in an ice cream maker according to the manufacturer's instructions.

Shopping Tip

Unsweetened shredded coconut is easy to find in the baking aisle of the supermarket. Look in health food stores or the natural foods aisle for brands that don't contain unwanted preservatives or chemical additives.

Nutrients per serving	
Calories	135
Fat	13 g
Carbohydrates	4 g
Protein	1 g

Star Fruit and Tofu Ice Cream

*Silken tofu and cream
pair up to make a
luscious, rich-tasting
ice cream that's packed
with nutrients.*

Tips

All parts of the star fruit
are edible, so there's no
need to peel it. Look
for fruits that are bright
yellow, with just a hint
of brown on the ridges.
They will be the ripest
and sweetest.

Look for pure vanilla
paste in health food
and gourmet stores. It's
a potent, alcohol- and
sugar-free way to add
flavor to recipes. It can
be pricey, but a little goes
a long way.

- Blender
- Ice cream maker

2	sheets gelatin (see tip, page 327)	2
2	star fruits (see tips, at left)	2
8 oz	silken tofu, drained	250 g
½ tsp	vanilla paste (see tips, at left)	2 mL
1 tbsp	raw cane sugar	15 mL
¼ cup	lemon juice (see tip, below)	60 mL
1 tbsp	fructose powder	15 mL
⅔ cup	heavy or whipping (35%) cream	150 mL
2 or 3	sprigs fresh lemon balm (see tip, page 183)	2 or 3

1. In a bowl, soak gelatin sheets in cold water for 5 minutes or until softened.

2. Meanwhile, cut 1 of the star fruits into 6 slices; set aside for garnish. Chop remaining star fruit. In a blender, purée together chopped star fruit, tofu and vanilla paste until smooth. Transfer to a bowl; set aside.

3. In a small saucepan, cook sugar over medium heat, stirring often, until melted and light caramel color. Stir in lemon juice until combined. Drain gelatin; stir into sugar mixture. Stir gelatin mixture and fructose into tofu mixture; refrigerate for 15 minutes.

4. In another bowl, beat cream until stiff peaks form; fold into tofu mixture. Pour mixture into an ice cream maker and freeze according to the manufacturer's instructions.

5. Scoop ice cream into dessert bowls; garnish with reserved star fruit and lemon balm.

Storage Tip

If you have a whole bunch of lemons, squeeze them and freeze the juice in recipe-size portions. It is a convenient way to avoid wasting extra lemons, and you'll always have freshly squeezed juice on hand.

Nutrients per serving	
Calories	150
Fat	10 g
Carbohydrates	10 g
Protein	5 g

Buttermilk Sorbet with Blueberries

Makes 4 to 6 servings

Prep time: 1 hour

Creamy buttermilk gives this sorbet a tangy taste that's really lovely. This dessert is especially delicious when wild blueberries are in season in the summer.

Tip

Full-fat (3.25%) buttermilk can be harder to find in North America, but it's worth looking for. Besides containing extra fat, which your body needs during cancer treatments, it's richer, thicker and more delicious in this dessert. If you can't find it, buy the highest-fat version you can find.

- **Ice cream maker**

2	sheets gelatin (see tip, opposite)	2
1	organic lemon	1
1⅔ cups	buttermilk (see tip, at left)	400 mL
5 tsp	fructose powder	25 mL
5 tsp	raw cane sugar	25 mL
1⅓ cups	blueberries	325 mL
1 tbsp	orange juice (see tip, below)	15 mL
1 tbsp	maple syrup	15 mL
	Fresh mint leaves	

1. In a bowl, soak gelatin sheets in cold water for 5 minutes or until softened.

2. Wash lemon well in hot water and pat dry; grate zest. Squeeze 2 tbsp (30 mL) lemon juice; save remainder for another use. In a bowl, stir together lemon zest, lemon juice, buttermilk, fructose and sugar.

3. Drain gelatin; transfer to a small saucepan. Cook gelatin, stirring, over low heat until dissolved. Whisk gelatin into buttermilk mixture. Pour mixture into an ice cream maker and freeze according to the manufacturer's instructions.

4. Meanwhile, place blueberries in a bowl; drizzle with orange juice and maple syrup. Let stand for about 10 minutes.

5. Divide sorbet between 4 or 6 dessert bowls; top with blueberry mixture. Wash mint leaves and pat dry. Garnish dessert with a few leaves; serve immediately.

Prep Tip

Freshly squeezed orange juice gives this dessert the brightest flavor. The best part: you need only about half of a small orange to yield the 1 tbsp (15 mL) of juice you need.

Nutrients per each of 6 servings	
Calories	72
Fat	1 g
Carbohydrates	13 g
Protein	3 g

Lime and Coconut Mousse

Makes 4 servings

**Prep time:
3½ hours**

There are few flavor pairings that go together better than lime and coconut. And just a splash of rum gives this mousse a sophisticated edge.

Tips

Check your can of coconut cream carefully. Many are sweetened, and this recipe requires the unsweetened version.

You can make this mousse a day ahead and refrigerate it overnight.

3	sheets gelatin (see tip, below)	3
2	eggs	2
1 tbsp	fructose powder	15 mL
	Zest and juice of 1 organic lime	
1²⁄₃ cups	canned unsweetened coconut cream (see tips, at left)	400 mL
1²⁄₃ cups	fresh strawberries, hulled	400 mL
2 tbsp	white rum	30 mL
1 tbsp	raw cane sugar	15 mL
	Unsweetened shredded coconut, toasted if desired	

1. In a bowl, soak gelatin sheets in cold water for 5 minutes or until softened.

2. In a heatproof bowl, whisk together eggs, fructose, lime zest and lime juice. Set over a saucepan of hot (not boiling) water; cook, beating constantly, until thick and creamy.

3. Drain gelatin; squeeze out excess water. Stir into egg mixture until dissolved. Remove bowl from heat; stir in coconut cream. Cover mixture, pressing plastic wrap onto surface to prevent condensation from forming, and refrigerate for 1 hour or until chilled and thickened.

4. Meanwhile, chop strawberries. In a bowl, stir together strawberries, rum and sugar. Divide between 4 dessert glasses or bowls.

5. Whisk coconut mixture; spoon over berry mixture. Cover and refrigerate for 2 hours or until chilled. Sprinkle with coconut just before serving.

Shopping Tip

Sheet gelatin is also called leaf gelatin. It comes in transparent sheets (hence the name). It's tricky to use powdered gelatin in place of the sheets, as the ratios for converting are different from brand to brand; your best bet is to stick to the number of sheets that are called for. Look for this type of gelatin at well-stocked supermarkets or online retailers that specialize in baking and cooking ingredients.

Nutrients per serving

Calories	845
Fat	79 g
Carbohydrates	19 g
Protein	11 g

Peach and Berry Salad with Fizzy Zabaglione

**Prep time:
20 minutes**

*A dessert like this tastes
a bit decadent, but it's
full of vitamin-rich
fruit. The pine nuts add
an appealing crunch to
each bite.*

Tip

If you'd prefer your
dessert without alcohol,
substitute kefir for the
wine and sugar, beating
as directed.

2 tbsp	pine nuts	30 mL
1	large ripe peach or nectarine	1
1 cup	red currants	250 mL
1 cup	fresh raspberries	250 mL
1 tbsp	lemon juice	15 mL
1 tbsp	maple syrup	15 mL
2	egg yolks	2
7 tbsp	dry sparkling wine (see tip, at left)	100 mL
1 tbsp	raw cane sugar	15 mL

1. In a dry skillet over medium heat, toast pine nuts, shaking pan often, for 3 to 5 minutes or until golden. Transfer to a bowl; let cool.

2. Halve and pit peach; cut into wedges. Pick through currants and raspberries and remove any bruised fruit or stems. In a bowl, gently toss together peaches, currants and raspberries; drizzle with lemon juice and maple syrup.

3. In a heatproof bowl set over a saucepan of boiling water, and using a hand mixer, beat together egg yolks, wine and sugar for 5 minutes or until creamy. Immediately spoon fruit salad and wine mixture into bowls. Sprinkle with pine nuts.

Nutrients per serving	
Calories	175
Fat	6 g
Carbohydrates	22 g
Protein	3 g

Melon Salad with Vanilla Mascarpone Cream

Fresh, juicy melon is a tasty partner for this vanilla-scented cream. You can also enjoy the cream with other combinations of healthy fruit for dessert. Check the Yellow-Light Foods list (page 148) for ideas and the carbohydrate content of different fruits.

Tip

Save the remaining half of the vanilla bean for making vanilla sugar. Bury the bean in raw cane sugar and let stand until the sugar absorbs the vanilla scent. Use the sugar in baking.

2 tbsp	lemon juice	30 mL
2 tsp	fructose powder	10 mL
12	fresh mint leaves	12
½	cantaloupe or honeydew melon (about 1 lb/500 g), seeded, peeled and cubed	½
½	vanilla bean (see tip, at left)	½
5 oz	mascarpone cheese	150 g
7 tbsp	plain yogurt	100 mL
2 tsp	raw cane sugar	10 mL

1. In a bowl, stir lemon juice with fructose. Wash mint leaves and pat dry; set aside 4 leaves for garnish. Cut remainder into fine shreds. Stir shredded mint into lemon juice mixture. Toss in melon to coat; let stand for 10 minutes to marinate.

2. Meanwhile, halve vanilla bean lengthwise; using the tip of a sharp paring knife, scrape the seeds into a bowl. Discard vanilla pod. Stir in cheese, yogurt and sugar until creamy.

3. Divide melon mixture between 4 dessert bowls; spoon mascarpone mixture over top. Garnish with reserved mint leaves.

Nutrients per serving	
Calories	262
Fat	19 g
Carbohydrates	19 g
Protein	3 g

Pear and Cranberry Compote

Makes 4 servings

**Prep time:
1¼ hours**

*Compotes are often
served over ice cream
or other dishes, but
they are so tasty on
their own. Try this
as a dessert around
the holidays, when
cranberries are
in season.*

Tip

Locust bean gum is also
called carob bean gum.
It is a natural plant
thickener that you can
use when you're on the
cancer-fighting diet (see
page 147). Look for it in
health food stores.

2 tbsp	chopped hazelnuts	30 mL
½ cup	pear juice	125 mL
1	cinnamon stick	1
2 cups	cranberries (fresh or thawed frozen), see spotlight, below	500 mL
1	ripe pear, peeled, cored and chopped	1
1 tsp	locust bean gum (see tip, at left)	5 mL
2 tbsp	pear nectar	30 mL
¾ cup + 2 tbsp	buttermilk (see tip, page 326)	200 mL
	Fresh mint leaves	

1. In a dry nonstick skillet over medium heat, toast hazelnuts, shaking pan often, for 5 minutes or until fragrant and golden brown. Transfer to a bowl; let cool.

2. In a saucepan, bring pear juice and cinnamon stick to a boil; stir in cranberries and pear. Reduce heat to low, cover and simmer for 2 to 3 minutes or until fruit is slightly softened. Stir in locust bean gum; simmer for 1 minute or until thickened. Remove from heat; stir in pear nectar. Let cool for 1 hour.

3. Spoon cranberry mixture into 4 dessert bowls; pour buttermilk over top. Sprinkle with hazelnuts. Wash mint leaves and pat dry; garnish dessert with a few leaves.

Spotlight

Cranberries in any form strengthen the immune system, no matter whether the berries are raw, cooked, dried or enjoyed as a juice. They are in season in the fall and early winter, so pick up multiple bags of cranberries then and freeze them for later. The berries are very tart, so they can be bracing. Pair them with sweeter fruits and juices for the most delicious results.

Nutrients per serving	
Calories	123
Fat	5 g
Carbohydrates	15 g
Protein	3 g

Ginger Panna Cotta on Papaya Purée

Panna cotta is creamy and decadent, and it contains plenty of the fat your body needs to fight cancer.

Tip

Check carefully before you buy pistachios. Many are salted, and you need unsalted ones for this recipe.

- Four ¾-cup (175 mL) ramekins or custard cups
- Blender

3	sheets gelatin (see tip, page 327)	3
2 cups	heavy or whipping (35%) cream	500 mL
1	piece (about 2½ inches/6 cm) gingerroot, finely grated	1
2 tsp	raw cane sugar	10 mL
2 tsp	fructose powder	10 mL
	Grated zest of ½ organic lime	
1	ripe papaya (about 8 oz/250 g)	1
2 tbsp	lime juice	30 mL
2 tbsp	chopped pistachios (see tip, at left)	30 mL

1. In a bowl, soak gelatin sheets in cold water for 5 minutes or until softened.

2. In a saucepan, bring cream, ginger, sugar, fructose and lime zest to a boil. Reduce heat to low and simmer, uncovered, for 5 minutes. Remove from heat.

3. Drain gelatin; squeeze out excess water. Stir into cream mixture until dissolved. Divide cream mixture between four ¾-cup (175 mL) ramekins. Cover and refrigerate for 5 hours or overnight, or until chilled.

4. Just before serving, halve and seed papaya. Peel papaya; dice two-thirds of the flesh. In a blender, blend diced papaya with lime juice, adding 2 to 3 tbsp (30 to 45 mL) water, to make smooth purée. Cut remaining papaya into wedges.

5. Pour papaya purée onto 4 dessert plates. Briefly dip ramekins into hot water; unmold panna cotta onto plates. Garnish with papaya wedges; sprinkle with pistachios.

Nutrients per serving	
Calories	462
Fat	42 g
Carbohydrates	11 g
Protein	6 g

Chilled Chocolate Pudding with Vanilla Sauce

Makes 4 servings		

| **Prep time: 3¾ hours** | | |

Chocolate pudding is such an old-fashioned treat. Here, it's topped with a creamy vanilla sauce that's just divine.

Tip

When you're choosing almond butter, look for pure versions that don't contain any added sweeteners, salt or other additives.

- **Four ¾-cup (175 mL) ramekins or custard cups**

3½ oz	dark chocolate (at least 70% cocoa content), chopped	100 g
1 cup	milk	250 mL
7 tbsp	heavy or whipping (35%) cream	100 mL
2 tbsp	almond butter (see tip, at left)	30 mL
2 tbsp	raw cane sugar	30 mL
¼ tsp	ground cinnamon	1 mL
Pinch	ground cloves	Pinch
⅓ cup	water	75 mL
1 tsp	agar-agar powder	5 mL
1 tbsp	chopped almonds	15 mL

Vanilla Sauce

2	egg yolks	2
1 tbsp	raw cane sugar	15 mL
1	vanilla bean	1
7 tbsp	milk	100 mL
7 tbsp	heavy or whipping (35%) cream	100 mL

1. In a saucepan, combine chocolate, milk, cream, almond butter, sugar, cinnamon and cloves; bring to a boil, stirring constantly, until chocolate is melted. Remove from heat.

2. In a small bowl, stir water with agar-agar until dissolved; stir into milk mixture. Return to a boil, stirring constantly. Reduce heat to low and simmer for 2 minutes. Pour mixture into ramekins; cover and refrigerate for 3 hours or until chilled.

3. **Vanilla Sauce:** Meanwhile, in a bowl, beat egg yolks with sugar until creamy. Set aside. Halve vanilla bean lengthwise; using the tip of a sharp paring knife, scrape the seeds into a saucepan. Add vanilla pod, milk and cream; bring to a boil. Remove vanilla pod. Gradually add hot milk mixture to egg mixture, whisking constantly. Return to saucepan; cook, stirring, for 5 minutes or until creamy and slightly thickened. Let cool.

4. Run knife around edges of puddings; invert onto 4 dessert plates. Sprinkle with almonds; serve with vanilla sauce.

Nutrients per serving	
Calories	483
Fat	38 g
Carbohydrates	27 g
Protein	9 g

Apple and Plum Gratin

Makes 4 servings

**Prep time:
30 minutes**

A puffy, creamy topping studded with golden almonds is the perfect way to show off fresh harvest fruits.

Tip

This gratin tastes equally delicious if you make it with mixed summer berries and fresh apricots instead of the apple and plums.

- Preheat oven to 475°F (240°C)
- 8-cup (2 L) gratin dish

1	tart apple (such as Granny Smith), cored and peeled (see tip, at left)	1
3	plums (about 7 oz/210 g), pitted	3
2 tbsp	dry white wine	30 mL
2	eggs, separated	2
1 tbsp	raw cane sugar	15 mL
7 tbsp	low-fat quark (see tip, below)	100 mL
1/3 cup	heavy or whipping (35%) cream	75 mL
1/2 tsp	ground cinnamon	2 mL
	Grated zest of 1 organic lemon	
2 tsp	lemon juice	10 mL
2 tbsp	sliced almonds	30 mL

1. Cut apple into thin wedges; quarter plums. Arrange apple and plums, alternating, in an 8-cup (2 L) gratin dish; drizzle wine over top.

2. In a bowl, beat egg yolks with sugar until creamy; stir in quark and cream until combined. Stir in cinnamon and lemon zest. In another bowl, beat egg whites with lemon juice until stiff peaks form; fold into quark mixture. Spread over fruit in gratin dish; sprinkle with almonds.

3. Bake in preheated oven for 10 minutes or until top is puffed and almonds are golden brown.

Substitution Tip

Quark is a German fresh cheese that is similar to a French fresh cheese called fromage frais. If you can't find either, you can drain plain yogurt to make yogurt cheese and use that instead.

Nutrients per serving	
Calories	184
Fat	10 g
Carbohydrates	14 g
Protein	8 g

Orange Tiramisu

Makes 4 servings

Prep time:
1¼ hours

Tiramisu usually involves a lot of carb-laden ladyfingers. This version has all the same flavors (plus a nice hit of orange), in a much healthier form.

Tip

No espresso maker? No problem. Either brew very strong coffee and let it cool to use in place of the espresso, or make the amount of espresso you need using instant espresso granules.

- Preheat oven to 350°F (180°C)
- 9-inch (23 cm) square glass baking dish, bottom lined with parchment paper

2	organic oranges	2
5 oz	mascarpone cheese	150 g
2 tbsp	raw cane sugar	30 mL
2	egg whites	2
¼ cup	cold espresso (see tip, at left)	60 mL
2 tbsp	orange liqueur	30 mL
1 oz	dark chocolate (at least 70% cocoa content), shaved	30 g

Almond Cake

2	eggs, separated	2
Pinch	salt	Pinch
1 tbsp	warm water	15 mL
1 tbsp	fructose powder	15 mL
½ cup	ground almonds	125 mL
¼ cup	chopped almonds	60 mL
½ tsp	vanilla paste (see tips, page 325)	2 mL

1. **Almond Cake:** In a bowl, beat egg whites with salt until stiff peaks form. In another bowl, whisk together egg yolks, warm water and fructose. Fold in ground and chopped almonds, vanilla paste and egg whites.

2. Spoon mixture into prepared baking dish; smooth top. Bake in preheated oven for 15 to 20 minutes or until cake is firm and golden. Run knife around edge of pan; turn cake out onto a wire rack. Peel off paper; let cool. Set baking dish aside to assemble tiramisu.

3. Meanwhile, wash oranges well in hot water and pat dry; finely grate zest. In a bowl, stir together cheese, sugar and orange zest. In another bowl, beat egg whites until stiff peaks form; fold into cheese mixture. Set aside.

4. Peel oranges, removing white pith; cut into slices. Halve slices. Cut almond cake into ¾- by 4½-inch (2 by 11 cm) strips; arrange in baking dish. In a small bowl, stir espresso with liqueur; drizzle over cake. Spoon cheese mixture over top; garnish with orange slices and shaved chocolate.

Nutrients per serving	
Calories	444
Fat	34 g
Carbohydrates	22 g
Protein	12 g

Cottage Cheese Cake

It's not the most luxurious dairy product, but cottage cheese becomes something really special in this cake. The nutty crust is a lower-carb, richer alternative to the usual graham cracker crust you find in cheesecakes.

Tip

Coconut flour is becoming more and more common now that an increasing number of people are following the Paleo Diet. You can usually find it in health food stores, but some supermarkets and food warehouse clubs carry it, too.

- Preheat oven to 350°F (180°C)
- 10-inch (25 cm) springform pan, greased or lined with parchment paper

4	eggs, separated	4
6 tbsp	raw cane sugar	90 mL
1¾ cups	cottage cheese	425 mL
1¾ cups	low-fat quark (see tip, page 333)	425 mL
2 tbsp	coconut flour (see tip, at left)	30 mL
	Zest of 1 organic lemon	
2 tbsp	lemon juice	30 mL

Nut Crust

1½ cups	pecans, finely chopped	375 mL
½ cup	ground almonds	125 mL
2	egg whites	2

1. **Nut Crust:** In a bowl, stir together pecans, almonds and egg whites until moistened. With moist hands, press nut mixture into prepared springform pan, pressing around edge to form a small lip. Refrigerate for 30 minutes.

2. Meanwhile, in a bowl, beat egg yolks with sugar until creamy; stir in cottage cheese, quark, flour, lemon zest and lemon juice. In another bowl, beat egg whites until stiff peaks form; fold into cheese mixture.

3. Spread cheese mixture over crust; smooth top. Bake in preheated oven for 50 to 60 minutes or until just firm in center. Let cool slightly.

4. Release side of pan; transfer cake to wire rack and let cool completely.

Nutrients per slice

Calories	249
Fat	17 g
Carbohydrates	9 g
Protein	15 g

Poppy Seed Soufflés

Makes 4 servings

Prep time: 1 hour

These mini soufflés are very pretty, so they make a lovely dessert when you're entertaining.

Tip

A clean coffee grinder or spice grinder is perfect for grinding tiny poppy seeds for this recipe. If you have one, an old-fashioned metal poppy seed grinder is a fabulous tool, too.

- Preheat oven to 350°F (180°C)
- Four ¾-cup (175 mL) ramekins, greased and sprinkled with raw cane sugar
- Large roasting pan

¼ cup	ground poppy seeds (see tip, at left)	60 mL
¼ cup	butter, softened	60 mL
¼ cup	raw cane sugar, divided	60 mL
3	eggs, separated	3
2 tbsp	white rum	30 mL
1 tbsp	chopped hazelnuts	15 mL
½ tsp	grated organic lemon zest	2 mL
Pinch	salt	Pinch
1 tsp	locust bean gum (see tip, page 330)	5 mL
1	pink grapefruit	1
2	fresh figs	2

1. In a dry nonstick skillet over medium heat, toast poppy seeds, shaking pan often, for about 1 minute or until fragrant. Transfer to a bowl; let cool.

2. In a large bowl, beat butter with 3 tbsp (45 mL) of the sugar for 2 to 3 minutes or until creamy. Stir in egg yolks; fold in poppy seeds, rum, hazelnuts and lemon zest. In another bowl, beat egg whites with salt, gradually adding remaining sugar, until stiff peaks form. Fold egg whites and locust bean gum into poppy seed mixture.

3. Spoon mixture into prepared ramekins; place in a large roasting pan. Pour in enough water to come halfway up sides of ramekins. Bake in preheated oven for 25 to 30 minutes or until puffed and golden.

4. Meanwhile, peel grapefruit, completely removing white pith. Using a sharp paring knife and working over a bowl to catch juice and segments, cut between membranes to separate flesh into segments. Drain off all but 2 tbsp (30 mL) of the juice (save drained juice for another recipe). Cut figs into wedges; add to bowl. Stir gently to combine.

5. Run knife around edge of each ramekin; turn soufflés out onto 4 dessert plates. Serve with grapefruit mixture.

Nutrients per serving	
Calories	373
Fat	25 g
Carbohydrates	25 g
Protein	8 g

Parsnip and Chocolate Cake

Makes 1 cake, about 16 slices

Prep time: 1½ hours

OK, parsnips aren't the first thing that come to mind when you think of cake. But they give this cake a wonderful, moist texture, and add plenty of vitamins and minerals.

Tips

Pear nectar makes this cake delicately sweet. Look for bottles of it in health food stores.

Defatted cocoa powder has some of the natural fat removed. It's great for baking, because it has a rich, very deep chocolaty flavor. Look for it in health food stores, too.

- Preheat oven to 350°F (180°C)
- 12- by 4-inch (30 by 10 cm) loaf pan, greased

6	eggs, separated	6
¼ cup	raw cane sugar	60 mL
3 tbsp + 1 tsp	pear nectar (see tips, at left)	50 mL
½ tsp	ground cinnamon	2 mL
½ tsp	vanilla paste (see tips, page 325)	2 mL
8 oz	parsnips (about 3), peeled and finely grated	250 g
3 cups	ground almonds	750 mL
3 tbsp	kirsch	45 mL
3½ oz	dark chocolate (at least 70% cocoa content), chopped	100 g
⅔ cup	whole-grain spelt flour	150 mL
⅓ cup	defatted cocoa powder (see tips, at left)	75 mL
1 tsp	cream of tartar	5 mL
Pinch	salt	Pinch
2 tbsp	chopped almonds	30 mL

1. In a bowl, beat together egg yolks, sugar, pear nectar, cinnamon and vanilla paste until creamy. Stir in parsnips, almonds and kirsch. In another bowl, whisk together chocolate, flour, cocoa powder and cream of tartar. Fold into egg mixture.

2. In another bowl, beat egg whites with salt until stiff peaks form; fold into egg yolk mixture. Scrape batter into prepared loaf pan; smooth top. Sprinkle with chopped almonds. Bake in preheated oven for 50 to 60 minutes or until tester inserted in center comes out clean.

3. Let cool in pan on rack for 10 minutes. Transfer cake to a wire rack; let cool completely.

Storage Tip

Wrap the cake tightly in foil and store for 1 or 2 days; it will stay lovely and moist.

Nutrients per slice

Calories	235
Fat	17 g
Carbohydrates	13 g
Protein	8 g

Apple and Coconut Squares

This is an excellent dessert to share with friends or family, especially at a party. The squares are sweet, fruity and nutty at the same time.

Tip

Agave nectar is a sweetener you can't use freely on the cancer-fighting diet. But here, just a tiny bit adds sweetness to a big batch of bars without raising the amount of carbs per serving too much.

- Preheat oven to 350°F (180°C)
- Baking sheet, greased

2 lbs	tart apples (such as Granny Smith), peeled and cored	1 kg
2 tbsp	lemon juice	30 mL
4	eggs, separated	4
Pinch	salt	Pinch
2 tbsp	fructose powder	30 mL
2 tbsp	agave nectar (see tip, at left)	30 mL
7 tbsp	butter, melted	100 mL
1¼ cups	ground hazelnuts	300 mL
1 cup	ground almonds	250 mL
1 cup	unsweetened shredded coconut	250 mL
¾ cup + 2 tbsp	whole-grain spelt flour	200 mL
2 tsp	cream of tartar	10 mL
1 tsp	locust bean gum (see tip, page 330)	5 mL
¾ cup	fresh or thawed frozen blackberries	175 mL

Garnish

2 tbsp	unsweetened shredded coconut	30 mL

1. Cut apples into thin wedges; drizzle immediately with lemon juice to prevent browning. Set aside.

2. In a bowl, beat egg whites with salt until stiff peaks form. In another bowl, whisk together egg yolks, fructose and agave nectar until thick and creamy. Stir in butter.

3. In another bowl, stir together hazelnuts, almonds, coconut, flour, cream of tartar and locust bean gum. Fold into egg yolk mixture; fold in egg whites. Spread over prepared baking sheet; top with apple slices and blackberries. Bake in preheated oven for 15 to 20 minutes.

4. **Garnish:** Sprinkle coconut over fruit mixture; bake for 5 minutes or until golden.

Nutrients per square

Calories	159
Fat	11 g
Carbohydrates	11 g
Protein	3 g

Index

Library and Archives Canada Cataloguing in Publication

Coy, Johannes F., 1963-
[Die neue anti-krebs Ernährung. English]
  The cancer fighting diet : diet and nutrition strategies to help weaken
cancer cells and improve treatment results / Dr. Johannes F. Coy, Maren Franz.

Includes index.
Translation of: Die neue anti-krebs Ernährung.
ISBN 978-0-7788-0508-3 (pbk.)

  1. Cancer—Diet therapy—Recipes. 2. Cancer—Nutritional aspects.
3. Cookbooks. I. Franz, Maren, 1968-, author II. Title. III. Title: Die
neue anti-krebs Ernährung. English.

RC271.D52C6913 2015   616.99'40654   C2014-908415-3